THE BRAIN & THE EYE

ATLAS *of* TUMOR RADIOLOGY

PHILIP J. HODES, M.D., *Editor-in-Chief*

Sponsored by

THE AMERICAN COLLEGE OF RADIOLOGY

—with the cooperation of:

AMERICAN CANCER SOCIETY
AMERICAN ROENTGEN RAY SOCIETY
CANCER CONTROL PROGRAM, USPHS
EASTMAN KODAK COMPANY
JAMES PICKER FOUNDATION
RADIOLOGICAL SOCIETY OF NORTH AMERICA

THE BRAIN
AND
THE EYE

by

ERNEST H. WOOD, M.D.

Late Professor of Radiology, College of Physicians and Surgeons,
Columbia University; Director of Neuroradiology, Neurological Institute of New York,
Columbia-Presbyterian Medical Center

JUAN M. TAVERAS, M.D.

Professor of Radiology, Harvard Medical School;
Radiologist-in-Chief, Massachusetts General Hospital, Boston

MICHAEL S. TENNER, M.D.

Associate Professor of Radiology, State University of New York,
Downstate Medical Center; Director of Neuroradiology
at the University Hospital, Downstate Medical Center,
and Kings County Hospital, Brooklyn

YEAR BOOK MEDICAL PUBLISHERS · INC.

35 EAST WACKER DRIVE · CHICAGO

Editor's Preface

IN 1960, the Committee on Radiology of the National Research Council began to consider the preparation of a tumor atlas for radiology similar in concept to the Armed Forces Institute of Pathology's "Atlas of Tumor Pathology." So successfully had the latter filled a need in pathology that it seemed reasonable to establish a similar resource for radiology. Therefore a subcommittee of the Committee on Radiology was appointed to study the concept and make recommendations.

That original committee, made up of Dr. Russell H. Morgan (Chairman), Dr. Marshall H. Brucer and Dr. Eugene P. Pendergrass, reported that a need did indeed exist and recommended that something be done about it. That report was unanimously accepted by the parent committee.

Soon thereafter, there occurred a normal change of the membership of the Committee on Radiology of the Council. This was followed by a change of the "Atlas" subcommittee, which now included Dr. E. Richard King (Chairman), Dr. Leo G. Rigler and Dr. Barton R. Young. To this new subcommittee was assigned the task of finding how the "Atlas" was to be published. Numerous avenues were explored; none seemed wholly satisfactory.

With the passing of time, it became increasingly apparent that the American College of Radiology had to be brought into the picture. It had prime teaching responsibilities; it had a Commission on Education; it seemed the logical responsible agent to launch the "Atlas." Confident of the merits of this approach, the entire Committee on Radiology of the Council became involved in focusing the attention of the American College of Radiology upon the matter.* In 1964, as the result of their persuasiveness, the Board of Chancellors of the American College of Radiology named an ad hoc committee to explore and define the scholarly scope of the "Atlas" and the probable costs. In 1965, the ad hoc committee recommended that the College sponsor and publish the "Atlas." Accordingly, an Editorial Advisory Committee was chosen to work within the Commission on Education with authority to select an Editor-in-Chief. At the same time, the College provided

---

* At that time, the Committee on Radiology included, in addition to the subcommittee, Drs. John A. Campbell, James B. Dealy, Jr., Melvin M. Figley, Hymer L. Friedell, Howard B. Latourette, Alexander Margulis, Ernest A. Mendelsohn, Charles M. Nice, Jr., and Edward W. Webster.

funds for starting the project and began representations for grants-in-aid without which the "Atlas" would never be published.

No history of the "Atlas of Tumor Radiology" would be complete without specific recording of the generous response of the several radiological societies, as well as the private and Federal granting institutions whose names appear on the title page and below among our acknowledgments. It was their tangible evidence of confidence in the project that provided everyone with enthusiasm and eagerness to achieve our goal.

The "Atlas of Tumor Radiology" includes all major organ systems. It is intended to be a systematic body of pictorial and written information dealing with the roentgen manifestations of tumors. No attempt has been made to provide an atlas equivalent of a medical encyclopedia. Nevertheless the "Atlas" is designed to serve as an important reference source and teaching file for all physicians, not radiologists alone.

The fourteen volumes of the "Atlas" are: *The Hemopoietic and Lymphatic Systems,* by Gerald D. Dodd and Sidney Wallace; *The Bones and Joints,* by Gwilym S. Lodwick (published); *The Chest,* by Roy R. Greening and J. Haynes Heslep (published); The Gastrointestinal Tract: *The Esophagus and Stomach* (published) and *The Duodenum, Small Intestine and Colon* (published) by George N. Stein and Arthur K. Finkelstein; *The Kidney,* by John A. Evans and Morton A. Bosniak (published); *The Adrenals, Retroperitoneum and Lower Urinary Tract,* by Morton A. Bosniak, Stanley S. Siegelman and John A. Evans; *The Breast,* by David M. Witten (published); *The Head and Neck,* by Gilbert H. Fletcher and Bao-Shan Jing (published); *The Brain and Eye,* by Ernest H. Wood, Juan M. Taveras and Michael S. Tenner (published); *The Female Reproductive System,* by G. Melvin Stevens (published); *The Endocrines,* by Howard L. Steinbach and Hideyo Minagi (published); *The Accessory Digestive Organs,* by Robert E. Wise and Austin P. O'Keeffe (published); and *The Spine,* by Bernard S. Epstein (published).

Some overlapping of material in several volumes is inevitable, for example, tumors of the female generative system, tumors of the endocrine glands and tumors of the urinary tract. This is considered to be an asset. It assures the specialist completeness in the volume or volumes that concern him and provides added breadth and depth of knowledge for those interested in the entire series.

The broad scope of the "Atlas of Tumor Radiology" has precluded its preparation by a single or even several authors. To maintain uniformity of format, rather rigid criteria were established early. These included manner of presentation, size of illustrations, as well as style of headings, subheadings and legends. The authors were encouraged to keep the text at a minimum, freeing as much space as possible for large illustrations and meaningful legends. The "Atlas" is to be just that, an "atlas," not a series of "texts." The authors were urged, also, to keep the bibliography brief.

The selection of suitable authors for the "Atlas" was extremely difficult, and to a degree invidious. For the final choice, the Editor-in-Chief accepts full responsibility. It is but fair to record, however, that his Editorial Advisory Committee accepted his recommendations. The format of the "Atlas," too, was the choice of the Editor-in-Chief, again with the concurrence of his advisory group. Should the "Atlas of Tumor Radiology" fall short of its goals, the fault will lie with the Editor-in-Chief alone; his Editorial Advisory Committee was selfless in its dedication to the purposes of the "Atlas," rendering invaluable advice and guidance whenever asked to do so.

As medical knowledge expands, medical concepts change. In medicine, the written word considered true today may not be so tomorrow. The text of the "Atlas," considered true today, therefore may not be true tomorrow. What may not change, what may ever remain true, may be the illustrations of the "Atlas of Tumor Radiology." Their legends may change as our conceptual levels advance. But the validity of the roentgen findings there recorded should endure. Thus, if the fidelity with which the roentgenograms have been reproduced is of superior order, the illustrations in the "Atlas" should long serve as sources for reference no matter what revisions of the text become necessary with advancing medical knowledge.

ACKNOWLEDGMENTS

The American College of Radiology, its Commission on Education, the Editorial Advisory Committee, the authors and the Editor-in-Chief wish to acknowledge their grateful appreciation:

1. For the grants-in-aid so willingly and repeatedly provided by The American Cancer Society, The American Roentgen Ray Society, The Cancer Control Program, National Center for Chronic Disease Control (USPHS Grant No. 59481), The James Picker Foundation, and the Radiological Society of North America.

2. For the superb glossy print reproductions provided by the Radiography Markets Division, Eastman Kodak Company. Special mention must be made of the sustained interest of Mr. George R. Struck, its Assistant Vice-President and General Manager. We applaud particularly Mr. William S. Cornwell, Technical Associate and Editor Emeritus of Kodak's *Medical*

Radiography and Photography, as well as his associates, Mr. Charles C. Heckman and Mr. David Edwards and others in the Photo Service Division whose expertise provided the "Atlas" with its incomparable photographic reproductions.

3. To Year Book Medical Publishers, for their personal involvement with and judicious guidance in the many problems of publication. There were occasions when the publisher questioned the quality of certain illustrations. Almost always the judgment of the authors and the Editor-in-Chief prevailed because of the importance of the original roentgenograms and the singular fidelity of their reproduction.

4. To the Associate Editors, particularly Mrs. Anabel I. Janssen, whose talents lightened the burden of the Editor-in-Chief and helped establish the style of presentation of the material.

5. To the Staff of the American College of Radiology, especially Messrs. William C. Stronach, Otha Linton, Keith Gundlach and William Melton, for continued conceptual and administrative efforts of unusual competence.

For the second time publication of a volume of the "Atlas" has been marred by death of an author. Galley and some page proofs were in hand when death struck Dr. Wood. In fact, he was at his desk working on his volume when the end came.

From the very beginning difficulties beset this work. It was Dr. Juan M. Taveras who first accepted its responsibility. Doctor Wood was to be his coauthor. Soon thereafter Dr. Taveras moved from St. Louis to Boston to assume new and demanding responsibilities. Realizing he no longer had time for his commitments to the Editorial Committee of the "Atlas," Dr. Taveras asked Dr. Wood to accept the senior authorship. Despite the fact that he already was heavily committed, Dr. Wood accepted this one more burden. Doctor Taveras would help, but it was now Dr. Wood who had the prime obligation to produce *The Brain and the Eye.* Fortunately Dr. Wood had a most able associate at the Neurological Institute, Dr. Michael Tenner. Just as Dr. Taveras turned to Dr. Wood, so did Dr. Wood turn to Dr. Tenner for the help he needed.

Doctor Tenner responded magnificently. Added impetus was given the work; the manuscript developed steadily. At about this time Dr. Tenner left Dr. Wood to become Associate Professor of Radiology and Director of Neuroradiology at State University of New York Downstate Medical Center. Despite all he faced in his new post, Dr. Tenner continued to press on trying constantly to lighten the burden for Dr. Wood. And when Dr. Wood died, it was Dr. Tenner who completed the work. The Editorial Committee of the "Atlas" is acutely aware of and thankful for the part he played in bringing this volume of the "Atlas" to its readers.

The "Atlas of Tumor Radiology" is being published at a time when massive scientific effort is taking place at an unprecedented rate and on an unprecedented scale. We hope that our final product will provide an authoritative summary of our current knowledge of the roentgen manifestations of tumors.

PHILIP J. HODES
Editor-in-Chief

Emeritus Professor of Radiology,
Thomas Jefferson University, Philadelphia
Professor of Radiology, University of Miami School
of Medicine, Miami, Florida

Editorial Advisory Committee

HARRY L. BERMAN   VINCENT P. COLLINS   E. RICHARD KING
LEO G. RIGLER   PHILIP RUBIN

Authors' Preface

THIS VOLUME was conceived in a manner somewhat different from the others in this series because of the different problems inherent in diagnosing disorders of the brain and eye. There are relatively few highly specific radiographic findings for a particular lesion. When a high degree of specificity in diagnosis is possible (for example, meningiomas), this has been dealt with in detail. Our energies have otherwise been directed to dealing with precise anatomic localization as this has far-reaching therapeutic implications especially when the therapy takes the form of surgical intervention or irradiation of the tumor-containing volume of brain. For this reason we have utilized a thoroughness in anatomic description beyond what would normally be done in a work surveying this field. Material has also been carefully selected so that anatomic representation of mass lesions is as complete as possible within space limitations dictated by this format.

Intracranial masses of all types are encountered, and the classic methods of plain film examination, pneumoencephalography and cerebral angiography in general only reveal the presence of a mass, which could be a neoplasm or some other type of space-occupying process such as an abscess, a hematoma or a cyst. Very commonly the morphology of the lesion did not allow us to determine by radiologic methods which specific disease process pertained in an individual case, and the final diagnosis and the therapeutic decision were ordinarily based on the radiologic findings coupled with the clinical history and the results of neurologic examination. The recent development of computerized tomography has brought us one step farther in our efforts to arrive at a nonoperative etiologic diagnosis on radiologic grounds alone. Computerized tomography can easily differentiate a hematoma from a tumor and a cyst from a solid mass. This could have significant implications in the management of patients suffering from neurologic disorders. Because the material for this volume had reached an advanced stage of readiness when computerized tomography became available, only representative examples of the usefulness of this technique in the diagnosis of brain tumors are illustrated in these pages.

We appreciate the support given by the Editor-in-Chief, Philip Hodes, and the personal efforts of his editorial associate Anabel Janssen. The exacting photographic requirements were satisfied by William Cornwell and his Eastman Kodak staff.

As this volume approached completion its senior author, Ernest H. Wood, suddenly passed away. The attentive and thorough manner which he brought to his work is an inspiration to those who follow him in neuroradiologic endeavors.

JUAN M. TAVERAS
MICHAEL S. TENNER

Table of Contents / XIII

PART 1

Neural Tumors and Radiologic Methods of Diagnosis

Characteristics and Diagnostic Techniques

RADIOLOGIC TECHNIQUES were first used extensively in neurosurgery during the Spanish-American War, a relatively few months after the discovery of the roentgen ray. Since then, physicians practicing the clinical neurologic sciences have become highly interested in, and dependent on, neuroradiology as a means of detecting, localizing and identifying the type of pathologic process with which the clinician is dealing. During the more than three-quarters of a century since discovery of the x-ray, numerous special procedures have been introduced until neuroradiology has become a full-fledged subspecialty. One of the more recent additions has been computerized transverse axial tomography, devised by Hounsfield (1973), or computerized photon absorption radiography. The computerization of radiologic data, which is a noninvasive technique, is considered in Part 2 with the discussion of plain film examination. The eye, considered an appendage of the brain, is discussed separately in Part 14.

NEURAL TUMORS

In most cases it is possible to detect and localize a brain tumor. Identification preoperatively is much more difficult unless the location of a tumor is characteristic, such as an acoustic neurinoma at the internal auditory meatus or a colloid cyst at the foramen of Monro. At times angiography will denote with certainty that a malignant tumor is present or that a tumor of characteristic vascular architecture, such as a hemangioblastoma, is observed. It is important, therefore, to have a working knowledge of the neuropathology of brain tumors and to interpret radiologic findings in view of the types of tumors being sought and their growth patterns.

SPECIAL FEATURES OF BRAIN TUMORS

Brain tumors have several characteristics not common to neoplasms growing elsewhere. (1) They are encountered at all ages and are not predominantly associated with degenerative changes occurring in the latter part of life. (2) Gliomas in particular have the unusual feature of changing their biologic nature with the passage of time. Many benign astrocytomas, for example, become malignant glioblastomas spontaneously or have malignant characteristics when they recur after treatment. (3) For all practical purposes, brain tumors do not metastasize outside of the central nervous system.

The term "brain tumor" is usually considered to include not only neoplasms arising from brain tissue itself but those of the meninges, blood vessels, endocrine glands and cranial nerves. Extraneous cells may give rise to intracranial masses, including metastatic tumors, congenital inclusions or rests, abscesses or granulomas, parasitic cysts and lymphomas. In addition, some neoplasms arising from the skull extend intracranially.

Little is known about the etiology of primary brain tumors. In some cases trauma, including irradiation, may be a causative factor. Cushing found that some meningiomas arose at a site of cranial injury. Heredity may be a factor in some cases, and tumors in multiple members of a family have been observed. In von Recklinghausen's disease, optic nerve tumors are common as well as tumors of cranial nerve sheaths and meningiomas. In tuberous sclerosis, relatively benign gangliogliomas may develop. Viral infections are thought to be a causative factor in some types of intracranial neoplasms.

The general incidence of brain tumors, and particularly of specific types, depends in large part on the institution where statistics are gathered. In some centers there is a large referral of some types of tumors to physicians especially interested in their treatment. If only autopsy data are examined, approximately 2% of patients coming to necropsy throughout the United States are found to have a brain tumor. On an average neurologic service the incidence of brain tumor is third in frequency behind cerebrovascular disease and infectious diseases of the nervous system.

As noted above, brain tumors are seen at any age and are common in infants and children. In the analysis of Michael (1964) gliomas are second only to leukemia among malignant lesions diagnosed at the Children's

TABLE 1.—TEN MOST COMMON INTRACRANIAL TUMORS IN ORDER OF FREQUENCY
Total Number of Cases: 5199

		No. of Cases	%
1.	Glioma	1633	31.4
2.	Metastatic tumor	1056	20.3
3.	Meningioma	802	15.4
4.	Inflammatory masses	334	6.4
5.	Vascular masses	305	5.9
6.	Pituitary adenoma	229	4.4
7.	Sarcoma	216	4.1
8.	Malignant lymphoma	168	3.2
9.	Craniopharyngioma	84	1.6
10.	Medulloblastoma	82	1.6
	All others	290	5.7

From Zimmerman, H. M.: Seminars in Roentgenol. 6:48, 1971.

TABLE 2.—RELATIVE INCIDENCE OF GLIOMAS
1727 cases, Neurological Institute of New York; 1633 cases, Zimmerman

	N.I.N.Y.	ZIMMERMAN*
Astrocytoma	36	25
Glioblastoma	31	51
Medulloblastoma (neuronal)	10	2
Ependymoma	4	6
Oligodendroglioma	3	5
All others and unclassified	16	11
Total	100%	100%

* Zimmerman, H. M.: Seminars in Roentgenol. 6:48, 1971.

Hospital of San Francisco. In an earlier study by Helmholz (1931) at the Mayo Clinic, central nervous system malignancies were by far the most common type on record, almost half of the cases reviewed being central nervous system lesions and these tumors being seen more than twice as often as leukemia and other lymphoid lesions. This probably reflects the referred nature of the material reviewed. On the other hand, gliomas were the most common tumor to cause death in children among an autopsy series of 37,000 cases at the Los Angeles County Hospital (Steiner, 1947).

The incidence of various types of intracranial tumors was given by Zimmerman (1971) from a review of pathologic material in 5199 cases of intracranial space-occupying lesions (Table 1). The relative frequency of gliomas shows that those arising from astrocytes are by far the most common. Table 2 gives the relative incidence of the five most common types among 1727 gliomas occurring at the Neurological Institute of New York and among 1633 gliomas in the pathologic material of Zimmerman.

With increasing longevity, the number of metastatic tumors of the central nervous system that are observed has been steadily increasing. The most common source, by far, is carcinoma of the lung. The incidence of metastatic

TABLE 3.—METASTATIC TUMORS

	%
Lung	40
Melanoblastic	12
Breast	11
G.I. tract	8
Retroperitoneal	7
Sarcomas	5
Female genital	4
Head and neck	3
Eyes and nose	3
Male genital	2
Primary not discovered	5

From Courville, C. B.: *Pathology of the Central Nervous System* (3rd ed.; Mountain View, Calif.: Pacific Press Publishing Association, 1950).

brain tumors by site of origin was studied by Courville (1950) and is shown in Table 3.

Intracranial tumors may be divided into two large categories: (1) intracerebral, and (2) extracerebral neoplasms. They may be considered first according to histologic type, as listed in Tables 1 and 2.

INTRACEREBRAL TUMORS

Most brain tumors are gliomas and grow in the cerebral hemispheres. Some grow within the ventricles and are usually referred to as intraventricular tumors. It is not uncommon for a glioma to extend to the cerebral surface and then grow in an exophytic manner; in these cases it is difficult at times to differentiate the lesion from an extracerebral tumor by radiologic examination.

In an early stage of embryologic development the neural tube derived from the ectoderm divides with the formation of (1) a layer of lining cells for the central cavity, the ependymal layer, which becomes the ependyma of the adult nervous system and (2) a mantle layer which becomes very cellular. Two types of cells develop in the mantle layer: (1) the germinal cells, which give rise to neuroblasts, which eventually become the neurons of the gray substance and ganglion cells, and (2) spongioblasts, which develop into the supporting glial cells. It is from the supporting glial cells that most primary brain tumors arise.

ASTROCYTOMA.—By far the most frequent tumor of the central nervous system is the astrocytoma. It constitutes approximately one-third of all intracranial tumors in most reported series, and approximately two-thirds of all gliomas are astrocytomas. In most institutions they are graded according to malignancy, grade I being the best differentiated, to grade IV which is poorly differentiated. Grade IV astrocytomas are also called glioblastomas, and the benign and malignant forms of the lesion occur with almost equal frequency (Table 2). Some neuropathologists like to add descriptive terms such as protoplasmic, fibrillary or piloid astrocytoma, or astrocytoma with glioblastomatous changes. As already noted, it is not unusual for glial tumors to change their nature in the course of growth and become more malignant. It should also be kept in mind that surgical specimens may not be fully representative of the entire tumor, so that a lesion classified as a benign astrocytoma from biopsy may follow a rapid downhill course because another portion of the tumor (even the greatest portion) may be a glioblastoma. Some astrocytomas become cystic; this group tends to occur in younger individuals and in the cerebellum, usually following a more benign course. Astrocytomas frequently undergo calcific as well as cystic degeneration.

The tumors that reach the ventricle or grow to the brain surface may then metastasize to other parts of the central nervous system through the cerebrospinal fluid, including the spinal cord. This occurs more often with glioblastoma than with astrocytoma.

MEDULLOBLASTOMA.—Strictly speaking, medulloblastomas are not gliomas but are tumors of the neuron series. They are derived from the germinal cells that give rise to neurons of the gray substance and the ganglion cells. They are the only common tumor of the neuron series and are usually considered with the gliomas in most pathologic classifications. Other tumors of the neuron series include neuroblastoma, ganglioneuroma and the ganglioglioma, which is a mixed neuronal and glial neoplasm. Almost all medulloblastomas arise in the cerebellum and are seldom seen in the cerebral hemispheres except as secondary metastatic deposits.

The medulloblastoma is usually found in childhood, more than 50% of patients being less than 10 years of age. The maximal incidence is between ages 5 and 9. The tumor occurs in boys three times as often as in girls.

Approximately 75% of medulloblastomas are midline tumors. They may arise near the fourth ventricle in the vermis from nests of primitive cells that may be retained in the posterior medullary velum. From here the tumors often present as intraventricular masses; those arising more posteriorly in the cerebellar vermis may encroach upon the cisterna magna as well as compromising the fourth ventricle. Because the tumor grows rapidly and is friable, fragments often circulate in the cerebrospinal fluid and produce implants on other portions of the brain and the spinal cord.

EPENDYMOMA.—The ependymal lining of the neural tube becomes differentiated early in its embryologic development. Most tumors arising from these lining cells grow within the ventricular lumen. Ependymal tissue is relatively abundant in the region of the fourth ventricle, and intraluminal growth of well-differentiated neoplasms of this type is common at this site. In supratentorial locations it is not uncommon to find ependymomas growing outward into the hemispheres with a relatively small intraventricular component. The tumors occur predominantly in childhood and adolescence but may also be found in adults.

OLIGODENDROGLIOMA.—These tumors arise from the smaller supporting cells of the neural stroma. They usually occur in the cerebral hemispheres. Their highest incidence is in middle adult life, although they are not uncommon in younger patients, and in the average case they are marked by a slow clinical progression. In some cases, however, the tumors are not made up of pure oligodendroglial cells, but astrocytes may be included which often accelerate the tempo of growth. Although chiefly neoplasms of the centrum semiovale, oligodendrogliomas may be found within the lateral ventricles and in the region of the third ventricle, the former probably arising from cells in the septum pellucidum. With such intraventricular lesions it is common to find the tumor growing through the septum pellucidum and involving both lateral ventricles.

PINEAL NEOPLASMS.—Several different types of tumors may be found in the pineal region and in the prepineal portion of the third ventricle. The most common type of pineal tumor is derived from the pineal parenchyma. These pinealomas constitute about two-thirds of the tumors of the pineal region. Teratomas form about 25% of pineal lesions; the third most common neoplasms in the area are gliomas arising in the posterior portion of the third ventricle, the majority being ependymomas. Dermoid and epidermoid cysts are also found in this area. More primitive types of pineal body cells are found in occasional tumors and are referred to as pinealoblastomas by some investigators. The majority of primary pineal tumors occur in adolescence or early adult life. What have been called ectopic pinealomas may be found in the suprasellar region, although it is now believed that many of these lesions are dermoids rather than tumors of pineal glia. Calcification often occurs in pineal tumors, and the observation of pineal calcification, especially calcification covering a large area, in a young child or adolescent, in whom the normal gland is not usually calcified, should alert the radiologist to the possibility of a pineal neoplasm.

CHOROID PLEXUS PAPILLOMA.—Although the general incidence is small, choroid plexus papillomas form between 3 and 5% of brain tumors in children. Papillomas occur most frequently during the first decade (45%), when they are seen most often in the lateral ventricle. Papillomas occurring in adults are found most often in the fourth ventricle. Occasionally such lesions are found in the third ventricle and in the cerebellopontine angle.

Most papillomas resemble normal choroid plexus in structure on histologic examination. Malignant changes are not found frequently but, if metaplasia does occur, adjacent neural structures become invaded. Often the tumors are pedunculated, having a distinct stalk, so that the masses move with gravity in the ventricular fluid. The tumors usually cause excessive formation of cerebrospinal fluid.

COLLOID CYST.—The cyst is a special type of benign tumor which is thought to arise from residual epithelial cells of the paraphysis in the anterior portion of the third ventricular roof. Colloid cysts are loosely attached to the choroid plexus of the third ventricular roof. They move to a limited extent with gravity, and when they attain a size of 1.5–2 cm they usually block the foramen of Monro. The cyst wall is a thin fibrous capsule, while the lining is compressed epithelium which produces the colloidlike material within the cyst. The lesion must be differentiated from ependyma-lined cysts which are occasionally seen in the body of the third ventricle.

GANGLIONEUROMA AND GANGLIOGLIOMA.—These lesions are benign tumors of the neuron series mentioned above under medulloblastoma. They contain mature ganglion cells and some glial elements. The tumors are seen most often in children and young adults, and the incidence is high in patients with tuberous sclerosis. Most often the lesions are found within one of the lateral ventricles or in a periventricular area. Occasionally they may arise in the third ventricle and hypothalamus. When such a tumor arises in a lateral ventricle it is most often found in the anterior portion of the ventricle, where it can produce an obstruction at the foramen of Monro. Connective tissue is abundant in such tumors and deposits of calcium frequently are found within the masses.

TERATOMATOUS TUMORS.—This group comprises true teratomas containing tissues derived from all of the three germinal layers, dermoids, which contain all of the dermal elements, and epidermoids, which differ from dermoids in that they do not contain hair and glandular elements. Teratomas and dermoids are usually midline tumors. They are found most frequently in midsagittal posterior fossa locations, in the region of the pineal, and in juxtasellar locations. Epidermoidomas, also called cholesteatomas, may be found off the midline, particularly in the lateral ventricles and in the cerebellopontine angles. It is thought that in the latter instances the lesions are not of "inclusion" origin but may begin as new growths from the epithelium of the choroid plexus. The dermoids and epidermoids expand very slowly, but the teratomas, especially those encountered in infancy, are often highly malignant.

Epidermoidomas begin as epidermoid cysts which, because of their refractile and nodular surface, have been called pearly tumors. As the lesion grows, however, the cyst often ruptures, and the tumor may then extend widely and in an irregular manner giving it its cauliflowerlike appearance. The dermoids are called buttery tumors because of the secretions they contain derived from glandular elements. Teratomas also often have a cystic component containing the buttery secretions. Because of their frequent midline locations dermoids are more often diagnosed when they are smaller and the capsule is still intact than is the case with epidermoids.

METASTATIC TUMORS.—Next in order of frequency behind the gliomas and related tumors listed above stand metastatic neoplasms among the intracerebral new growth (see Table 1). The sources of the secondary central nervous system tumors are listed in Table 3. The great majority of metastatic tumors are carcinomas (83%), and almost one-half of these begin in the lung. Melanomas account for a surprisingly high percentage of secondary deposits. The majority of metastatic tumors arrive from other organs by way of the blood stream. Some tumors invade the central nervous system by direct extension; this is particularly true of nasopharyngeal carcinoma and other tumors of the head and neck. The most characteristic radiologic feature of metastatic tumors is their multiplicity, although on rare occasions multiple primary gliomas may be encountered.

INFLAMMATORY AND VASCULAR MASSES.—A surprisingly large number of inflammatory lesions appear in the statistical data of many neuropathologists dealing with the relative incidence of mass lesions of the brain. In many cases the statistics embrace the pre-antibiotic days when abscesses and tuberculomas were seen more frequently than at present. On the other hand, there seems to have been an increase in certain types of infections that are not drug sensitive and can cause local mass effects such as herpes simplex encephalitis, the occurrence of toruloma, and so on. While an overall incidence of approximately 10% for inflammatory and vascular mass lesions appears rather excessive, the possibility of such a pathologic process must be kept in mind when diagnosing any intracerebral mass lesion.

Some vascular masses are neoplasms, but the majority are not. The most important true blood vessel neoplasms are the hemangioblastomas, which are usually a combined cystic and solid tumor occurring in one cerebellar hemisphere. The tumors are usually seen in middle and later adult life and affect men more often than women. The incidence may be as high as 10% of all cerebellar tumors in adults. A paramedian position is common, and extension to the opposite hemisphere or to the cerebellar vermis may occur. The size of the cystic component varies greatly, and in some cases a small vascular mural nodule is situated inside of a very large cerebellar cyst. When small, the cystic and solid components may be almost equal in size. In many cases other vascular lesions are present in the brain or meninges, and in some syndromes there is angiomatosis of the retina, and in others non-neoplastic cysts of other organs. Polycythemia is often associated with cerebellar hemangioblastoma.

The supratentorial vascular masses are chiefly congenital malformations, sometimes called arteriovenous angiomas. In arteriovenous malformations the arteries and veins making up the lesions are enlarged in caliber and length. Because of the ectasia and elongation a tortuous vascular mass develops. The majority of such lesions are in the middle cerebral artery territory and the overall configuration is often wedge shaped. Because of the abnormal capillary development and arteriovenous shunting there is usually great enlargement of the afferent arteries and the efferent draining veins. With centrally situated malformations there may be marked deformity of the ventricular system by the many enlarged tributaries of the Galenic veins. Both arterial and venous aneurysms may develop within the malformation. When the vein of Galen is involved in such an aneurysmal dilatation it is often so great that it compresses the midbrain and aqueduct of Sylvius and must be differentiated from true tumors of the quadrigeminal region, such as pinealomas and tentorial meningiomas.

EXTRACEREBRAL TUMORS

As with intracerebral lesions, the extracerebral neoplasms may be benign or malignant, solid or cystic, primary or secondary, and large or small. The benign tumors have in common noninvasiveness of the brain itself as a growth characteristic. Instead the tumors displace cerebral structures away from them as they enlarge and frequently locally indent the brain, forming a niche, until the lesion may be largely enveloped by cerebral substance. As with other neoplasms, however, some forms of benign extracerebral tumors do have locally invasive qualities, while at other times meningeal hemorrhagic or inflammatory changes may cause adherence of the tumor to the cerebral surface. Other extracerebral tumors such as chordomas and sarcomas are frankly invasive from the outset.

MENINGIOMA.—The most common extracerebral tumor is the meningioma, and this lesion accounts for approximately 15% of all intracranial masses (see Table 1). They are discussed in detail in Part 2 dealing with plain skull radiographic changes.

NEURINOMA.—Nerve sheath tumors (schwannomas or neurilemmomas or neurinomas) are the solitary encapsulated lesions of the nerve roots. The other principal nerve sheath lesions are the multiple neurofibromas of von Recklinghausen's disease. The most commonly encountered extracerebral tumor of this type is the neurinoma arising from the eighth cranial nerve. In addition to acoustic neurinomas, however, similar lesions may be found on the trigeminal, glossopharyngeal, hypoglossal and other cranial nerves. Occasionally malignant neurinomas may be found. The majority of acoustic neurinomas erode bone which, through tomography, may be demonstrated on plain skull radiographs in a high percentage of cases.

Neurofibromas occur most commonly on the peripheral nerves, but central neurofibromatosis is frequently associated. Bilateral acoustic neurinomas are common in von Recklinghausen's disease, as well as tumors of other cranial nerves. In addition, tumors other than neurofibromas may be found. Meningiomas occur much more frequently in von Recklinghausen's disease than on the average, and glial tumors, especially astrocytomas of the optic nerve, are often seen in conjunction with neurofibromatosis. Tumors of other systems may also be found in neurofibromatosis; an example is the association in approximately 5% of cases of pheochromocytoma.

The solitary neurinomas have a strong tendency to involve sensory nerves. They occur during the middle years of life and are twice as common in women as in men.

BASAL TUMORS.—A large number of extracerebral tumors, including the neurinomas, are found at the base of the brain. A high percentage occur in juxtasellar locations and they are presented in Part 3, "Sellar and Parasellar Tumors." The most common lesions of the area are the tumors of pituitary origin, which were considered by Steinbach and Minagi in *The Endocrines* (An Atlas of Tumor Radiology, 1969). Following pituitary tumors, craniopharyngiomas, meningiomas, optic gliomas and aneurysms acting as basal mass lesions are encountered in that order of frequency. Optic gliomas may be extracerebral (when they involve only the nerve) or intracerebral as well. The majority of these lesions produce a mass effect on the visual pathways and the hypothalamus.

CHORDOMA.—Chordomas are malignant tumors arising from notochordal rests in or near the midline. The most common site of origin is the basisphenoid area, but they may arise at an even more rostral site. The tumors erode bone and grow first in an extradural location, displacing and compressing the brain stem from the ventral side. The tumors also frequently occur in the nasopharynx from which biopsy confirmation can often be obtained. Diagnostic changes can frequently be found on routine radiographs through evidence of bone erosion and sequestrated pieces of bone contained within the mass of the tumor. Other local tumors that secondarily involve the nervous system by direct extension are the glomus jugulare tumors, osteomas, osteochondromas and the malignant carcinomas of the nasopharynx and ear, and orbital tumors.

SARCOMA.—Sarcomas may arise from any of the cellular elements of the meninges, including the fibrous dura, the meningeal blood vessels and perivascular structures. Primary meningeal sarcomas are not rare, and secondary sarcomas occur with surprising frequency (see Table 3). Many of the latter are extensions of lymphosarcoma, Hodgkin's disease, multiple myeloma and osteogenic sarcoma. Orbital tumors often extend intracranially.

Fibrosarcomas are the commonest form of primary meningeal sarcoma, and although they are most often seen over the frontoparietal convexity or in the posterior fossa, they may occur within the brain itself, arising from elements of the pia arachnoid which follow blood vessels into the substance of the brain. In some cases meningiomas are, or become, malignant. Other types of more frequently encountered primary sarcomas are hemangiopericytomas and the reticulum cell group. A miscellaneous group includes tumors arising from muscular and cartilaginous elements, tumors of mixed cellular types and some classified only as small cell or giant cell sarcomas, the small cell lesions being most often seen in the posterior fossa. Radiolucent destructive bony changes are often found on routine radiographs. Hemangiopericytomas are highly vascular, and enlargement and proliferation of meningeal arteries and veins may be seen on plain films. In some cases fibrosarcomas or osteogenic sarcomas may develop in children who have received heavy radiation for the treatment of retinoblastoma. Further consideration of this type of lesion is given in Part 14, "The Eye and the Orbit."

METHODS OF DIAGNOSIS

Since a variety of procedures is available for the examination of patients suspected of having a brain tumor, not all involving radiologic methods, an orderly approach using groups of tests is necessary. It is generally accepted that procedures involving instrumentation, particularly the direct insertion of needles into the brain, and the disturbance of cerebrospinal fluid dynamics should be avoided whenever possible. A logical beginning would appear to be the use of studies that are painless and essentially harmless to the patient before resort to angiography, pneumoencephalography, positive contrast cisternography and especially ventriculography, as well as other techniques that carry with them some morbidity and a definite complication rate.

This concept entails for the neuroradiologist first plain skull radiography, high-definition tomographic filming and computerized tomography. In some cases sonography and radioactive nuclide imaging are also involved. Skull radiographs can be expected to show a shift of the calcified pineal gland in 10–15% of patients who have a supratentorial tumor. A direct diagnosis of certain tumors affecting bone, such as meningiomas, pituitary adenomas and acoustic neurinomas, can be expected in a high percentage of cases, especially when tomographic radiographs of good detail are included. At other times, pathologic calcification affords diagnosis from the plain films.

CRANIOCEREBRAL RADIOGRAPHY WITHOUT CONTRAST MEDIUM

The roentgenograms should be made in accordance with a good routine, and any additional views that might conceivably shed light on the clinical problem at hand should be obtained. It has been suggested that all patients admitted to hospitals have a single lateral skull radiograph as well as a routine chest radiograph. Although the value of such a routine has not been established, it might well prove worth while inasmuch as approximately 15% of hospital admissions have neurologic disorders.

Because the skull is a rounded object it is necessary to examine it from more than one side. The lateral view and the mentovertical base view are the anatomic projections. All of the frontal views are distortions, depending on the angulation of the x-ray beam with the base of the skull. The minimal examination consists of right-angle views, usually in lateral and frontal projections. It is our practice to obtain stereoscopic lateral views in order to have a three-dimensional depiction in every case. This is not always possible in children and after head injuries, but in such cases it is essential to obtain both right and left lateral views. Two exposures are usually made in postero-anterior projection; one is straight in relation to the orbitomeatal line, as described below, and the other is inclined so that portions of the upper facial bones are included. It is also important to obtain a third frontal exposure in anteroposterior half-axial projection (Towne view).

At this point it is necessary to define certain points, lines and planes with which neuroradiology deals (Fig. 1). The nasion is the midpoint of the frontonasal suture. The supraorbital and infraorbital points are the highest and lowest points respectively along the orbital rim. The center of the orbit anteriorly, sometimes called the pupillary point, is the center of the generally

Figure 1.—Reference points and lines used in radiography of the skull. **1,** Nasion; **2,** supraorbital point; **3,** center of the circular orbital rim; **4,** infraorbital point; **5,** center or axis of the external auditory meatus; **6,** inion; **7,** bregma; **8,** vertex. **A,** Anthropologic basal line; **B,** orbitomeatal basal line, and **C,** auricular line.

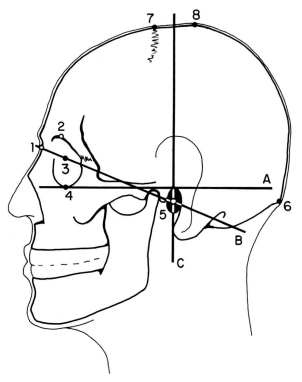

circular orbital rim. The external auditory meatus is another important land-mark; at times the center of the meatus (axis of the external auditory canal) is used for some reference lines while the superior border of the meatus is used for others. The inion is the external occipital protuberance. The bregma is the point of junction of the sagittal and coronal sutures. The vertex is the highest point of the calvaria when the skull is viewed with the anthropologic basal line horizontal.

The anthropologic basal line (Reid's baseline) is a line that joins the infraorbital point with the superior border of the external auditory meatus.* The orbitomeatal basal line is drawn from the palpable tubercle of the fron-tosphenoidal process of the zygomatic bone, which is near the posterior ex-tremity of the orbital rim (on the lateral rim and 1 cm below the frontozy-gomatic suture), to the center of the external auditory meatus. The anterior point of the line usually coincides with the outer canthus of the eye (cantho-meatal line) and the center of the orbit. Extended forward the orbitomeatal line passes through or very near the nasion. The anthropologic and orbito-meatal basal lines form an angle of approximately 10 degrees. The other line of importance on the lateral surface of the skull is the auricular line. This line is perpendicular to the anthropologic basal line; it is drawn through the center of the external auditory meatus and usually passes midway between the bregma and the vertex.

As indicated above, the lateral view is the most anatomic and the most informative of the plain craniocerebral radiographs. The lateral projection is made with the median sagittal plane parallel to the film; the central ray is directly perpendicular to the median sagittal plane and centered on the auric-ular line 3–4 cm above the external auditory meatus. For the basal or axial projection the head is placed in hyperextension and the anthropologic plane (the plane containing the two anthropologic basal lines) is parallel to the film. The central ray is perpendicular to the anthropologic plane and passes along the biauricular plane (a plane perpendicular to the anthropologic plane and containing the two auricular lines). The straight posteroanterior projection is made with the orbitomeatal lines perpendicular to the film (usually the forehead and nose touch the film). The central ray is directed perpendicular to the film and its point of exit from the skull is the nasion. The inclined posteroanterior projection also has the orbitomeatal line per-pendicular to the film. The tube is angled 15 degrees craniocaudally to form a similar angle with the orbitomeatal line, and the exit of the central ray is again at the nasion. The projection is quite similar to the Caldwell view. The

* International Commission on Neuroradiology of the World Federation of Neurology, Brit. J. Radiol. 35:501, 1962.

final exposure of the routine skull series is the anteroposterior half-axial projection. For this the occiput is against the film and the orbitomeatal plane is perpendicular to the film. The central ray makes an angle of 25–30 degrees craniocaudally with the orbitomeatal plane and passes through the center of the axis joining the two external auditory meati.

TOMOGRAPHIC FILMING may be carried out using a variety of motions of the tube and film. Laminagraphy or planigraphy is the simplest form of tomographic study. In general, however, there are many parasite shadows which often interfere with the areas of special interest. Better tomograms are obtained using a circular or elliptical movement. The motion for best detail is the hypocycloidal, generally referred to as polytomography.

COMPUTERIZED TOMOGRAPHY is a means of defining intracranial structures and lesions by the differences in absorption by various tissues of radiation passing through the head. Cerebral tissue has an absorption coefficient approximately 8% greater than that of cerebrospinal fluid, with the result that the ventricular system and the subarachnoid space can be graphically depicted in contrast to the more absorptive soft tissue and highly absorptive bone. Any collection of intracranial calcium or of fat gives highly contrasting absorption values.

The computerized tomographic apparatus employs a narrow beam of radiation to scan the patient's head in a series of 1-cm wide transverse sections. The x-rays passing through the head activate two scintillation detectors pointing toward the radiation source. Both the x-ray tube and the detector move in a linear manner, making 160 recordings of radiation transmitted with each sweep. The system is then rotated 1 degree in relation to the head and the scanning process is repeated until a semicircle of 180 scans has been described. The procedure results in 28,000 readings taken for each section, which are processed on a computer which calculates the absorption value for the material within the brain section at 12,000 points. A picture can be built up from the absorption values calculated and displayed on an oscilloscope as an image in black, white and gray tones. The image can also be displayed on a television monitor and color added to represent different absorption values. A numerical computer printout is also obtained. Currently an area 1.5 mm square in size as seen face-on can be depicted as an individual shadow on the oscilloscope matrix. Although this definition of fluid-containing cavities and the margins of abnormal intracerebral densities is not as sharp as in intracranial pneumography, the safety and atraumatic nature of the computerized tomography technique makes it an important adjunct in neuroradiologic examination. The equipment is being continuously improved and images of higher resolution are thus being made available.

Computerized tomography demonstrates better than any other atraumatic survey technique the position of the pineal gland, third ventricle and other structures normally in the midline (see Fig. 24). The method gives a useful outline of the lateral cerebral ventricles and subarachnoid space, providing information about ventricular size and configuration, local ventricular enlargement or porencephaly, and deformities of ventricular outlines in the planes examined (see Fig. 14). The actual outline of deep and superficial tumors can be depicted on the oscilloscope owing to the difference in radiation absorption by a tumor and the normal adjacent cerebral tissue (see Fig. 25). The multiplicity of metastatic tumors can often be shown (see Fig. 34). In addition, intracerebral hematomas are readily shown and a cystic component of a neoplasm may be demonstrated, especially if it contains lipid material, such as a craniopharyngioma (see Fig. 33).

CONTRAST EXAMINATIONS

The choice of a special neuroradiologic procedure is concerned with the more important indications and contraindications for examinations requiring instrumentation. It is now widely held among neuroradiologists that angiography should be performed in the vast majority of cases prior to pneumoencephalography unless the patient is suspected of having a condition in which the complication rate is very high. Almost all patients suspected of having a supratentorial tumor have angiography as their first special procedure. By this approach, some patients may be spared intracranial pneumography altogether, as in the case of a convexity meningioma. Although intracranial pneumography may be required for a definitive diagnosis in many patients, prior angiography often gives important information as to the choice of the proper type of pneumographic procedure; for example, ventriculography rather than pneumoencephalography would be carried out if an angiogram disclosed ventricular dilatation and evidence of cerebral or cerebellar herniation.

In the past it was generally believed, with considerable validity, that pneumographic examination was the procedure of choice in any patient with a clinical syndrome suggesting disease in the posterior fossa, especially an infratentorial tumor. Improved angiography has introduced a new era. Through the use of bibrachial angiography or the use of selective vertebral catheterization, excellent delineation of the vasculature of the posterior fossa can be obtained. In some instances the angiographic architecture may give valuable information even about the type of tumor that is present. However, vertebral angiography is often inconclusive for tumor diagnosis, in which case a follow-up air study is required. Even in these cases some indication can be gained as to whether or not pneumography by the lumbar route will be safe and successful.

CEREBRAL ANGIOGRAPHY.—Certain standardized views have come into acceptance for initial investigation of supratentorial and infratentorial lesions. A frontal view (somewhat similar to a reverse Granger 107° projection), which is a view with the tops of the petrous bones superimposed on the tops of the orbits, and a true lateral view are the two standard projections for supratentorial lesions (Fig. 2). The Sylvian fissure is displayed with an acceptable degree of foreshortening while the floor of the anterior fossa is seen nearly end-on over the orbital roofs. Other views tailored for a particular location of the lesion may then be taken, and it is obvious that

Figure 2.—Angiographic projections. In the standard angiographic projections the occiput is against the film and the orbitomeatal plane (D) is perpendicular to the film. The lateral view is made with a horizontal beam directed toward a point on the auricular line 3–4 cm above the external auditory meatus, usually near the top of the ear, shown here as a dot. The frontal carotid angulation (A) is 12° craniocaudal to the orbito-meatal plane, the vertebral angulation (B) is 30°, and for the reverse Caldwell view the beam is angled 15° caudocranially (C). Each frontal beam is directed toward a midline point on the biauricular plane, corresponding to the point above the external auditory meatus used for the lateral view.

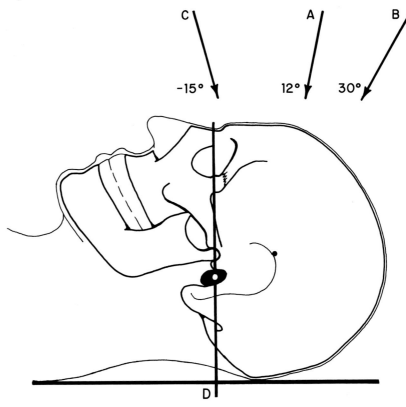

the variations are innumerable. A commonly used additional view is an inclined anteroposterior projection (reverse Caldwell view) to see the middle fossa contents through the orbit. Oblique views may be made in head injury cases to see the frontal and occipital poles, as well as a tangential view for a mass effect near the surface to ascertain if it is extracerebral in position. Lesions on the tentorial surface and infratentorial lesions are well displayed in a Caldwell-like view in which the posterior cerebral vessels above and the superior cerebellar vessels below the tentorium are seen clearly. This also requires the use of subtraction techniques in order to work out the vasculature through the facial structures. The Towne projection and a lateral view centered over the posterior fossa are the other standard views for infratentorial lesions. Magnification films are made liberally to demonstrate small vessel details.

The technique required for selective angiography may be either direct puncture or catheterization. When more than one cerebral vessel needs to be opacified it is usually easier for the patient to be catheterized. Catheterization techniques are standard procedure for opacification of the vertebral arteries. The exception to this is the elderly patient, in whom the vertebral-basilar system is more safely opacified by simultaneous bilateral brachial injections.

CEREBRAL PNEUMOGRAPHY.—There are relatively few contraindications to the intracranial use of gas in the study of neurologic disorders. The majority are acute processes such as infections or subarachnoid hemorrhage and recent craniocerebral trauma. It is generally believed that pneumography serves to spread infection, and the alterations in cerebrospinal fluid dynamics produced by the replacement of cerebrospinal fluid by gas may evoke pressure changes that can result in the rebleeding of an aneurysm.

Properly performed, pneumoencephalography should produce very few complications and almost always results in a more definitive examination than ventriculography. Any method that does not require the insertion of needles into the brain is better if the technique is considered safe. When clinical findings are marginal as to whether ventriculography or pneumoencephalography should be performed, it is common practice for the neurosurgeon to make burr holes in preparation for ventriculography but a needle is not actually inserted into the ventricles. Pneumoencephalography is then carried out by the lumbar route and the burr holes can be used to decompress the ventricles if this should become necessary. Dexamethasone (Decadron) is often given prophylactically before pneumoencephalography.

Pneumoencephalography rather than ventriculography is now carried out by preference even in the presence of certain known tumors. As noted above, tumors of the posterior fossa occurring in the forward portion of this compartment are safely and more effectively investigated by pneumoencephalography than by ventriculography. Intra-axial tumors of the brain stem are usually found clinically when the mass is still relatively small because of the important tracts and cranial nerve nuclei that are present in this region.

Ventriculography is usually carried out in the study of any cause of obstructive hydrocephalus, especially for cerebellar tumors and for intraventricular tumors producing obstruction. It may be necessary to perform ventriculography on patients with central tumors, as of the thalamus, or with hemispheric tumors when angiography has given insufficient information for diagnosis. Ventriculography may also be required when lumbar pneumoencephalography has failed to fill the ventricular system.

Complete failure of ventricular filling (but with good subarachnoid space demonstration) is not always an indication for ventriculography. Although a high percentage of the patients have a tumor, ventricular filling can sometimes be achieved after placing the patient on large daily doses (10–20 mg) of dexamethasone for two to three days and then performing a second examination. Combined ventriculography-pneumoencephalography is required in some cases; ventriculography is normally performed first when an aqueductal or posterior fossa obstruction is suspected.

Positive contrast media are not employed extensively in the United States for ventriculography. Water-soluble agents such as meglumine iothalamate (Conray) are recommended by some. Pantopaque is often used in small quantities (0.5–2.0 cc) to delineate points of ventricular obstruction which are difficult to define by air. One of the main advantages of intraventricular injection of Pantopaque is that it is not necessary to remove a significant amount of cerebrospinal fluid through the ventricular needle. Very often Pantopaque is injected after formal ventriculography has failed to give all of the information required for diagnosis. Obstruction of the aqueduct and collapse of the fourth ventricle, when these structures are ill-defined by air, are the conditions in which positive contrast ventriculography has been found most useful.

Cerebral pneumography is not commonly used today as a primary procedure to diagnose *supratentorial* neoplasms. Cerebral angiography is almost invariably carried out as the first procedure and a pneumographic procedure performed when the diagnosis may be in question following angiography. In general the tumors that are more deeply situated (such as the central tumors in the thalamus, basal ganglia and corpus callosum) are more easily and clearly demonstrated by cerebral pneumography. The more superficially placed tumors and those neoplasms which have a characteristic pattern of circulation are more easily demonstrated by angiography.

An orbiting or somersaulting chair is necessary for satisfactory cerebral pneumography. The chair should have the capability of completely immobilizing the patient in a comfortable manner and of orbiting 360 degrees in either direction. It should also be possible to rotate the patient on his own axis. Tomographic facilities in connection with the orbiting chair are essential for good pneumography. It should be possible to have tomographic movement in two planes and to use a motion transverse to the object of interest.

If it is possible, it is desirable to have a somersaulting device that orbits the patient and the radiographic apparatus around a fixed horizontal axis. The lateral and the frontal x-ray beams can then be made to pass through an isocenter. This assures minimal distortion since the frontal film in addition to the lateral, can be kept at an angle of 90 degrees to the central ray. The lateral x-ray tube is usually detached and separately mounted so that isocentral lateral projections can be made with the patient in any position of the orbit. This lateral tube should be coupled with a fixed image intensifier and a television monitor to provide gravitational control of air in the ventricular system during the examination.

Pneumoencephalography is usually carried out in two parts. The first is for examination of the posterior fossa and third ventricle. The second is for investigation of the lateral ventricles. The first part is carried out after the introduction of a relatively small amount of air (a total of 15 cc), only a few drops of cerebrospinal fluid having been removed for cell count. This is injected after the patient has been rotated forward 30 degrees from the orbitomeatal line horizontal position shown in Figure 3. This traps air in the fourth ventricle, aqueduct and posterior part of the third ventricle. The patient is then rotated backward until the orbitomeatal line is 30 degrees beyond the vertical plane (hanging-head position). This delineates to best advantage the anterior part of the third ventricle and equalizes the gas that has entered the anterior parts of the lateral ventricles.

The second part of the examination is carried out only after the areas mentioned above have been adequately seen. The patient is then returned to the filling position (orbitomeatal line 30 degrees below horizontal) and sufficient additional gas is injected to outline the lateral ventricles, the size of the ventricles having been estimated from the radiographs at the end of the first series. Some air is also injected with the patient straight upright, or with the head extended, to fill the basal cisterns and other portions of the subarachnoid space. The patient is usually again rotated backward to the

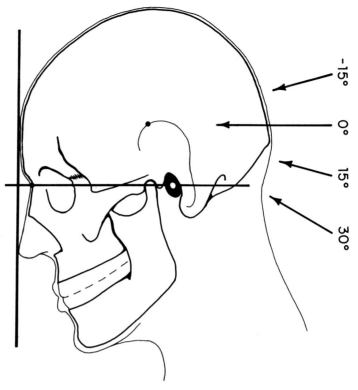

Figure 3.—Pneumographic projections. The sketch shows the patient in straight upright position with the orbitomeatal line horizontal. The lateral views are made with a horizontal beam directed toward a point on the auricular line, as in angiography (Fig. 2). As the patient is somersaulted, the orbitomeatal line remains perpendicular to the film for the frontal views, regardless of his station in orbit. Straight frontal views are made with the central ray parallel to the orbitomeatal line and directed toward a midline point on the biauricular plane, analogous to the point near the top of the ear used for the lateral view. Additional frontal exposures are made at different degrees of angulation off parallel, still directed toward the midline point described above, as required to demonstrate various cerebral structures (see text).

supine (brow-up) or hanging-head position to equalize the lateral ventricular air by exchange at the foramen of Monro and to obtain views of the frontal horns. A complete forward somersault is then carried out, stopping at upright, brow-down, inverted and finally back to brow-up position. In this way the air and ventricular fluid move with gravity so that all portions of the lateral ventricles are outlined piecemeal by filming at the various stops listed. With the patient in the brow-up position after the forward somersault, air should fill both temporal horns, including the anterior temporal tips.

Ventriculography is essentially the reverse of pneumoencephalography. Air is introduced into the lateral ventricles and these cavities are studied first. Since most patients undergoing ventriculography have hydrocephalus resulting from a central lesion blocking the third ventricle or aqueduct, or a cerebellar tumor, it is necessary to move the air caudad to prove ventricular patency or to show a ventricular obstruction or deformity. For this a backward somersault is required. The patient is carried from the upright to the supine (brow-up), hanging-head, inverted and over to the brow-down posture, exposures being made at each station of the orbit. With the patient brow-down, maximal gas should be available to fill the posterior third ventricle, the aqueduct and fourth ventricle or to outline an abnormality of these areas.

Filming at pneumography is somewhat more tailor-made than at angiography. Nevertheless a good routine is necessary, and precise centering and coning are required. Most of the lateral exposures are made with the x-ray beam centered on a point on the auricular line 3–4 cm above the external auditory meatus. This will usually fall near the top of the ear and the central ray will pass near the center of the ventricular system in the prepineal portion of the third ventricle (Fig. 3). For the posterior fossa and the anterior third ventricular views, the central ray of the lateral beam may be positioned behind the external auditory meatus over the posterior fossa, or above the temporomandibular joint in the suprasellar region, respectively. The frontal beam is usually directed toward a midline point on the auricular plane, corresponding to the point above the meatus mentioned above. Frontal radiographs are usually made in more than one projection. With the patient in each position, an exposure should be made with the beam parallel to the orbitomeatal line; it is usually helpful to have one or more additional frontal views made with different degrees of caudocranial angulation and occasionally to have a frontal view with craniocaudal angulation (Caldwell projection). With most somersaulting devices it is more convenient to obtain the frontal views in posteroanterior projection, but when it is necessary to improvise, anteroposterior projections can be satisfactory.

BIBLIOGRAPHY

1. Courville, C. B.: *Pathology of the Central Nervous System* (3rd ed.; Mountain View, Calif.: Pacific Press Publishing Association, 1950).
2. Helmholz, H. F.: Malignant neoplasms in childhood. Proc. Interstate Postgrad. M. Assembly North America, p. 209, 1931.
3. Hounsfield, G. N.: Computerized transverse axial scanning (tomography): Part 1: Description of system, Brit. J. Radiol. 46:1016, 1973.
4. Michael, P.: *Tumors of Infancy and Childhood* (Philadelphia: J. B. Lippincott Company, 1964).
5. Steiner, P.: Los Angeles County Hospital files, 1947.
6. Zimmerman, H. M.: The ten most common types of brain tumor, Seminars in Roentgenol. 6:48, 1971.

PART 2

Craniocerebral Radiography

Craniocerebral Radiography

THE CRANIOCEREBRAL RADIOGRAPHIC EXAMINATION, described in Part 1, is designed to demonstrate primary cerebral evidence of disease and secondary cranial evidence of an intracranial tumor. There are three levels of information that may be obtained: (1) the presence of an intracranial expanding lesion may be recognized; (2) the presence and localization of an expanding intracranial process may be determined; and (3) the presence, localization and identification of a brain tumor may be established.

INCREASED INTRACRANIAL PRESSURE

Intracranial hypertension beyond infancy is most often caused by a brain tumor. In infancy and childhood plumbism, hydrocephalus from any cause, and a number of inflammatory processes may expand the cranium.

In early life increased intracranial pressure is manifested by *enlargement of the head* and *widening of the major sutures*. It is possible for the head to enlarge gradually so that there is no suture widening, only meg-

Figure 4.—Acute suture widening. A 2½-year-old boy had headache and lethargy for 1 month and vomiting for 10 days before hospitalization. Bilateral papilledema was found, and routine skull radiographs revealed widening of the major sutures, the sagittal suture showing the greatest widening without sclerotic margins or evidence of bridging of the gap. The changes were caused by a large cystic glioma of the right cerebral hemisphere.

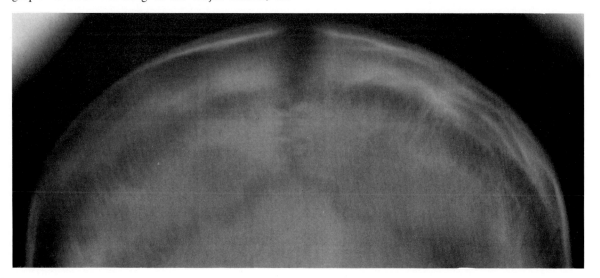

alocephaly. Widening of the major sutures is much more common. Increased intracranial pressure may be manifested as suture widening up to age 20. After the second decade, suture widening is rarely seen except as a manifestation of diastasis resulting from trauma.

The anterior fontanelle is open for the first 1½ years of life and radiologic as well as clinical evidence of bulging may be found. On lateral radiographs a soft tissue convexity may be seen that tapers to normal only beyond the bone edges; this does not vary with the patient's physiologic state as does the bulging seen clinically. Adjacent to an open fontanelle the sutures are wide normally. The younger the child, the greater the suture widening with intracranial hypertension, in most cases. The severity of

Figure 5.—Types of suture widening. In acute widening (**A**), separation of the bones may be great and there is no evidence of reaction along the serrated edges of the separated bones. When widening is less acute (**B**), bony condensation develops along the serrated bone edges and the digitations of the sutures begin to elongate. After a longer period of time (**C**), there is bridging of portions of the gap. With lower grades of prolonged intracranial hypertension (**D**) the suture widening usually is not as great and there may be considerable bridging of the intraosseous space.

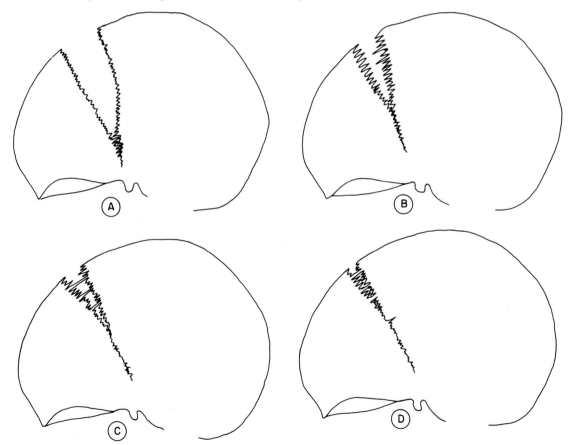

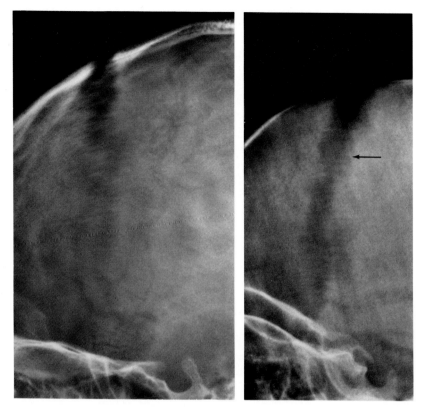

Figure 6 (left).—Elongation of digitations of the coronal suture. The digitations on both sides of the coronal suture show some increase in density and have become elongated, extending into the space between the frontal and parietal bones. The changes occurred in a 6-year-old boy who had progressive ataxia for five weeks and vomiting for one week. On hospitalization a large head, papilledema and truncal ataxia were found. Angiographic and pneumographic studies demonstrated a fourth ventricular tumor producing obstructive hydrocephalus, and at operation a large medulloblastoma was found.

Figure 7 (right).—Bridging of widened suture. A 1½-year-old infant became irritable, cried frequently and moved his extremities poorly for three weeks. He then began to sleep for prolonged periods and for a week before hospitalization vomited two or three times a day. Although the coronal suture is quite wide, numerous elongated digitations (**arrow**) extend completely across the gap between the separated cranial bones. The patient had a cerebellar medulloblastoma.

the pressure is, of course, also a factor. After the age of 3 years, a suture may be considered abnormal if the bones are separated more than 2 mm.

In infants and young children acute suture widening may develop overnight when sudden occlusion of the aqueduct of Sylvius develops, producing hydrocephalus. The coronal and sagittal sutures are most often affected (Fig. 4). The lambdoidal suture is also widened in some cases but is usually affected by more prolonged pressure. By acute suture widening is meant a large gap between the bones of the vault with no evidence of bridging, or attempted bridging, of the space between the serrated edges of the bones (Fig. 5). When the widening has continued for a longer period the serrated edges of the sutures (or the digitations) become sclerotic, elongate and extend into the space between the separated cranial bones. At first they may not bridge the entire gap produced by the separation (Fig. 6). In the subacute stage of suture diastasis bony bridges can be seen to extend across the gap between the separated cranial bones (Fig. 7). This indicates that a decompression of the intracranial expansion has been accomplished, at least for the time being. With lower grades of more prolonged intracranial hypertension the suture widening may be only a slight separation of the bones, and there is often complete bridging of the interosseous space, denoting equilibrium with an abnormally large intracranial volume (Fig. 5).

Figure 8.—Chronic intracranial hypertension. A 13-year-old girl had intermittent headache for many years. More recently, headache had become more frequent and more severe and blurring of vision developed. The skull film reveals pressure changes of both vault and base. The head is large, and slight widening of the cranial sutures is shown with areas of sclerosis around the suture edges and bridging at many points indicating the chronic nature of the intracranial hypertension. The convolutional markings are prominent over the entire vault, especially in the parietal areas where normally few impressions are seen. The dorsum sellae and posterior clinoid processes are absent and the anterior clinoid processes are demineralized. The severe hydrocephalus, including marked enlargement of the hypothalamic portion of the third ventricle, was caused by a glioma of the posterior part of the third ventricle.

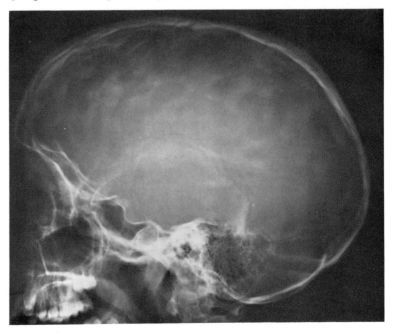

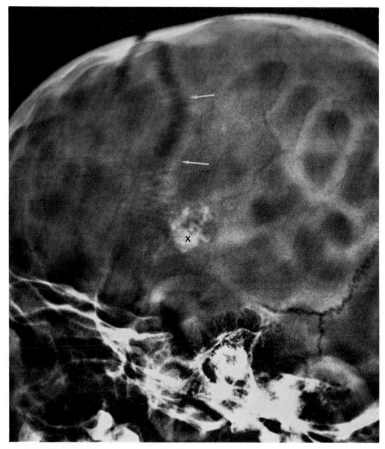

Figure 9.—Chronic pressure changes. In the second decade, prolonged increased intracranial pressure may cause changes in the vault as well as atrophy of the sella turcica. There is moderate widening of the coronal suture with numerous bridges across the gap (**arrows**). There is marked deepening of the convolutional markings in the frontal area, and unusually prominent markings are present in the parietal region where they are seldom found normally. The patient, a girl of 16, who had headache for many years, and more recently blurred vision, was found to have a partially calcified oligodendroglioma (**X**) involving the septum pellucidum and extending into the third ventricle.

Increased convolutional markings are seen most often in patients with prolonged increased intracranial pressure. The markings, or digital impressions, are most significant when found in the parietal area (Fig. 8). Prominent markings may be seen normally in the frontal and occipital regions, especially between age 2 and 10. The markings can occur in normal children in the temporal and in the parietal regions but they are less numerous than at the poles of the brain. An increase in the number, depth and overall prominence of the markings should raise a suspicion of abnormal pressure. However, they should not be used as the only basis for diagnosis of intracranial hypertension except in the presence of craniostenosis. Abnormal convolutional markings are a better indication of the chronicity of intracranial hypertension rather than being absolute secondary evidence of increased intracranial pressure (Fig. 9).

Increased vascularity, either generalized or localized, may be seen in some cases of increased intracranial pressure. This must be differentiated from the increase in number and size of arterial markings occurring with meningiomas and the enlargement of arterial grooves and diploic veins seen with some vascular lesions, particularly arteriovenous malformations. In some cases of intracranial hypertension there may be hypertrophy of the Pacchionian granulations so that the Pacchionian impressions enlarge. The venous tributaries of the dural sinuses along which Pacchionian bodies are

Figure 10.—Enlarged emissary veins. With prolonged intracranial hypertension the emissary veins (**arrows**) of the occipital region and their foramina may become greatly enlarged. The changes shown occurred in a patient with a frontoparietal astrocytoma (same case as Figs. 15 and 70).

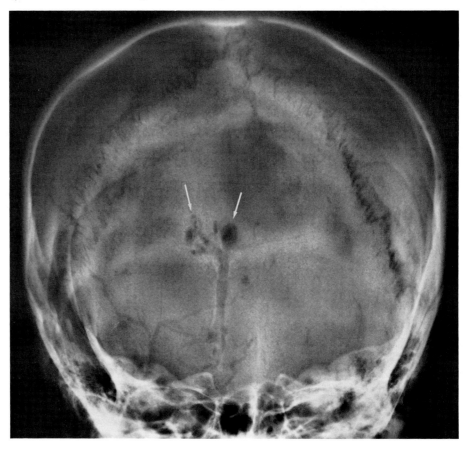

found may also dilate. These changes are seen more often with congenital hydrocephalus than as evidence of a tumor. However, in the occipital region the emissary veins and their tributaries may enlarge and result in marked prominence of the vessel grooves and emissary foramina (Fig. 10). The principal vein in this region is directed vertically near the midline below the torcular Herophili, and normally the foramen does not exceed 2 mm diameter. Other emissary veins and their foramina, such as the mastoid emissary, may also enlarge with long-standing increased intracranial pressure, probably resulting from an interference with the drainage of external vessels into the dural sinuses.

Diffuse atrophy of cranial bones may result from intracranial hypertension, particularly in infants and children, but may also be found in adults. When the vault is affected the bony architecture may become indistinct, with loss of definition of the inner table and pronounced thinning or absence of the diploic space (Fig. 11). In young patients there may be expansion of the cranial cavity in an area markedly affected by such a change. Such atrophy must be differentiated from that sometimes seen with porencephalic cavities or cysts, occasional chronic subdural hematomas and hygromas, and other non-neoplastic processes.

Local atrophy of individual or adjacent cranial bones is much more common than diffuse atrophy, particularly in adults. Atrophy of individual bones or local erosion of portions of bones may result from generalized increased intracranial pressure. The superior portion of the sphenoid bone, particularly the sella turcica, is most vulnerable because of its intracranial extension. By reason of its easy radiographic visibility it is the most important single structure for the detection of intracranial disease after the age of 12. Changes in the sella turcica can be found in the routine radiographs of one-third of patients having brain tumors, even at a distance from the sella itself.

The mechanisms of production of pressure atrophy of the sella turcica have been a subject for extensive study and speculation. Some investigators have considered the pulsations of the carotid and basilar arteries and the circle of Willis to be important when there is increased pressure. The role of enlargement of the third ventricle was stressed by Twining (1939). A more recent study and classification of pressure atrophy and erosion of the sella turcica was made by El Gammal and Allen (1972).

The most common finding is loss of definition of the bony cortex forming the anterior wall of the dorsum sellae. This area is continuous with the cortex forming the sellar floor, but normally the cortex of the floor is thinner. With continued increased intracranial pressure the floor of the

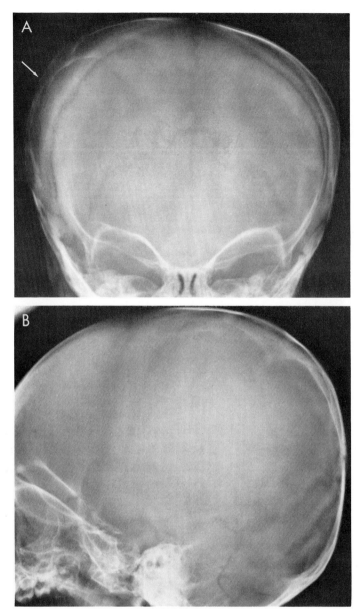

Figure 11.—Extensive hemicranial pressure atrophy. A 6-month-old infant was hospitalized for evaluation of progressive enlargement of the right side of the head. In the frontal view (**A**) the sutures are not too remarkable for the patient's age but there are enlargement and outward bulging of the right hemicranium (**arrow**). Large areas suggesting scalloping are seen along the lateral wall of the vault on the right where the bone is very thin with loss of definition of the inner table and diploic space. In the lateral view (**B**) marked thinning from diffuse atrophy involves the entire parietal bone and upper half of the occipital bone. The patient had a choroid plexus papilloma of the right lateral ventricle filling the atrium and extending into the temporal and occipital horns. While the right ventricle was larger than the left, there was diffuse enlargement from overproduction of cerebrospinal fluid.

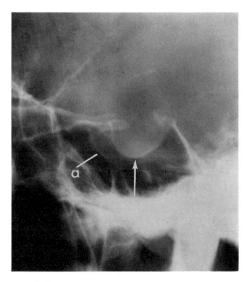

Figure 12.—Increased intracranial pressure in the adult. The interior cortex of the sella turcica (**arrow**) is thin, both in the region of the dorsum and along the sellar floor. The pneumatized dorsum, seen through the laterally situated clinoid processes, appears pointed. The posterior clinoid processes have lost their cortical boundary and the carotid arterial groove (**a**) is prominent along the side of the sella turcica in the cavernous sinus. The patient had a frontal meningioma.

sella also becomes eroded, and eventually the bony cortex of the anterior wall appears to be quite atrophic (Fig. 12). It is thought that these changes of the inner cortex of the pituitary fossa are facilitated when there is a large opening in the diaphragma sellae for the pituitary stalk through which an extension of the subarachnoid space can develop. With the subarachnoid fluid under increased pressure the tongue of arachnoid projecting beneath the diaphragma sellae enlarges and its pulsation erodes the inner cortex of the dorsum. As the space further enlarges, erosion of the top of the dorsum, the sellar floor and eventually the back of the dorsum will take place. Occasionally a very wide diaphragm opening allows a broad arachnoid extension to occur, and in these cases there may be enlargement of the sella turcica without appreciable cortical erosion if the fluid pressure is only slightly elevated (Fig. 13).

When there is ventricular obstruction in the posterior part of the third ventricle, in the aqueduct or in the posterior fossa, the hypothalamic portion of the third ventricle may become greatly dilated (Fig. 14). In these cases the ballooned infundibular recess may rest on the dorsum sellae and erode the top of the dorsum. With time and as the third ventricle enlarges further, the infundibular recess straddles the dorsum and erodes it both internally and externally (Fig. 13). The dorsum may become short and pointed and

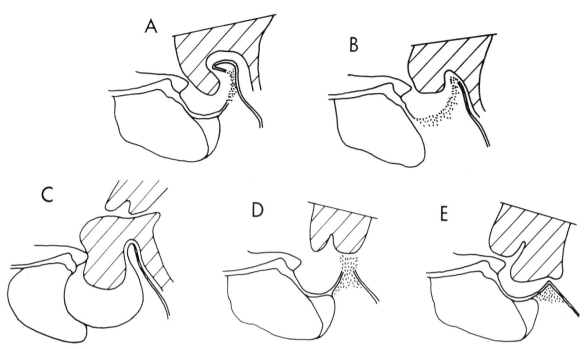

Figure 13.—Pressure erosion of the sella turcica. The probable mechanism of early erosion of the anterior wall of the dorsum is shown in **A.** A tongue of arachnoid projects through the opening in the diaphragma sellae and its pulsations erode the dorsum. With prolonged pressure there is further dilatation of the basal cisterns with erosion of the sellar floor as well as the top of the dorsum (**B**). With a very large opening in the diaphragma sellae there may be generalized sellar enlargement without a high grade of intracranial hypertension (**C**). When the anterior part of the third ventricle enlarges, the infundibular recess often rests on the top of the dorsum, which becomes eroded (**D**). With further dilatation of the anterior third ventricle, the dorsum is further worn away until it is short and pointed. The dilated recesses also erode sellar floor and anterior part of the sella (**E**).

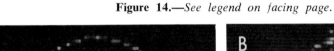

Figure 14.—*See legend on facing page.*

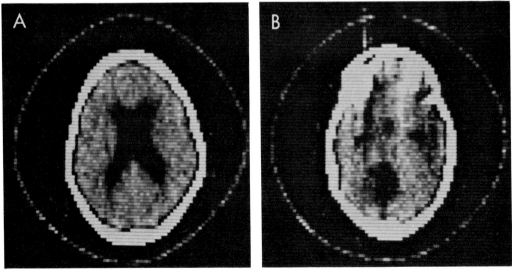

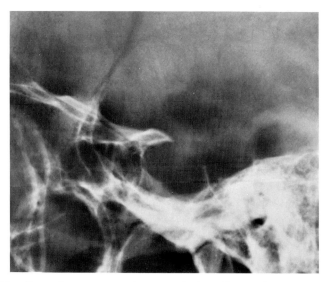

Figure 15.—Extensive pressure damage of the sella turcica. With prolonged increased intracranial pressure, the sella is enlarged, and the increase in depth is often at the expense of the sphenoid sinus into which the floor of the sella is depressed. When there is cancellous bone rather than pneumatized sinus beneath the sella, the erosion of the floor progresses more rapidly. The posterior clinoids have disappeared and the dorsum is very thin and pointed (same case as Figs. 10 and 70).

then disappear altogether. By this time, third ventricular pressure is being transmitted to the floor of the pituitary fossa, so that atrophy occurs here also. When the third ventricle is wide the anterior and posterior clinoid processes may exhibit atrophy and the dimensions of the sella may be enlarged. In advanced cases the floor of the sella may be depressed and the sphenoid sinus partially obliterated (Fig. 15). In some cases the shadow of the pituitary gland herniates through the tissue-thin sellar floor and can be seen against the air contained in the sinus (see Figs. 27 and 37). A cerebrospinal fluid fistula can develop if pressure is not relieved.

Changes along the anterior part of the sella turcica in the region of the tuberculum and planum sphenoidale may be found, indicating pressure

Figure 14.—Cerebellar astrocytoma with hydrocephalus. Obstructive hydrocephalus can be readily diagnosed by computerized tomography. In **A** the oscilloscope display of a computerized transverse axial tomogram of the head in the plane of the lateral ventricles is shown. The display is a crown view of the structures in the body plane for which the section is made. The lateral ventricles, appearing black because of less radiation absorption than the surrounding brain, are obviously enlarged. In another section, the third ventricle was shown to be dilated. In a lower plane through the cerebellar chamber (**B**) a cystic astrocytoma is demonstrated as the round dark area in the lower part of the figure, with a marginal less radiolucent area on the left edge representing the solid part of the lesion.

Increased Intracranial Pressure / 37

atrophy from a greatly ballooned optic recess of the third ventricle. Atrophy along the superior surface of the lesser wings can occur from frontal horn enlargement. In some cases there may be marked atrophy of the greater sphenoid wing from generalized increased intracranial pressure, and the lateral borders of the superior orbital fissure may become indistinct. More commonly, thinning of the greater sphenoid wing and floor of the middle fossa may be found on one side, owing to the presence of a slowly growing tumor of the temporal lobe or an extracerebral expanding lesion of the middle fossa on the corresponding side. In some cases the margins of the optic foramina lose their sharp definition because of elevated intracranial pressure which could be mistaken for erosion of the canal by an optic glioma.

In the anterior fossa it is common for the ethmoid plate to become markedly thinned. This can be produced by enlargement of the anterior horns of the lateral ventricles in cases of long-standing ventricular obstruction, such as may occur with an ependymoma of the fourth ventricle. At times the cribriform plate is markedly depressed into the ethmoid air sinuses and the plate may become almost invisible because of its thinness. Similar atrophy and deformity can occur with slowly growing anterior fossa tumors, such as a frontal meningioma. A cerebrospinal fluid fistula to the ethmoid sinuses is not uncommon, resulting in spontaneous rhinorrhea. In a similar manner, the horizontal portions of the frontal bone forming the supraorbital ridges may become atrophic. Less frequently the vertical portion of the frontal bone is involved.

Figure 16.—Occipital thinning. In the frontal projection (**A**) the horizontal portion of the occipital bone is thin bilaterally with the right side expanded downward (**arrows**). In the lateral view (**B**) the right occipital squama (**arrow**) exhibits marked thinning and outward bowing beyond the normal line of the posterior fossa floor. The patient, a 26-month-old boy, had a history of unsteadiness for six months and projectile vomiting just before admission. Cerebellar signs were found on neurologic examination. At operation a large cystic astrocytoma containing 70 cc of fluid was removed.

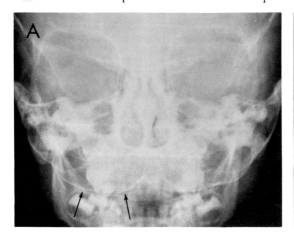
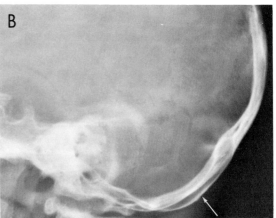

In the middle fossa, in addition to the changes of the sphenoid wing described above, it is not uncommon to find the tips of the petrous pyramids poorly defined as a result of atrophy from generalized increased intracranial pressure. The appearance is not easily confused with erosion by an acoustic neurinoma and other tumors adjacent to the pyramid because the cortex is only thinned and a ghost of the normal structure remains. With pressure atrophy the changes are usually symmetrical on the two sides. There may be thinning of the basal portion of the temporal bone forming the lateral floor of the middle fossa, and rarely there may be some thinning of the temporal squama as well. In young patients there can be thinning and molding, often expansion, by a slowly growing middle fossa lesion such as a cystic temporal glioma or an extracerebral cystic lesion.

In the posterior fossa thinning of the occipital squama is often seen. In both frontal and lateral views the floor of the posterior fossa may be extremely thin (Fig. 16). Such changes are most often found with cystic astrocytomas of the cerebellar hemispheres. If a cystic astrocytoma affects one hemisphere, an ipsilateral change is seen; there may be bilateral changes, greater on the side of the tumor. It is not rare for such lesions to affect both hemispheres. There is often outward and downward bowing of the occipital bone between the foramen magnum and the lateral sinuses. In some cases, especially with anterolateral extra-axial tumors, there may be thinning and concavity or scalloping of the clivus. The posterior fossa may be generally enlarged, especially in the horizontal direction, by cystic tumors in young patients. Other examples of diffuse and local atrophy will be shown along with contrast studies in connection with tumors of various specific sites.

LOCAL BONE EROSIONS

The words "erosion" and "atrophy" are often used interchangeably in neuroradiology. However, the word "erosion" is derived from the same Latin root as rodent and literally translated means "a gnawing away." In this sense a more local and active process is implied. On the other hand, erosion and atrophy can be considered to be an interference with bone metabolism involving concomitantly an excessive wearing away of existing bone and failure of normal replacement. Erosion does not usually imply bone destruction, which is caused by direct invasion of bone by a tumor. After surgical relief of generalized or localized pressure atrophy and erosion the bony structures frequently return to normal density with slight remodeling.

The cranial structures most often affected by local bone erosions are the sella turcica, the petrous pyramids, the optic and jugular foramina or canals, and the inner table of the vault. Radiographs of high detail are required for thorough evaluation of erosive changes. Tomograms are required in most instances for a full appreciation of the extent and nature of the changes.

SELLA TURCICA.—This is again the intracranial structure most commonly exhibiting local erosion. The changes most frequently come from within the sella turcica, and enlargement of the sella as well as alteration of its contour, boundaries and mineral content are important. In practice, linear measurements of the sella turcica are usually satisfactory to determine whether the size of the pituitary fossa is within normal limits. On the lateral skull radiograph the maximal measurements of 17 mm length and 12 mm depth are usually applied (see Fig. 47). Some authors believe that the area of the sella turcica as determined from the lateral view is more accurate to detect enlargement. The figure of 130 sq mm is considered to be the maximal size for a normal sella turcica. An even more scientific evaluation is possible through a calculation of the volume of the pituitary fossa. A simplified formula for the volume of an ellipsoid was worked out by Di Chiro (1960).

$$\text{Volume} = \frac{\frac{1}{2} \ (\text{length} \times \text{width} \times \text{height in mm})}{1000}$$

A mean value of approximately 600 cu mm and a maximal value of approximately 1100 cu mm was found in normal adults by Di Chiro and Nelson (1962). The width of the sella turcica can usually be ascertained from frontal views in which the floor of the normal sella turcica is a plateau, and measurements can be taken from the points where the bony cortex begins to slope down and laterally to the parasellar region (see Fig. 47D). At other times the base view of the skull may be helpful because the anterior portion of the sella turcica can be seen, and with enlargement the anterior wall often exhibits changes (see Fig. 48).

The chromophobe pituitary adenoma is the most frequently encountered lesion eroding the sella turcica from within. In the average case the sella is obviously enlarged in length or depth on the lateral view (see Fig. 48). In the vast majority of cases the enlargement is asymmetrical and more extensive on one side of the midline. This is usually manifested radiographically as a difference in depth of the sella on the two sides, so that a "double floor" exists. This indicates deeper erosion of the floor of the sella on the side ipsilateral to the bulk of the adenoma. An asymmetry in length can also be appreciated in many cases especially on base views, and in tomograms (see Fig. 47). The sella has a ballooned appearance in most cases, caused by enlargement in all directions. There is often erosion in the region of the tuberculum sellae and along the inferior aspect of the anterior clinoid processes, giving the processes an "undercut" appearance. In some cases a pituitary adenoma will herniate through the eroded floor of the sella to become visible against the sphenoidal sinus air shadow, and in rare cases it may extend into the nasopharynx.

It is not necessary always to have enlargement of the sella turcica with a pituitary adenoma. The so-called microadenomas are now being sought as hormonal assays have become more readily available and trans-sphenoidal hypophysectomy has become popular. Chromophobe microadenomas usually cause some asymmetry of the sellar floor on the two sides, and any sloping of the floor revealed by tomography should be regarded with suspicion. The radiologic diagnosis is often confirmed by pneumoencephalography, at which time a slight upward sloping of the diaphragma sellae may be seen and there may be thickening or tilting of the pituitary stalk, as outlined by air in the suprasellar cistern.

Eosinophilic adenomas also produce a rounded enlargement (ballooning) of the sella turcica. If they occur before epiphyseal closure of the long bones they result in gigantism. More often, however, they are seen in middle-aged individuals with acromegaly. The skull radiographs will show, in addition to enlargement of the sella, hypertrophy of the paranasal sinuses and an increase in thickness of the bones (see Fig. 45), especially of the cranial vault, and enlargement and elongation of the mandible. Enlargement of the hands is usually seen, especially in the width of the soft tissues, which can be appreciated clinically as well as radiologically. There is usually enlargement of the ungual tufts of the terminal phalanges in radiographs of the hand. The vertebral column may be affected in some cases. There is an increase in the anteroposterior width of the vertebral bodies with associated anterior wedging and thoracic kyphosis. In some cases the growth of such an adenoma becomes arrested spontaneously and a portion of the tumor may then calcify.

Basophilic adenomas are uncommon. When they do occur they are usually small and do not enlarge the sella turcica. Cushing's syndrome is more often caused by adrenal tumors, and in these cases there is hypophyseal hypertrophy without true adenoma formation. Osteoporosis is a common manifestation which also affects the sella turcica, and the decalcification may be so marked that the sella appears to be enlarged when there is no true erosion.

In some cases pituitary tumors are mixed in cell type. Rarely multiple endocrine adenomatosis is encountered, a hereditary condition in which tumors develop in the hypophysis, the parathyroid glands, the pancreas and the adrenal cortex. In approximately 1% of pituitary adenomas, malignant changes can be found. An adenocarcinoma may develop primarily in the hypophysis, or there may be malignant metaplasia of a previously benign pituitary adenoma.

The *empty sella* is a relatively common cause of enlargement of the pituitary fossa. The condition is found approximately 10 times as often in women as in men. Because the condition is observed most often in women of middle age and beyond, it has been thought that the basis is dynamic changes in the pituitary gland related to the reproductive cycle. The gland is thought to enlarge and then regress repeatedly; during the enlargement phase there is also some enlargement of the sella turcica and later, with regression, the hypophysis does not fill its fossa. In some cases, however, an empty sella is found in young women and it is occasionally seen in men. It may be caused by an open type sella with a large passage in the diaphragm for the pituitary stalk. In such cases a diverticulumlike extension of the subarachnoid space may invade the sella turcica and produce erosion, as occurs with increased intracranial pressure. At pneumography air can be shown to fill the intrasellar subarachnoid space, which may occupy most

Figure 17.—Suprasellar dermoid. The sella turcica is open with a short stubby dorsum and no posterior clinoid processes. The sella is also shallow with considerable increase in density of the cortex of the sellar floor. The patient, a 17-year-old boy with vision loss, had a suprasellar and retrosellar dermoid cyst.

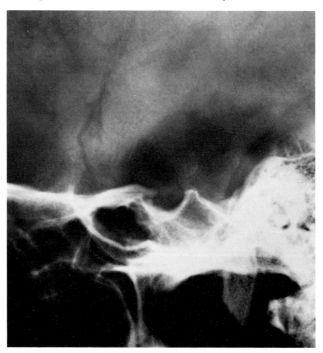

of the pituitary fossa, while the gland fills only a fraction of the space. It is important to carry out pneumography before any treatment, such as radiation therapy, for a presumed pituitary adenoma which may be thought to exist from the plain film finding of an enlarged pituitary fossa.

Craniopharyngiomas are seen most often in the first two decades of life, since the tumors arise from remnants of the craniopharyngeal duct or Rathke's pouch. The tumors may occasionally be seen, however, late in life. In children there is almost always calcification in the cellular part of the tumor or in the capsule of the associated cyst. In later life, however, calcification may not be seen in more than 50% of cases.

Radiologically the sella turcica is enlarged in approximately 75% of craniopharyngiomas. It is usually of the "open" type with poorly developed clinoid processes. The sella is relatively shallow, although often enlongated. The dorsum sellae is usually short or stubby. There is a peculiar increase in density of the cortex of the floor of the sella turcica with craniopharyngioma and certain other suprasellar cysts (see Fig. 52). Similar changes in the sella turcica may be found with suprasellar epidermoid and dermoid tumors, but calcification in these lesions is seldom present (Fig. 17). Although pituitary adenoma and craniopharyngioma are the most commonly occurring lesions in and around the sella turcica, other juxtasellar tumors that can produce erosion include meningioma, optic glioma, hypothalamic tumors including ectopic pinealoma, metastatic deposits and tumors of the cranial and extracranial soft tissues. The possibility of an aneurysm must be considered with all juxtasellar masses.

PETROUS PYRAMIDS.—The petrous pyramids require very painstaking examination since it is easy to overlook an erosion because of the density of the structures involved. It is important to have an accurate history and knowledge of neurologic findings. If the findings suggest a cerebellopontine angle tumor, examination is concentrated on the petrous tips and internal auditory canals. If the clinical findings indicate involvement of more caudal cranial nerves, the examination has to be centered on the posterior fossa, the jugular foramen and condylar foramen. Radiographs obtained in connection with the routine skull examination give cursory demonstration of the petrous bones. These structures can be seen in the modified half-axial projection (Towne view) and the two posteroanterior views, one of which usually projects the pyramids through the orbits. Radiographs of the skull base are helpful, and views in the Stenvers projection are essential. Tomograms should also be made in almost every suspected case to determine whether erosion is present and its extent. The erosion produced by small lesions may be demonstrated only in one of the several views that are taken.

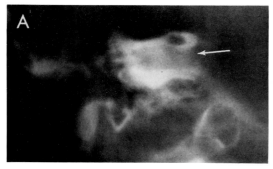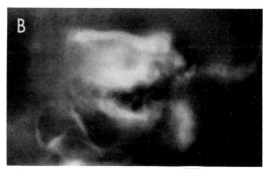

Figure 18.—Left acoustic neurinoma. **A,** on the right side the tomogram shows a canal (**arrow**) of almost even height throughout, with well-defined superior and inferior walls. The internal auditory meatus is well mineralized and the superior wall curves only slightly upward at the meatus. **B,** on the side of the tumor the inner cortex of the superior wall bows slightly upward in the midportion of the canal and, medial to this, it becomes less well defined and, at points, irregular. There is flaring at the internal auditory meatus with thinning of the superior margin of the meatus as compared with the normal side. On the original radiographs the width or height of the meatus on the left measured twice that of the internal opening on the right, the actual measurement being 10 mm. The changes occurred in a 46-year-old man who had progressive loss of hearing in the left ear for six years; more recently, he had suffered vertigo.

Neurinomas arising from the sheath of the eighth cranial nerve are the tumors that most often cause erosion of the petrous bones. In some cases the tumor arises in the internal auditory canal and is still intracanalicular when the patient is seen. Eventually, however, the tumor will grow outside of the canal into the subarachnoid space of the cerebellopontine angle. As the tumor reaches the internal auditory meatus there is less resistance to its growth. The meatus is usually enlarged to a greater degree than the deeper portions of the canal so that the canal takes on a funnel-shaped appearance. Enlargement of the meatus and canal usually occurs at the expense of the superior wall, but the inferior margin of the meatus is also frequently involved. The inferior wall is more characteristically eroded by a tumor of the glomus jugulare.

In addition to the enlargement of the internal auditory meatus and the canal, the sharpness of the superior border of the canal is often lost. In many cases the posterior wall of the canal is involved, along with the superior margin. In advanced cases the meatus and medial portion of the canal may be completely eroded so that the canal appears to be shorter on the involved side. Although there is frequently a variation in appearance on the two sides and the width of the canals may vary slightly, a difference of 2 mm or more is always considered abnormal (Fig. 18). A vertical measurement of the meatal opening greater than 8 mm should always be regarded as suggestive of the presence of an acoustic neurinoma. Employing polytomography, the presence of an acoustic neurinoma should be suspected 90%

of the time from the plain film examination. The size of the tumor and the extent of compression of neural structures are determined by the use of contrast material, either air or Pantopaque cisternography. Angiography will often give a good indication of the tumor size and give valuable information about its vascularity (see Part 12, under Extra-axial Tumors). Neurinomas of the fifth cranial nerve often erode the petrous tip but do not enlarge the canal. In these cases the canal is shortened and the medial end of the eroded canal is frequently sharply defined.

Pituitary adenomas extending laterally may erode the petrous tip in a similar manner, but these are readily recognized because of changes in the sella turcica. Meningiomas of the cerebellopontine angle often produce hyperostosis or sclerosis along with bone erosion of the pyramid. In the case of epidermoid tumors of the cerebellopontine angle, pure erosion of the medial portion of the petrous bone is produced without sclerotic changes or enlargement of the canal.

JUGULAR FORAMEN AND FOSSA.—Routine base views of the skull do not show the foramina of the posterior fossa as well as those of the middle fossa. Various angle views have been devised to delineate these structures, and good tomography is essential to demonstrate the extent of erosive processes. The ninth, tenth and eleventh cranial nerves all pass through the jugular foramen, and it is not unusual for patients with a neurinoma of one of the nerves to have multiple cranial nerve deficits from compression of others. The hypoglossal, although a motor nerve, occasionally develops a nerve sheath tumor.

With tumors of the last four cranial nerves, the jugular foramen or the hypoglossal canal slowly enlarges, depending on the origin of the neurinoma. Either of the apertures may be enlarged to two or three times its normal size, yet a well-defined boundary of bone remains around the periphery of the opening. The jugular foramen may be even more extensively eroded by glomus jugulare tumors (chemodectomas). These tumors arise from chemoreceptive tissue and develop as small bodies in the immediate vicinity of the jugular bulb and just beneath the petrous bone and the jugular foramen. Multiple cranial nerve palsies are often present and most patients complain of tinnitus and loss of hearing. Women are affected approximately five times as often as men. The tumors are highly vascular, and both carotid and vertebral angiography are usually required to outline completely the sources of vascular supply. Growth can occur relatively rapidly, and intracranial invasion and local destruction in the region of the jugular fossa and the petrous pyramid are the common findings. The tumors erode the inferior wall of the internal auditory canal, as contrasted with more frequent erosion

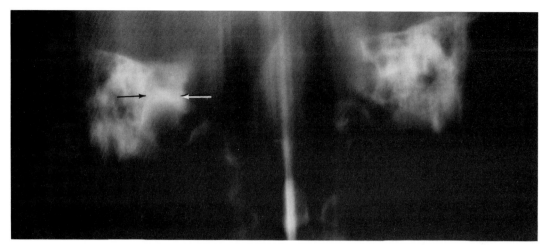

Figure 19.—Right glomus jugulare tumor. Erosion of the medial portion of the petrous pyramid is present on the right. The erosion has involved the inferior wall of the internal auditory canal **(arrows)**. Considerable clouding of the mastoid air cells on the right side was shown by standard mastoid projections. The patient, a 53-year-old woman, had complained of tinnitus and progressive hearing loss in the right ear for 10 months.

of the superior wall with acoustic neurinomas (Fig. 19). As the tumor extends laterally, a large portion of the inferior aspect of the petrous bone may be eroded. Further extension produces destruction of mastoid cells, which are usually clouded on the involved side, and the tumor then may grow into the middle ear. Angiography is usually required to define the tumor's blood supply and its vascular architecture. Examination of the posterior fossa subarachnoid space with air and tomography or with Pantopaque may be needed to determine the degree of intracranial extension. Similar studies should be carried out in the case of tumors of the last four cranial nerves.

Erosions of the optic canals or foramina are common in the presence of an optic glioma arising in the orbit which extends intracranially and vice versa. Routine radiographs as well as contrast studies are presented in Part 14 dealing with tumors of the orbit.

INNER TABLE OF THE SKULL.—Superficially located gliomas, especially cystic tumors, and hemispheric tumors that become exophytic can produce localized erosion of the inner table of the vault. Local thinning results most often from a slowly growing tumor such as an oligodendroglioma or a cystic astrocytoma. The bony changes are most frequently found in children (Fig. 20). The erosions are thought to be the result of pulsations transmitted through gyri that are enlarged and flattened because of the tumor and the close contact of the abnormal cerebral surface with the inner table of the skull through the relatively thin meninges of children. As with diffuse

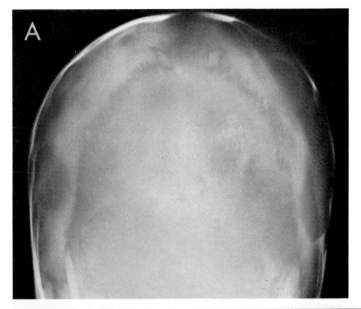

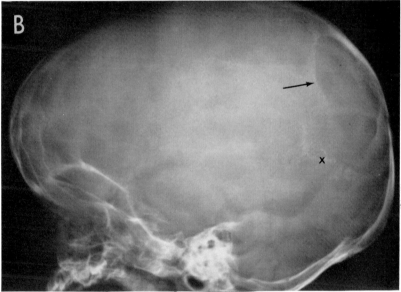

Figure 20.—Erosion of the inner table of the vault. The head is large and the major sutures are widened. In **A,** frontal view, an area of bone thinning is present in the posterior parietal region. The thinning has occurred at the expense of the inner table and diploic space, leaving only a thin shell overlying the outer table. Enlarged occipital emissary veins are evident. In **B,** lateral view, the anterior margin of the thin area (**arrow**) appears fairly well defined and it is more localized than the change shown in Figure 11. A conglomerate collection of granular calcification (**X**) is present deep in the parieto-occipital area. The patient had a large cystic astrocytoma (angiogram shown in Fig. 75).

thinning of the vault, the changes are at the expense of the inner table and diploic space and eventually the outer table, leaving just a thin shell of bone over the site of the superficial tumor.

Similar changes may be found in the middle cranial fossa. The cystic tumors of the temporal lobe not infrequently thin the temporal squama. As noted in the discussion of generalized increased intracranial pressure, there may be thinning of the floor of the middle fossa and its anterior wall, the sphenoid ridge. Enlargement and molding of the middle fossa boundaries may be seen in some cases.

The cranial changes, particularly those occurring in the vault, must be differentiated from various osseous lesions. These include epidermoid tumors of the skull in the diploic space, cavernous hemangioma, eosinophilic granuloma, fibrous dysplasia and other cranial conditions that are not secondary to intracranial disease.

Erosions of the base of the skull, other than those described above, are for the most part caused by malignant tumors and could more properly be called bone destruction. These include carcinomas arising in the nasopharynx and the paranasal air sinuses, chordomas, metastatic tumors, and so on. Some of these destructive processes can be difficult to differentiate from chronic inflammatory conditions progressing to osteomyelitis and mucoceles. As with the osseous tumors of the vault, these processes are extradural in origin rather than cerebral, and involvement of the basal meninges, cranial nerves and base of the brain is secondary to destruction and extension of the tumor.

INTRACRANIAL CALCIFICATION

Calcifications in the brain may be helpful in the diagnosis of tumor in two ways. First, there may be physiologic intracranial calcification that is displaced from its normal position by tumor (secondary evidence of the lesion). Second, there may be direct evidence of a neoplasm by the occurrence of calcific degeneration in the tumor itself. Calcification is commonly seen in normal individuals in the falx cerebri and along the walls of the dural sinuses, in the falx cerebelli, in the tentorium cerebelli and the petroclinoid ligaments, in the diaphragma sellae, as plaques in the dura, and some arachnoid granulations become calcified. In the depths of the brain, calcification may be found in the pineal gland, in the habenular commissure and in the choroid plexus, particularly in the glomera. Vascular calcification is often seen later in life as a result of atherosclerosis of the internal carotid arteries. In some cases of nuclear calcification, such as in the basal ganglia and dentate nuclei, symptoms and signs of disease may be absent.

The pineal gland is the most frequent intracranial structure to calcify

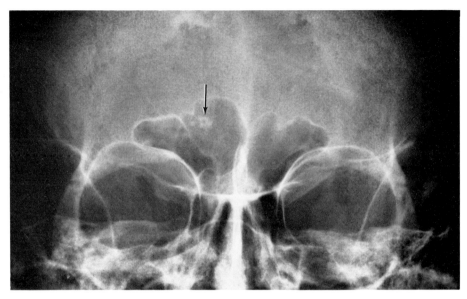

Figure 21.—Lateral pineal shift. The calcified pineal is seen through the right frontal sinus situated slightly more than 1 cm to the right of the midline (**arrow**). The displacement was caused by a left posterior temporal astrocytoma.

sufficiently to be visible on plain skull radiographs. A calcified pineal is identifiable in more than 50% of adult patients. The pineal can be demonstrated by computerized tomography without calcification because of the regressive changes and fibrosis that begin early in life (see Fig. 24).

Since the pineal body is normally situated in the midline, a lateral dislocation is often found when there is a tumor of one of the cerebral hemispheres (Fig. 21). There are several methods of determining whether the pineal gland is in normal or abnormal position in the sagittal plane. Some of the methods employ the distance of the pineal from the frontal bone in relation to its distance from the occipital bone to ascertain anteroposterior position. It is also possible to determine whether the pineal is displaced upward or downward by its measurements from the vertex and from the plane of the foramen magnum (Fig. 22). In addition, the following mathematical formula can be used to estimate anteroposterior displacement, again referring to the measurements shown in Figure 22:

$$\frac{2(A+B)-5}{3} = A \pm 0.5 \text{ cm}$$

As noted above, the pineal is most often displaced laterally by a hemispheric tumor. At times, however, it is displaced in the sagittal plane without lateral displacement. This may occur owing to a tumor of the pineal itself.

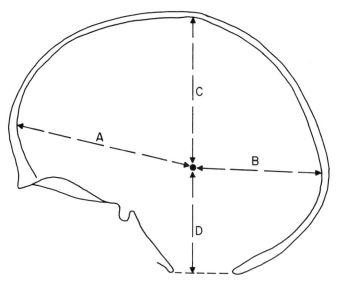

Figure 22.—Method of measuring the pineal in sagittal plane. The anteroposterior position of the pineal is determined by measuring the greatest distance from the inner table of the frontal bone to the pineal (**A**) and then the greatest distance from the pineal to the inner table of the occipital bone (**B**). For the vertical position, the distance from the pineal to the vertex (**C**) and to the plane of the foramen magnum (**D**) is measured. The normal or abnormal pineal position can then be estimated from graphs such as those described by Dyke (1930). An equation can also be used to determine if the pineal position is normal or abnormal in anteroposterior direction (see text). The anteroposterior measurements are usually made to the anterior part of the calcified pineal shadow to avoid errors due to normal variation.

Backward and downward displacement without a midline shift is often seen with bifrontal tumors and bilateral subdural hematomas and as a result of hydrocephalus.

At times, calcification in the tela choroidea overlying the habenular commissure may occur without pineal calcification. This can usually be recognized by its having the shape of the letter "C." When the two calcifications occur together, there is usually a distinct separation of the habenular from the pineal shadow (see Figs. 29 and 35). The habenular calcification is situated approximately 6 mm anterior to the center of the pineal. If only habenular calcification is present, this should be recognized since application of pineal measurements to the habenular commissure could result in a figure anterior to the normal zone.

In some individuals who have a relatively flat skull posteriorly (brachycephaly) the pineal measurement may fall posterior to the normal zone without the gland actually being displaced. It has been found that if measurements are made to the anterior part of the calcified pineal (not habenular), the false-positive measurement will be largely eliminated. Also, a measurement 2 mm beyond the normal zone is usually allowed in the anteroposterior direction as a normal variation. On the other hand, any deviation from the normal zone in a vertical direction is usually abnormal, and for this determination measurements to the center of the gland are ordinarily used. It should be noted that it is unusual to find pineal calcification in normal children under the age of 10 years; if it is observed in this age group, the possibility of pineal tumor must be considered, as pointed out further in Part 10, Intraventricular Tumors.

Figure 23.—Displaced pineal and choroid. An astrocytoma with extensive convoluted calcific degeneration is present on the right (**X**). The pineal (**a**) is displaced 5 mm to the left. The calcified right choroid glomus (**b**) is 1 cm closer to the midline than normal, displaced medially by the mass which was in the posterior temporal region. The general triangular relationship between the choroid and pineal calcifications is maintained.

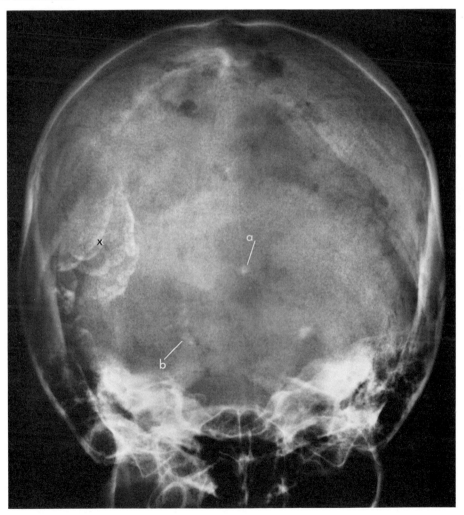

Approximately 10% of patients have calcification in the choroid plexus. The glomus of the choroid plexus of the lateral ventricle is the most common portion to become calcified. The calcification may appear as a collection of punctate shadows which form an aggregate that may measure more than 1 cm in diameter. At other times the calcification may be ringlike or amorphous. In the typical case, calcification is bilateral and the choroid shadows are usually superimposed on lateral views. In frontal views the choroid calcium deposits are usually symmetrically projected lateral to and below the pineal calcification and they maintain a triangular relationship with the pineal.

Both the pineal and choroid deposits may be displaced by a brain tumor (Fig. 23). In some cases only the choroid may be displaced or the triangular relationship with the pineal may be disturbed. Caution must be taken, however, in the interpretation of choroid displacement. In the first place, calcification does not always occur symmetrically in the two glomera; instead, it may be eccentric in one. The two choroid glomera may not be attached at exactly the same level on the two sides. In addition, it is not rare to find one

Figure 24.—Pineal localization by computerized tomography. **A,** axial scanning has been carried out in the plane of the pineal. The pineal is represented by the dense white square just behind the center of the cranial cavity in the biparietal plane. Just behind the pineal is the quadrigeminal cistern and rostral to it are a normal-appearing third ventricle and the inferior margins of the frontal horns.

In this case the pineal was only faintly calcified and could not be seen in frontal view. In **B,** the pineal is slightly to the left of the midline. No evidence of a tumor was found on angiography or pneumography, but the head was slightly asymmetrical, smaller on the right, and the corresponding lateral ventricle was slightly larger than normal.

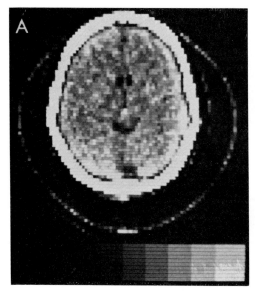 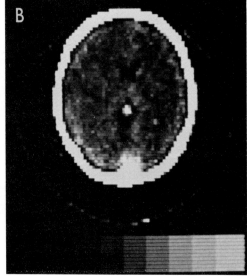

choroid glomus pedunculated so that it moves with gravity in the cerebrospinal fluid with change in position of the head. In rare instances, minimal displacement of the pineal gland and choroid plexus may be caused by cerebral atrophy or hypoplasia (Fig. 24). Still, the utility of the calcified pineal and choroid to give secondary evidence of a tumor, because of displacement, should not be underestimated.

GLIAL CALCIFICATION

Direct evidence of a tumor on routine radiographs through calcific degeneration in the neoplasm is most often observed with gliomas (Table 4). This is true because the most common intracranial tumors are gliomas, and astrocytomas and oligodendrogliomas constitute 80% of glial neoplasms, according to the figures of Zimmerman (1971). Gliomas often undergo cystic or calcific degeneration (Fig. 25). Approximately one-third of gliomas can be shown to have some calcification on histologic examination if a representative specimen is chosen. In the past, it was thought that perhaps one patient in ten with a glioma could be found to have some visible calcium in the lesion by stereoscopic study of plain films (Sosman, 1927). With the earlier clinical presentation of patients with tumors and the increase in metastatic tumors because of increased longevity, it is highly doubtful that such a high percentage is seen today, even with improved techniques. On the other hand, it is now possible to detect tumors containing calcium that cannot be seen on

TABLE 4.—BRAIN TUMOR CALCIFICATION

GLIAL	
Oligodendroglioma	50%
Pineal glia	50%
Ganglioglioma	50%
Astrocytoma	20%
Ependymoma	20%
Medulloblastoma	2%
NON-GLIAL	
Chondroma & osteochondroma	Almost all
Chordoma	80%
Craniopharyngioma	80%
Lipoma	30%
Meningioma	15%
Choroid papilloma	5%
Pituitary adenoma	4%
Metastatic carcinoma	2%
Teratoma	Often
Dermoid	Often
Epidermoid	Rarely
Neurinoma	Rarely

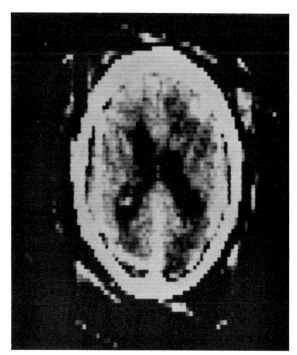

Figure 25.—Right frontal glioma. A computerized tomogram through the plane of the anterior horns, bodies and atria of the lateral ventricles shows a "low density" area in the right frontal lobe. Such reduced radiation absorption may be related to the cellular structure of the tumor, edema or cystic degeneration, all of which played a role in the case illustrated. The right frontal horn has been collapsed by the tumor and its shadow is largely absent.

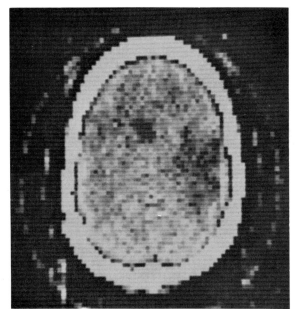

Figure 26.—Posterior supra-Sylvian astrocytoma. There is a large abnormal area in the right hemisphere consisting of irregular decreased density, scattered among which are some smaller areas of increased density (high absorption coefficient due to calcification not visible on conventional radiographs). The tumor was a large astrocytoma with some areas of malignant metaplasia. The radioactive isotope brain scan was negative.

conventional radiographs with the use of computerized tomography because of the greater absorption of x-rays (Fig. 26).

Calcification usually takes place in one or more of three places. First, the calcification may be found in the perivascular fibrous stroma of the tumor; the deposits may also occur in the blood vessel walls themselves. Second, the

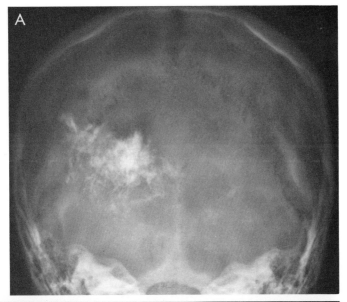

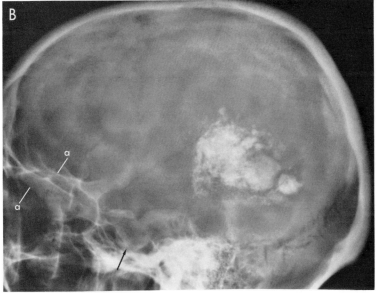

Figure 27.—Calcified oligodendroglioma. In **A,** frontal view, a large conglomerate shadow of calcium density is present in the right cerebral hemisphere. Near the margins of the tumor there are linear and curvilinear collections. In **B,** lateral view, the calcification is even more dense and many nodular elements are seen. The sella turcica (**arrow**) exhibits evidence of long-standing increased intracranial pressure. There is also pressure atrophy farther forward along the floor of the anterior fossa with cortical thinning (**a**) of the planum sphenoidale, cribriform plate and supraorbital plates. The patient, a 41-year-old woman, for nine years had suffered from a convulsive disorder. Several months before admission she complained of blurred vision and on examination was found to have bilateral papilledema and left homonymous hemianopia. At operation, the tumor extended from the parietal cortex into the atrium of the right lateral ventricle, which it filled. The lesion was largely resected.

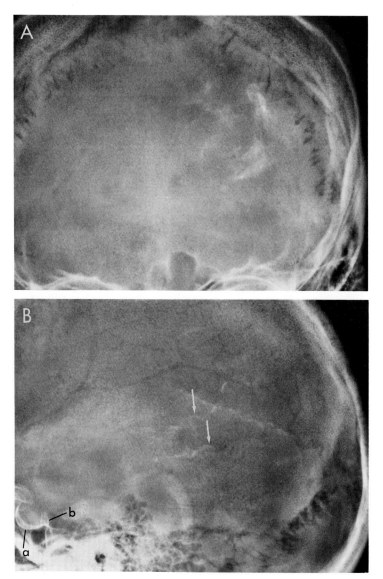

Figure 28.—Retro-Sylvian oligodendroglioma. In **A,** frontal view, curvilinear, trabecular and amorphous calcium deposits are present deep in the left cerebral hemisphere. In **B,** lateral view, some of the collections suggest convolutions (**arrows**). The calcification is shown to extend well back into the occipital lobe. There is deepening of the sella turcica (**a**) with thinning of the floor, absence of the posterior clinoid processes and a short dorsum (**b**). The patient, a 44-year-old man, had no complaints until six weeks previously, when he developed increasingly severe bilateral frontal headaches with nausea. For four weeks he had episodes of visual disturbance characterized as "electric flashing." For two weeks he had been aware of vision loss in the visual field on the right side. Examination revealed papilledema and right homonymous hemianopia. Intracranial exploration disclosed a large cystic component of the tumor beneath the cortex, deep to which the solid and calcified portions of the lesion were found.

lime salts may be found in areas of hemorrhagic and ischemic necrosis. Third, in the case of encapsulated lesions, which are usually not gliomas, the deposits may be in the walls of the lesions with the result that they are usually curvilinear. Additionally, some nonglial lesions become infected so that the entire mass may become calcified.

Of the glioma series, the *oligodendroglioma* exhibits the highest incidence of gross calcification. Nevertheless, because astrocytomas are more common tumors than oligodendrogliomas by a factor of more than 10:1, the chance is highest that any intracerebral tumor containing calcium is an astrocytoma. Oligodendrogliomas have more extensive and more dense calcification than other gliomas (Fig. 27). The collections are often conglomerate masses of heavy nodular and amorphous calcium. Trabecular and curvilinear calcium collections may be found near the margin of the tumor (Fig. 28). Since oligodendrogliomas occur most often in the deep central white matter, they do not show the convoluted pattern of calcium that occurs with more superficial astrocytomas.

Astrocytomas, particularly those of grades I and II, which are of the common fibrillary or of the rare protoplasmic type, often contain enough calcium to be visible on plain films because the tumors frequently undergo cystic or calcific degeneration (Fig. 29). Portions of an astrocytoma may be densely calcified while other areas may be only lightly calcified. Although many of the deposits are amorphous and granular, as well as trabecular, same have a convoluted pattern (see Fig. 23). At times astrocytomas may be found within the ventricular lumen and the calcification may appear as a cast of one ventricle (Fig. 30).

It is not unusual to find tumors of *mixed types* containing astrocytes and oligodendroglia. Most of these tumors grow slowly. It would appear that the majority of glioblastomas that are listed as being calcified actually represent malignant metaplasia in a well-differentiated astrocytoma that underwent calcific degeneration early in its course.

The *ganglioglioma* is a mixed tumor of adult ganglion cells and astrocytes. It has an abundant connective tissue stroma and grossly nodular calcific deposits are frequently found in portions of the tumor. The tumors are often seen in patients with tuberous sclerosis.

Ependymomas are not common gliomas, but a fairly high percentage contain calcium. The incidence has been given from 15–20%. The tumors occurring above the tentorium more often contain lime salts than those arising in the fourth ventricle, although the lesions are found with approximately equal frequency in the two locations. The tumors that invade the central white matter apparently have a great tendency to cystic and calcareous

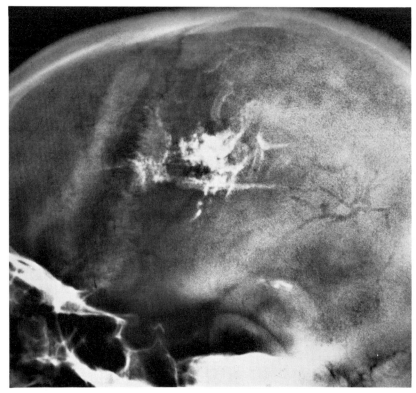

Figure 29.—Calcified supra-Sylvian astrocytoma. Calcification extends over a large part of the frontoparietal region. The central portion of the tumor is a conglomerate mass of dense calcium, many of the elements appearing to be granular and nodular. Along all of the margins the calcification has a tapered linear or curvilinear configuration indicating the infiltrative nature of the lesion. The calcified pineal is displaced downward, and the dorsum sellae shows some cortical thinning. The sella turcica is rounded, and measurements were at the upper limits of normal on the original radiograph, suggesting some enlargement caused by long-standing increased pressure of relatively low grade. The tumor proved to be a fibrillary astrocytoma, largely infiltrating and replacing normal brain.

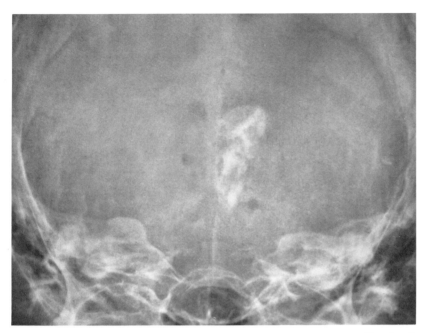

Figure 30.—Calcified intraventricular astrocytoma. An area of calcification is apparent in the frontal film which, from its configuration, suggests that the lesion has formed a cast of the left ventricular body. The patient, a 63-year-old woman, had no complaints until 10 days previously when, after a day of blurred vision in the right eye, she discovered that she could not see straight ahead with that eye. Peripheral vision remained intact, as did the total vision in the left eye. She had no other symptoms. Neurologic examination was completely unremarkable except for papilledema in the right eye and a large central scotoma on the right. By left frontal craniotomy, subtotal removal of the intraventricular astrocytoma was accomplished.

change. In young patients a large tumor of one hemisphere that contains a small nodular or curvilinear calcium shadow, sometimes a solitary deposit, is usually an ependymoma.

Pinealomas, although relatively uncommon, contain calcium deposits in a high percentage of cases. Tumor calcification is seen most often in children and adolescents. Physiologic calcification of the pineal is unusual under the age of 10, and well-developed calcification in the younger age group should suggest the possibility of a pinealoma. This is especially true when large amounts of calcium in the pineal region extend beyond the usual limits of the pineal body (Fig. 31). In many cases the calcification is seen as a collection of granular and finely nodular shadows. At other times the calcium is laid down in curvilinear streaks, but it is rare for the whole tumor to calcify.

It is often possible to make the diagnosis of a pinealoma from the plain

Figure 31.—Pinealoma. Abnormal calcification is present above and behind the sella, which covered a 2 × 3 cm area on the original radiograph. The frontal view showed the calcification to be in the midline. No shadow definitely identifiable as the pineal could be made out. In this lateral view the sella turcica shows changes of chronic intracranial hypertension. The atrophic dorsum has a flat top and no posterior clinoid processes are visible, the changes suggesting erosion by an enlarged anterior third ventricle. The patient, a 22-year-old man, had had intermittent headache for many years and recently developed Parinaud's syndrome.

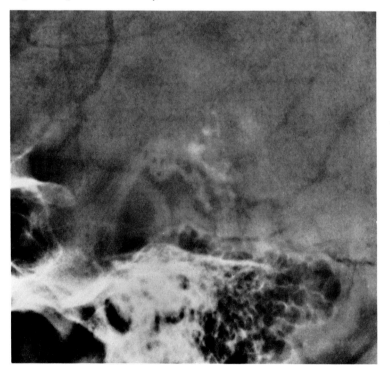

radiographs. The location of the abnormal calcification, especially if it is displacing a partially calcified normal gland, together with evidence of increased intracranial pressure should suggest such a diagnosis. The evidence of increased pressure may appear as chronic suture widening with increased convolutional markings in a young patient. After the sutures have closed, abnormal calcification in the pineal region together with sella turcica changes of the type associated with erosion from an enlarged third ventricle should strongly suggest pinealoma.

NON-GLIAL TUMORS

Tumors arising from the base of the skull such as *chondromas* and *osteochondromas* usually produce bone or undergo calcification. Osteomas and fibromas are also found along the skull base, although osteomas are common over the vault, especially the temporal and frontal areas. The osteochondromas growing intracranially resemble those found in other parts of the body in that they contain small islands of radiolucent cartilage remaining in a global, largely calcified mass (Fig. 32). Differentiation of these cranial tumors from a meningioma may be a problem and angiography may be required.

Chordomas characteristically arise along the clivus and produce destructive changes of the basisphenoid. The sella turcica is often involved. Calcium in varying amounts is found in most instances. Often, however, many of the visible calcium shadows are the result of inclusion of sequestrated bone within the mass, bone destruction being the most characteristic feature of a chordoma and serving to differentiate it from a meningioma.

Craniopharyngioma is the most common tumor to produce suprasellar calcification. Virtually all craniopharyngiomas, both cystic and solid, occurring in children exhibit calcification radiologically and one-half of adult patients have calcification. As discussed above, when curvilinear capsular calcification or calcification in the cellular portion of the lesion is associated with a shallow sella turcica with a dense floor and stubby dorsum, an accurate diagnosis can be made in almost all cases from the routine radiographs (see Fig. 51). Computerized tomography often gives a characteristic pattern of increased absorption from the calcified portion of the tumor and increased radiability produced by the lipid material in the cyst cavity (Fig. 33).

Lipomas of the corpus callosum usually contain calcium in the capsule of the mass. This together with the characteristic reduced density of adult fat in the mass make it possible to make the diagnosis from ordinary skull radiographs. Only one-third of lipomas of the brain are found in the corpus callosum, however, and elsewhere the lesions may not calcify or the thin

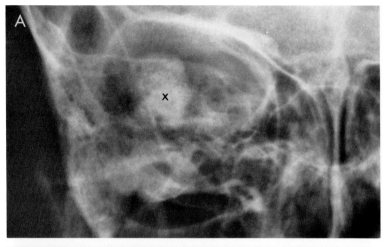

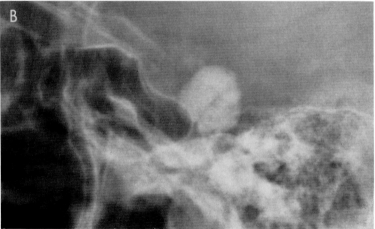

Figure 32.—Middle fossa osteochondroma. **A,** frontal view, reveals a rounded, almost completely calcified mass (**X**) which is projected through the petrous ridge. In **B,** lateral view, the lesion appears to be arising from the anterior aspect of the petrous bone. Numerous small areas of relative radiolucency are present indicating cartilaginous islands. The tumor, which measured 2 cm diameter on the original radiographs, was an incidental finding in a 41-year-old woman with a glioblastoma of the left frontal lobe.

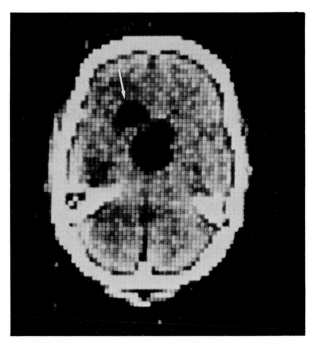

Figure 33.—Craniopharyngioma. A computerized tomogram was taken through the plane of the petrous pyramids, which are shown as triangular shadows of high absorption coefficient in the lower portion of the figure. In the central and anterior portions, a large, rounded radiolucency is present in the midline with a large loculation extending into the left anterior fossa **(arrow)**. The blackness of the tumor denotes high radiability caused by cholesterol in the cystic craniopharyngioma. Around the margin of the central shadow are small areas of increased density representing calcification in the cyst wall. (Courtesy of Dr. James Ambrose, London, England.)

capsular calcification may be impossible to see, as in the posterior fossa.

Except for meningiomas, which are described separately below, the other more commonly encountered brain tumors contain gross calcium in only a small percentage of cases (see Table 4). Choroid papillomas were found to exhibit calcium of diagnostic value in less than 5% of the 234 cases reviewed by Rovit *et al.* (1970). It is possible that the higher percentages given by many authors result from the frequent occurrence of calcification in adjacent normal choroid plexus tissue. Large pituitary adenomas, especially those extending well above the sella turcica, with cystic degeneration may contain a curvilinear deposit of calcium in the capsule (see Fig. 49).

It is surprising that a figure as high as 2% is given by those who have examined the frequency of calcification in *metastatic neoplasms* seen on plain radiographs. The multiplicity and relative density of secondary deposits can often be demonstrated by computerized tomography. In some cases the metastases absorb less radiation than the surrounding brain, while at other times, as with metastases from a carcinoma of the breast, there may be increased radiation absorption (Fig. 34).

Tumors of the *teratoma* group are relatively infrequent, so that large series for a single observer's analysis are not available. From case reports and the descriptions of small series, as well as personal observations, it can be said that teratomas and dermoid tumors often exhibit calcification. The calcification of teratomas may be extensive in some instances, and the presence of bone and dental elements has been described. At times fat may also be present, producing shadows of diminished density. Dermoids, as well as epidermoids, are avascular lesions; however, capsular calcification of a curvilinear type may be seen with dermoid tumors, but it is infrequent with epidermoidomas. Some apparently completely calcified dermoid and epidermoid lesions have been described; since some of these tumors are related to dermal sinuses it seems probable that internal calcifications are the result of infection.

Whenever a calcified intracranial mass is encountered it is necessary to consider among the diagnoses entertained the possibility of an inflammatory or vascular mass (see Table 1). An intracranial calcification resulting from a healed *brain abscess* is seen infrequently now that the antibiotic control of many infections is possible. The majority of calcified abscesses do not exceed 1–2 cm diameter. The calcification is most dense in the capsule, which is well defined although often irregular, and the central area of the lesion may remain radiolucent. The temporal and cerebellar locations adjacent to an abnormal mastoid are good clues to the correct diagnosis. Granulomatous

Figure 34.—Metastatic carcinoma. A computerized tomogram displays two distinct rounded areas of high absorption coefficient. The patient, a 52-year-old woman, had a scirrhous carcinoma of the breast.

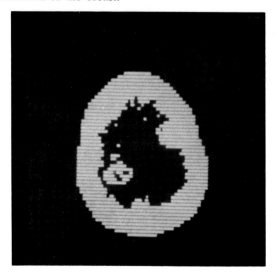

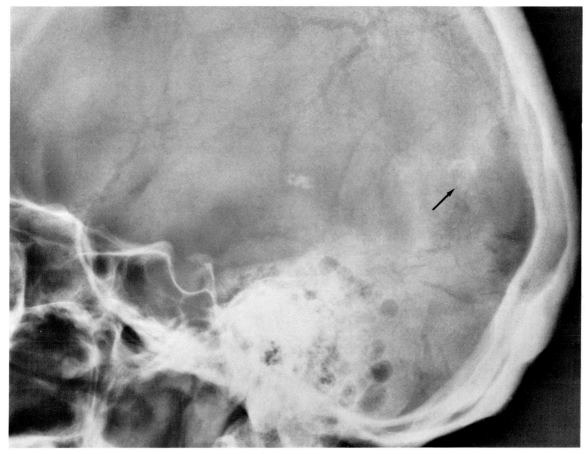

Figure 35.—Occipital hemangioma. An abnormal crescentic calcium shadow is present, open inferiorly (**arrow**), where there are several clumped deposits of calcium. The over-all area of calcification measured slightly over 1 cm diameter on the original radiograph. The calcified pineal gland and well-calcified habenular commissure are not displaced and there is no evidence of increased intracranial pressure. The patient, a 41-year-old man, for six years had episodes of numbness and tingling of the face and left shoulder lasting only a few seconds. During the week before admission he had two grand mal seizures. Neurologic examination was entirely normal except for almost total left homonymous hemianopia. At operation the posterior two-thirds of the right occipital lobe was occupied by a vascular mass which contained scarred and calcified tissue. There was considerable cortical involvement. Pathologic examination revealed numerous vascular channels of widely varying size whose walls also varied considerably in thickness.

lesions, such as tuberculosis, may present an appearance not unlike that of a pyogenic abscess when it is healed and calcified. The lesions of sarcoidosis and histocytosis-X usually do not calcify.

Calcification in angiomas or true vascular neoplasms of the brain, such as hemangioblastomas, is unusual (Fig. 35). *Arteriovenous malformations,* on the other hand, frequently contain calcium. This results from repeated

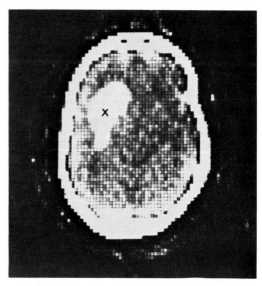

Figure 36.—Intracerebral hematoma. A computerized tomogram shows a large mass (**X**) in the left hemisphere with a very high absorption coefficient. A high coefficient of radiation absorption is a common finding with hematomas.

leakage of blood with perivascular fibrosis and from ischemia of the brain surrounding the lesion from an inadequate capillary blood supply. The calcifications may be punctate, nodular trabecular or curvilinear. It is not unusual for the calcification and the mass of such an arteriovenous malformation to lead to an erroneous diagnosis of a glioma unless adequate angiography is performed. Angiography and even intracranial exploration may not result in the correct diagnosis in occasional cases if there has been extensive thrombosis, necrosis and gliosis. If the lesion has a dural blood supply, then the presence of deep channels in the bone caused by dilatation of meningeal vessels and enlargement of diploic channels are a great help in diagnosis.

A solitary gross *intracerebral hemorrhage* is not often mistaken for a tumor. A capsule usually does not develop around an intracerebral hematoma, and for this reason a gross connective tissue scar is not the common end-result, as is the case with abscess. There are exceptions, however, and amorphous calcium deposits up to 2 cm diameter and even larger can be the result of an intracerebral hematoma. In the acute stage an intracerebral hematoma can usually be diagnosed by computerized tomography because of the high absorption coefficient of the hemorrhagic mass (Fig. 36).

Meningiomas arise from the arachnoid villi although they are generally attached to the dura. The majority of arachnoid villi are concentrated along the walls of the major dural sinuses. They are also found widely disposed in relation to tributary veins and clusters of arachnoid cells are located in the basal dura. The occurrence of meningiomas at certain specific intracranial sites in relation to the anatomic occurrence of these groups of arachnoid cells is of considerable diagnostic importance (Table 5). The greatest number of meningiomas arise in the parasagittal region and are attached either to the falx or to the superior longitudinal sinus. The next most common location is the cerebral convexity, probably related to the occurrence of arachnoid villi associated with tributaries of the sinus. The sphenoid ridge, olfactory groove and suprasellar areas are the next most common sites, and when these numbers are added together they account for approximately 80% of all meningiomas. Other sites of predilection are the posterior fossa, the tentorial edges and the peritorcular area. A small number arise in the floor of the middle fossa and elsewhere. Infrequently meningiomas may be found within the ventricles, presumably arising from leptomeningeal extensions into the interior of the brain to provide blood supply and stroma of the choroid plexus. Rarely extradural meningiomas may be found as cranial or extracranial lesions. Presumably such tumors arise from ectopic arachnoid cells which become incorporated in the bony skull during its growth.

Meningiomas evoke cranial changes of hyperostosis and increased vascularity in a high percentage of cases, so that the lesions can be suspected from routine examination of the skull in approximately 50% of cases. In addition, 10–15% of meningiomas contain enough calcium to be visible on plain skull radiographs.

A high percentage of patients with meningioma have indirect evidence of a tumor. The pressure changes occurring in the region of the sella turcica

TABLE 5.—TEN MOST COMMON LOCATIONS OF INTRACRANIAL MENINGIOMAS

Parasagittal	22%
Cerebral convexity	18
Sphenoid ridge	18
Olfactory	10
Suprasellar	10
Tentorial & posterior fossa	8
Peritorcular	4
Middle fossa	4
Falx	2
Intraventricular	2
Multiple or with neurinoma	2
	100%

do not differ basically from those occurring with other types of intracranial neoplasms except that the atrophy may be more pronounced because of the chronic course of these slowly growing neoplasms (Fig. 37). In approximately two-thirds of patients with a supratentorial meningioma who have pineal calcification visible in the frontal view, there will be displacement of the pineal shadow. It is not uncommon for a meningioma of the superior surface of the tentorium to displace one calcified choroid glomus upward and medially and sometimes forward as well. Even more important, however, are

Figure 37.—Occipital meningioma. This lateral radiograph demonstrates chronic changes of increased intracranial pressure with the dorsum sellae and posterior clinoids absent and the floor of the sella depressed. Herniation of the sellar contents into the sphenoid sinus is apparent, and there is some general sellar enlargement. Numerous large arterial grooves (**arrows**) of the bony skull extend backward and slightly upward to a radiolucent area in the upper part of the occipital bone that measured 2 × 3 cm on the original films. Within and just below the radiolucent area are numerous rounded shadows of diminished density (**X**), some punctate, that produce a stippled appearance caused by new vessels perforating the skull to supply the tumor at its attachment. The patient, a 23-year-old woman, had suffered from headache for two years. Three weeks previously her vision became blurred and she was aware that the field of vision was markedly narrowed. Chronic papilledema was present bilaterally and right homonymous hemianopia was elicited. Operation revealed a large meningioma of the left occipital pole which had invaded the bone and the left transverse sinus.

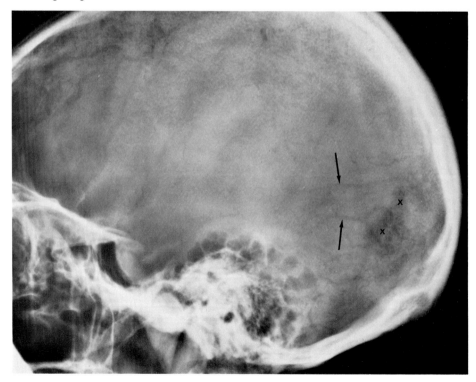

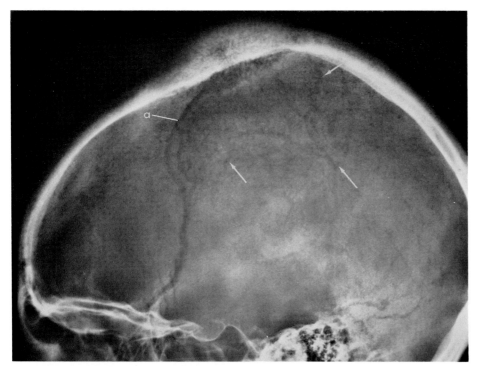

Figure 38.—Parasagittal meningioma. The diploic space is greatly widened and has a spongy appearance. An external mound of bony tissue is present, and along the former line of the outer table new bone has been laid down in a perpendicular manner. There is a marked increase in the vascular grooves of the inner table, especially the right middle meningeal groove (**a**), which is tortuous and has many branches. There is also enlargement of the diploic veins (**arrows**), and their tributaries leading to a large posterior trunk draining the tumor. The dorsum sellae is atrophic. The patient, a 47-year-old woman, had had seizures for many years following a fall which had been blamed for her difficulty. At operation, a large and very vascular meningioma was excised.

the specific changes in plain skull radiographs secondary to meningiomas that constitute direct evidence of the lesion as noted above. In addition, computerized tomography increases the diagnostic accuracy appreciably.

HYPEROSTOSIS.—Thickening of the skull resulting from hyperostosis adjacent to a meningioma occurs in about 50% of cases. The inner table of the skull, the diploic space and the outer table may all be involved. The inner table is by far the most common cranial layer to be affected (see Fig. 125). The hyperostotic process results from the laying down of bone in multiple sheets parallel to the plane of the inner table. When viewed tangentially, it can be seen that the change is an enostosis with the newly formed bone actually encroaching on the intracranial space. With a pure enostosis, the diploic space and outer table may be virtually uninvolved in the process.

At other times, there is also evidence of diploic sclerosis and an exostosis. The diploic space may become only hypertrophic, but more often the spongy appearance is obliterated by the development of more compact bone. Hypertrophy of the diploic space with preservation of the spongy appearance is thought to be related to increased vascularity within the space. This is often associated with involvement of the outer table and the production of an external mound of bony tissue which may be detectable clinically (Fig. 38). Although in most cases the laying down of new bone along both the inner and the outer table is parallel, occasionally perpendicular changes occur resulting in spicule formation. The laying down of bone at right angles to the skull occurs most often with tumors of the cerebral convexity or of the parasagittal region.

A somewhat similar bony change occurs with tumors of the planum sphenoidale. In some cases there is a brushlike area of hyperostosis. A unique change found in tumors adjacent to an air sinus is upward bulging of the cortex. This most often is seen in bone overlying the posterior ethmoid cells and the anterior portion of the sphenoid sinus. The change is referred to as "blistering" (Figs. 39 and 128). There is usually hyperostosis associated with this upward bowing of the overlying cortex of the sinuses as seen in the lateral view.

When hyperostosis involves the inner third of the sphenoid wing, it may produce narrowing of the optic canal and deformity of the superior orbital fissure (see Fig. 130). Tumors growing along the floor of the middle fossa may encroach on other foramina. In the case of hyperostosis produced by frontal meningioma, the changes should not be mistaken for benign hyperostosis often seen in women. Frontal meningiomas occurring near the midsagittal plane frequently extend across the midline, obliterating the slightly radiolucent zone of attachment of the falx cerebri, whereas with benign hyperostosis this zone is always spared (see Fig. 125).

Bone destruction may occur in a small percentage of patients, and this often develops in combination with hyperostotic changes. This does not always indicate a malignant type of neoplasm, but it is thought to be evidence of heavy infiltration of the bone by tumor (see Fig. 37). Pure osteolytic or destructive changes are more suggestive of a sarcomatous meningioma. At times a meningioma of the convexity which has not extended through the dura may cause pressure erosion of the inner table of the skull such as that seen with a superficially placed cystic tumor or a porencephalic cyst, as described earlier.

INCREASED VASCULARITY.—The second of the cardinal manifestations of a meningioma is increased vascularity, which also occurs in approximately

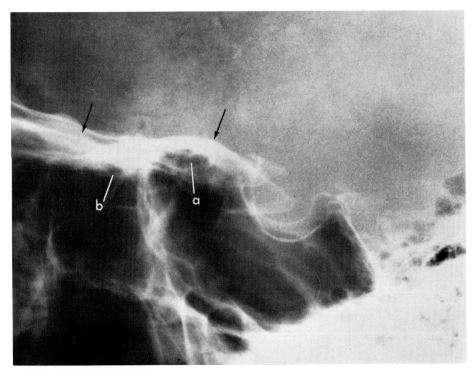

Figure 39.—Meningioma of the planum sphenoidale. Hyperostosis **(arrows)** extends forward from the tuberculum sellae along the planum sphenoidale to the posterior part of the cribriform plate. Only a few small brushlike vertical perpendicular spicules are present near the middle of the planum. The anterior part of the sphenoid sinus **(a)** and a few of the posterior ethmoid cells **(b)** extend up into the hyperostosis, well above the normal level of the planum. These changes of "blistering" are most often found with planum meningiomas. Nodular calcific deposits are present above the planum in the depths of the tumor. There are marked thinning and depression of the floor of the sella turcica, and the dorsum is eroded and the posterior clinoids absent. The patient, a 55-year-old woman, complained of vision loss and was found to have optic atrophy and prechiasmal type visual field defects. At operation a meningioma of 5 cm diameter was found.

50% of cases. First, there may be an area of localized increased vascularity, either hypervascularity or neovascularity, of the bone in the region of the tumor. Second, there may be enlargement of the vascular channels, either supplying or draining the tumor area. The majority of tumors exhibiting increased vascularity are those of the cerebral convexity and parasagittal areas since there is a better opportunity to delineate vascular changes of the vault than along the skull base.

Neovascularity occurs in a relatively small area beneath the tumor and may be associated with hyperostotic or osteolytic changes. In occasional cases the neovascularity may be so abundant that it gives the impression of an osteolytic process. The decreased density is then caused by perforation of

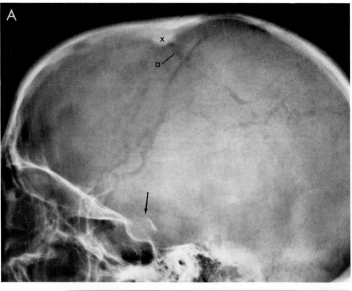

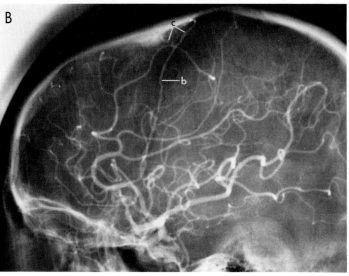

Figure 40.—Meningioma at the bregma. **A** shows the anterior cortex of the dorsum sellae to be markedly eroded (**arrow**). There is also thinning of the cortex of the floor of the sella and of all of the clinoid processes, secondary to increased intracranial pressure. A widened meningeal groove is seen ascending the convexity of the skull. Near its termination a large tortuous branch (**a**) is given off which extends to the hyperostotic button (**X**) to which the meningioma was attached. The main meningeal arterial groove turns forward to enter the posterior part of the hyperostotic area at the bregma. **B,** a common carotid angiogram, shows an enlarged middle meningeal artery (**b**) within the meningeal groove. Two terminal branches (**c**) are given off which course forward to the hyperostotic area of attachment of the tumor. The configurations of the main arterial trunk and the forward branches conform to the channels seen on the plain skull radiograph (**A**). A large anterior supra-Sylvian mass effect is present, especially affecting the callosomarginal branches and the pericallosal branch of the anterior cerebral artery. The patient, a 50-year-old woman, had a five-year history of occasional convulsive seizures. There were only minimal neurologic findings consisting of slight right hyperreflexia and early papilledema. At operation a global tumor of 4 cm diameter was found in the parasagittal region extending downward beside the falx almost to its free edge.

the skull by many small arteries and veins extending to and from the tumor at its point of attachment. These new perforating channels result in the presence of many small rounded radiolucent areas referred to as "stippling" (see Fig. 37).

Enlargement of the meningeal vascular grooves of the skull occurs more often than stippling. The middle meningeal arterial groove is frequently enlarged with parasagittal and convexity meningiomas. The middle meningeal groove, which carries both the meningeal artery and veins, often undergoes unilateral enlargement when there is a tumor of the convexity. It is not unusual for a meningioma near the midline to receive its blood supply from branches of both external carotid arteries. The enlarged groove may appear tortuous as does the artery at angiography. Abnormal meningeal branches are also seen in a high percentage of cases (Fig. 40). The abnormal branch vessels entering the tumor may be larger than the parent artery because of a "steal" of blood by the tumor. This causes retrograde flow from branch arteries into the main trunk and into abnormal tumor vessels. For the same reason, the middle meningeal groove usually does not become smaller as it ascends the vault and arborizes but instead may actually enlarge after branching.

Frontal meningiomas frequently cause abnormal branching of the middle meningeal artery. There are usually no visible straight anterior branches of the middle meningeal artery or, if one is occasionally seen, it is quite inconspicuous. In the case of frontal meningiomas, however, there are often large abnormal branches extending straight forward or forward and upward from the main middle meningeal trunk. They may be tortuous and quite large (Figs. 41 and 125). In some cases the artery may be shown to be large as it enters the skull at the foramen spinosum, the foramen itself being enlarged (more than 2 mm in diameter). More important than the size of the foramen is a widened and tortuous middle meningeal groove extending forward and laterally as the vessel courses toward the pterion where it begins to ascend the lateral wall of the vault. This change is seen best in axial views, the submentovertical projection of the skull base (see Fig. 131). This is the only opportunity to demonstrate increased vascularity with meningiomas along or near the base, such as a tumor of the sphenoid wing.

Other branches of the external carotid artery also enlarge and become tortuous when they contribute to the blood supply of a meningioma. The changes in some are reflected in skull radiographs, while others contributing to neovascularity, such as the superficial temporal artery, may be observed only in angiograms. In some cases localized enlargement of diploic veins or a very conspicuous regional trunk may occur with a meningioma.

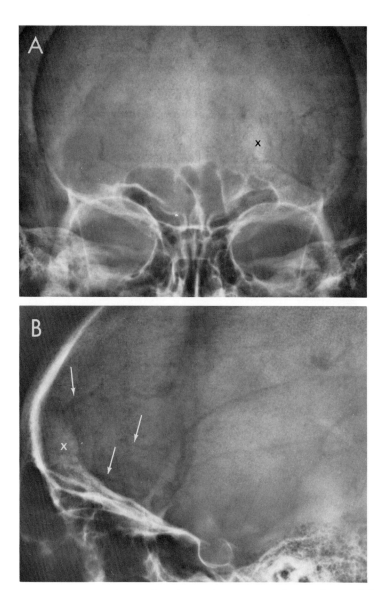

Figure 41.—Frontal pole meningioma. In **A,** frontal view, a localized rounded area of markedly increased density (**X**) is demonstrated just above the lateral aspect of the left frontal sinus. This is surrounded by a halo of less dense hyperostosis. At least three prominent vascular channels are seen coursing along the lateral aspect of the left frontal bone to the area of abnormal density where branching occurs. In **B,** lateral view, the area of abnormal density (**X**) is visible along the inferior aspect of the vertical portion of the frontal bone. The three vascular grooves (**arrows**) noted in **A** are seen to be large branches of the middle meningeal artery, the highest branch coursing to the superior aspect of the hyperostosis being quite wide and tortuous. The changes occurred in a 55-year-old woman who had had one seizure. Results of the neurologic examination were normal, but electroencephalography and a radioactive isotope brain scan indicated a lesion in the left frontal region. At operation, total gross removal of the tumor was achieved. (An angiogram of this case is shown in Fig. 127.)

CALCIFICATION.—The occurrence of calcification in a meningioma has been variously reported from as low as 7% to more than 20%. With some of the higher figures it appears probable that hyperostosis is being regarded as tumor calcification in some cases. A reasonable figure appears to be about 15% (see Table 4).

The extent of calcification in the tumors varies markedly radiologically, as it does pathologically. The most common type of calcification is a cloud-like, globular shadow of increased density. In some instances the entire tumor is calcified, and in these cases one segment of the lesion is shown to

Figure 42.—Calcified meningioma of the planum sphenoidale. A densely calcified mass (**X**) is present at the planum sphenoidale extending along its entire length and then back over the diaphragma sellae to the dorsum. On the original radiographs the calcified tumor measured 2 cm thick above the planum sphenoidale. The sella turcica is slightly deeper than normal, and there is extensive benign hyperostosis of the inner table of the skull. The patient, a 60-year-old woman with failing vision, was found to have greatly reduced visual acuity on both sides, more marked on the right, and a prechiasmal type of visual field pattern. At operation, it was found that the over-all size of the meningioma was 50% larger than the visible calcified portion, and decompression of the optic nerves and chiasm was accomplished.

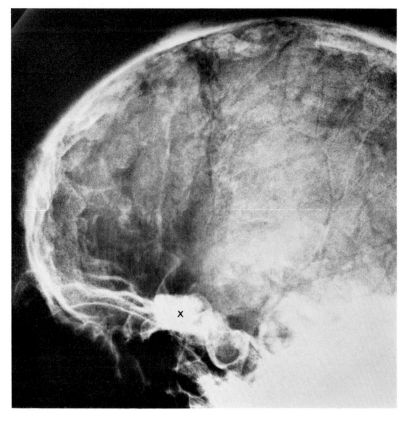

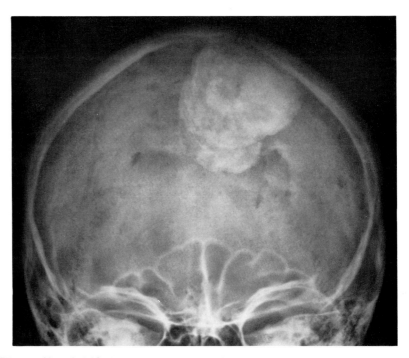

Figure 43.—Calcified parasagittal meningioma. A large cloud of calcium is present in the left parasagittal region which bulges across the midline. The calcium abuts the inner table of the parietal bone and is attached along a wide base, measuring 5 cm on the original radiographs. The tumor is fairly densely calcified, but there are a number of incompletely calcified areas so that it is not altogether homogeneous. The patient was a 32-year-old woman who had suffered from seizures since the age of 12. A diagnosis of idiopathic epilepsy had been made by her family physician and she had been treated with anticonvulsive medication for 20 years without a radiographic examination having been carried out until the present study just before hospitalization. At operation the tumor was found to be a psammomatous meningioma identical in size to the globular calcium shadow observed radiologically.

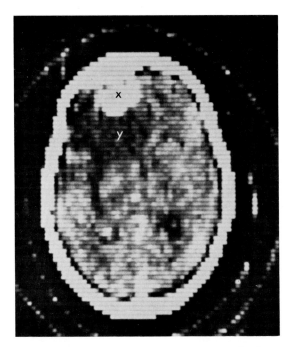

Figure 44.—Left frontal meningioma. The computerized tomogram shows a rounded area (**X**) with a high radiation absorption coefficient abutting the inner table of the frontal bone just to the left of the midline. Behind the dense meningioma is a large area of reduced density, appearing dark (**y**), which is the result of edema of the adjacent portion of the frontal lobe.

abut the bony skull or a dural septum such as the falx or the tentorium (Figs. 42 and 43). At other times the calcification may occur chiefly about the margin of the tumor or in one quadrant, in which case the calcified lesion may not clearly abut the skull. Occasionally the calcification may be atypical and consist of branching plaques of calcium resembling that found in a glial tumor or granuloma.

The basis for the calcification is a conglomeration of psammoma bodies which are usually most abundant in fibrous meningiomas. Fibrous tumors may occur at any of the characteristic meningioma sites (see Table 5). Although the incidence of calcified meningiomas is low, the fibrous lesions may be seen as areas of high radiation absorption by computerized tomography (Fig. 44). In some cases they appear as global masses against the inner table of the skull, just as in radiographs.

BIBLIOGRAPHY

1. Di Chiro, G.: The width (third dimension) of the sella turcica, Am. J. Roentgenol. 84:26, 1960.
2. Di Chiro, G., and Nelson, K. B.: The volume of the sella turcica, Am. J. Roentgenol. 87:989, 1962.

3. Dyke, C. G.: Indirect signs of brain tumor as noted in routine roentgen examinations; displacement of pineal shadow: A survey of 3000 consecutive skull examinations, Am. J. Roentgenol. 23:598, 1930.
4. El Gammal, T., and Allen, M. B., Jr.: Further consideration of sellar changes associated with increased intracranial pressure, Brit. J. Radiol. 45:561, 1972.
5. Rovit, R. L.; Schechter, M. M., and Chodroff, P.: Choroid plexus papillomas: Observations on radiographic diagnosis, Am. J. Roentgenol. 110:608, 1970.
6. Sosman, M. C.: Radiology as an aid in diagnosis of skull and intracranial lesions, Radiology 9:396, 1927.
7. Twining, E. W.: Radiology of the third and fourth ventricles; Part I and Part II, Brit. J. Radiol. 12:385 and 569, 1939.
8. Zimmerman, H. M.: The ten most common types of brain tumor, Seminars in Roentgenol. 6:48, 1971.

PART 3

Sellar and Parasellar Tumors

General Considerations

THE NEOPLASMS of the sellar, parasellar or juxtasellar area have rather predictable origins. Many produce disorders of function of the pituitary gland and hypothalamus. The neurologic changes depend on whether the tumor grows primarily into the suprasellar or retrosellar area or into the middle fossa.

The most common tumor is the pituitary adenoma; this type of sellar lesion is also presented in the Atlas of Tumor Radiology, *The Endocrines,* by Steinbach and Minagi (Chicago: Year Book Medical Publishers, 1969). The craniopharyngioma is a tumor found most often in childhood and has a second incidence peak during middle age. For some reason the tumor in the adult does not contain calcification as frequently as that seen in the child. Meningiomas may take origin from the planum sphenoidale, tuberculum, diaphragma or dorsum sellae. A meningioma may also appear within this area from origins in the cavernous sinus region or medial third of the sphenoid wing.

Orbital and intracanalicular optic gliomas can extend into the suprasellar area. Lesions arising from the intracranial portion of the optic nerve and optic chiasm are primary in the suprasellar region. The gliomas involving the optic tracts and hypothalamus are often difficult to differentiate from one another because of the frequent aggressive behavior of the lesions with involvement of contiguous structures. Primary bone tumors and chordomas may also be found. Congenital tumors such as epidermoids, dermoids, teratomas and ectopic pinealomas, although rare, arise in this region. Aneurysms may appear as suprasellar mass lesions and therefore should be excluded angiographically.

Clinical presentation of this group of tumors is most often related to involvement of the visual pathways. Hypothalamic dysfunction is seen most often with an infiltrating glioma but is a common finding postoperatively and an occasional finding preoperatively with craniopharyngioma. As a mass extends upward to the foramen of Monro, obstructive hydrocephalus and its resultant signs and symptoms occur. Compression of the brain stem may be caused by retrosellar extension of the tumors.

RADIOLOGIC DIAGNOSIS

Changes observed on pneumoencephalography are related to expansion of the lesion into the suprasellar cistern as well as its lateral extensions.

Occasionally lateral growth is sufficient to displace the temporal horn. Posteriorly the mass extends into the interpeduncular fossa. Changes in the ventricular system are primarily effacement of the optic and infundibular recesses of the third ventricle. With larger lesions the mass impinges upon the foramen of Monro or frontal horns.

Angiographic diagnosis may be difficult even in large lesions because the space surrounded by the circle of Willis is such that it does not permit angiographic detection early. The lesion must reach laterally enough to straighten or reverse the convex curves of the anterior choroidal, posterior communicating and internal carotid arteries. Lateral extension of intrasellar lesions causes a characteristic lateral displacement of the cavernous portion of the carotid artery. Often the posterior portion of the carotid artery will be displaced away from its normally medial position where it is related to the dorsum sellae in comparison to the normally more laterally positioned anterior part of the cavernous carotid artery related to the more laterally located anterior clinoid process.

Lateral retrosellar extension displaces the thalamocinereal branches of the posterior communicating artery laterally. Displacement of the basilar artery or its perforating thalamic branches occurs posteriorly. Local venous changes may also be seen with posterior displacement of the crural and pontomesencephalic veins.

If the lesion extends directly superiorly, or superiorly and anteriorly, the horizontal portion of the anterior cerebral artery is often elevated. In one-third of patients, however, the proximal anterior cerebral arteries retain their developmental configuration, being directed upward and forward away from the sella. With larger lesions lateral displacement of the uncal vein and upward displacement of the septal or internal cerebral vein may be found.

Figure 45.—Eosinophilic pituitary adenoma and acromegaly.

The patient had headache and typical signs of acromegaly. Laboratory examination revealed an elevated growth hormone level which was indicative of an active tumor.

Lateral projection: This reveals moderate enlargement of the sella turcica, which measured 23 mm in length by 17 mm in depth. It exhibits a rounded (ballooned) configuration. There is a concavity of the anterior sellar wall, which has been called undermining of the tuberculum sellae, most typical of intrasellar masses.

The frontal sinuses are enlarged and there is increased thickness of the calvaria. The lower jaw shows an increase in the angle between the horizontal and vertical portions but there is no prognathism, although the patient is edentulous.

The patient underwent a trans-sphenoidal cryohypophysectomy. Postoperatively she did well and is being followed.

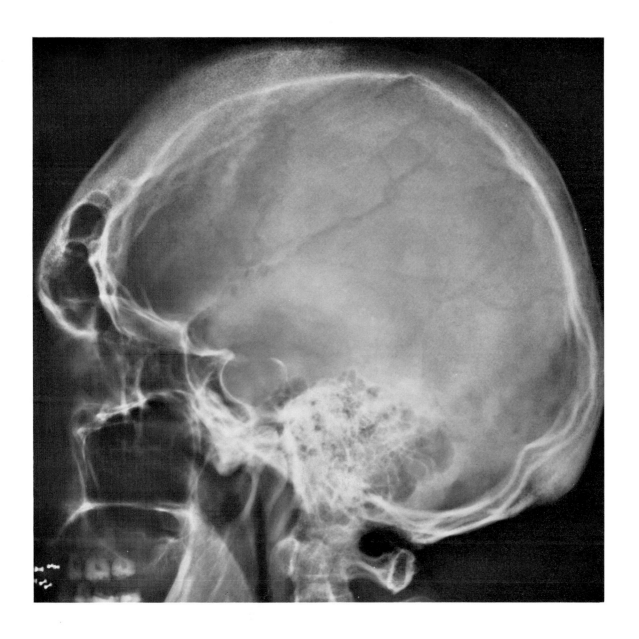

Figure 45 · **Pituitary Adenoma & Acromegaly / 83**

Figure 46.—Eosinophilic pituitary adenoma.

A 52-year-old woman had a five-year history of enlargement of the feet and hands. On examination there was a puffy appearance to her eyelids and cheeks. The optic fundi were normal and there was no evidence of a visual field defect.

A, sagittal tomogram of the sella turcica taken to the left of the midline: This shows a deep sella without an increase in the anteroposterior diameter. This cut was taken through the enlarged portion of the sella.

B, tomogram, frontal projection: An asymmetrical sella turcica with marked depression of the floor on the left side (**arrow**) is demonstrated.

C, thick tomographic cut taken during pneumoencephalography: No upward extension of the intrasellar contents is evident. The double floor of the sella turcica (**arrow**) is well demonstrated in this view.

D, anteroposterior projection made after injection of contrast material into the inferior petrosal sinus via a catheter inserted into the jugular vein: There is bulging of the sellar contents laterally (**arrow**) on the left side encroaching upon the cavernous sinus. The right side is normal.

The patient underwent a trans-sphenoidal cryohypophysectomy. Postoperatively the growth hormone levels were found to have returned to normal after having been elevated prior to operation.

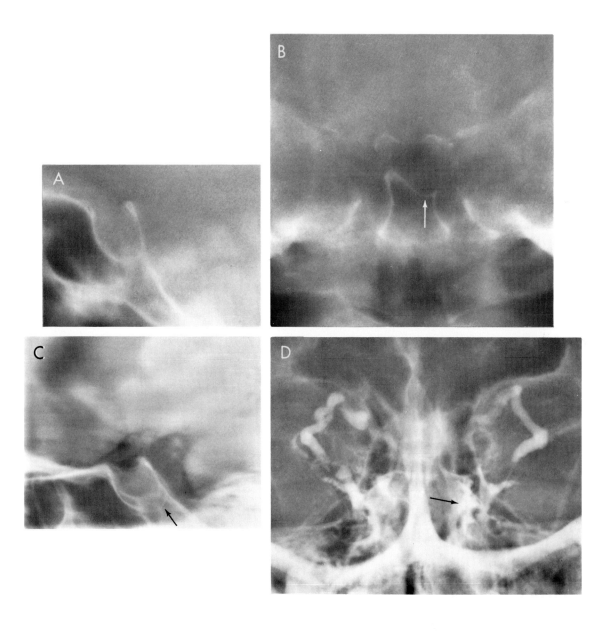

Figure 46 · Pituitary Adenoma / 85

Figure 47.—Asymmetrical enlargement of sella turcica with pituitary adenoma.

An 18-year-old girl complained of headache and absence of menstruation. From age 13 she had noticed that her hair was not as thick as it should have been. The results of neurologic examination were completely normal and there was no evidence of a visual field defect. Laboratory examinations were noncontributory.

A, tomogram: There is evidence of sella enlargement on the right side. Actual measurements were 20.5 mm in length and 19 mm in depth.

B, tomogram: The left side of the sella is almost normal in size, measuring 19 mm in length (which is slightly above the normal) and 10 mm in depth (which is within normal limits). The configuration is somewhat rounded, however, which should raise the question of an intrasellar mass.

C, tomogram, basal projection: This shows the asymmetrical enlargement of the sella (**x**) with a ballooned right side and displacement of both the anterior (**a**) and the posterior (**b**) wall. The walls curve toward each other normally on the left side (**c**). Pneumoencephalography showed no evidence of suprasellar extension.

D, drawing of the sella turcica to show how the length is determined by measuring the greatest distance from the anterior wall to the dorsum. For the height, a line is taken from the tuberculum sellae to the top of the dorsum; a perpendicular line to the deepest part of the sella is constructed. The width is the span of the sellar floor to the points where the bone begins to slope downward and lateralward away from the sella.

The patient received a dose of 5000 r in six weeks to the pituitary region. She tolerated the treatment well and the headache disappeared. Hormonal therapy was instituted.

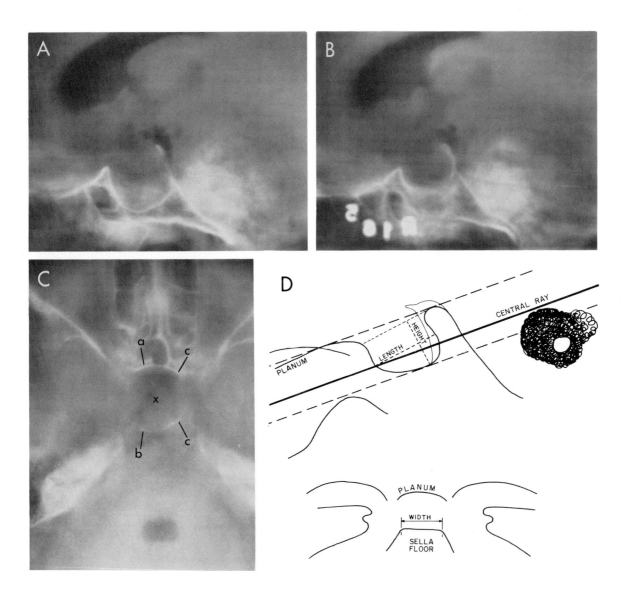

Figure 47 · Pituitary Adenoma / 87

Figure 48.—Chromophobe pituitary adenoma.

A 22-year-old man noted difficulty in reading for three months. On examination, he had bitemporal hemianopia with slightly reduced visual acuity bilaterally. One month prior to admission he began to have nocturia once nightly and some increase in water requirements. He had also noted a tendency to gain weight during the past four years.

A, frontal projection: The sellar floor slopes downward on the left, indicating greater deepening of the pituitary fossa on that side (**arrow**).

B, lateral view: This reveals enlargement and ballooning of the sella turcica. There is a double floor with the local erosion extending into the anterior wall on the same side. The cortical boundary of the interior of the sella is demineralized and thin (**arrow**).

C, base view: The anterior wall of the sella is thin and farther forward on the left than on the right (**arrows**).

D, right brachial angiogram, frontal view: This shows elevation of the horizontal portion of the anterior cerebral artery (**arrow**), indicating suprasellar extension of the mass. Similar suprasellar expansion of the mass was present on the left.

E, angiogram, lateral projection: No definite displacement of the siphon and no tumor vessels are noted.

F, angiogram, base view: There is lateral displacement of the intracavernous portion of the internal carotid artery (**arrow**). The frontal view (**D**) does not clearly demonstrate this lateral displacement with the angulation used here.

Partial surgical removal of the tumor was accomplished. After operation diabetes insipidus developed, which was controlled with pituitary snuff. At the time of discharge the polyuria and polydipsia were disappearing.

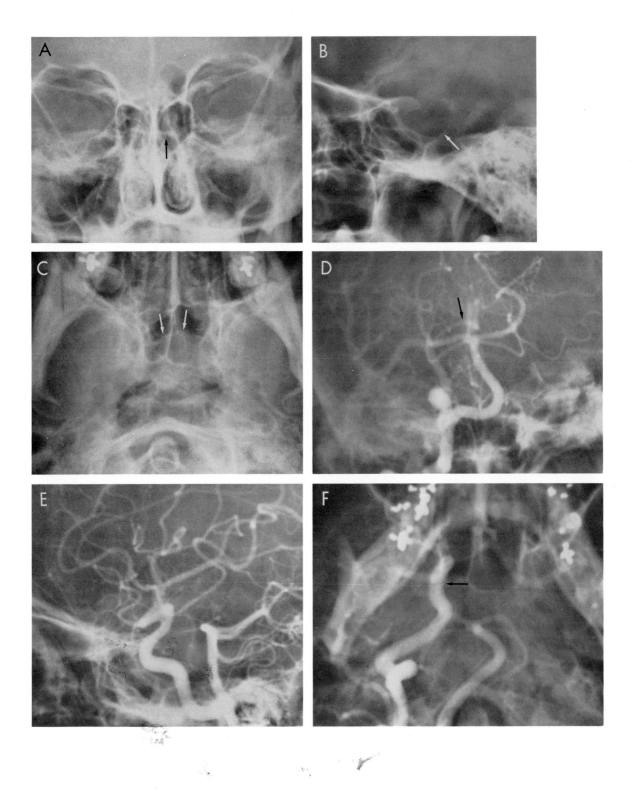

Figure 48 · Pituitary Adenoma / 89

Figure 49.—Calcification in chromophobe pituitary adenoma with suprasellar extension.

A 29-year-old man complained of some impairment of vision for eight months. One month prior to this examination a peripheral field defect in the left eye was discovered by an ophthalmologist. On admission he had early optic atrophy on the left with some pallor of the disc on the right. There was marked constriction of the visual field in the left eye with a residual temporal island of vision and a quadrantal temporal defect in the right visual field.

A, skull radiograph, lateral projection: This shows a demineralized sella turcica which has a double floor. The dorsum sellae can no longer be made out. There is herniation of the pituitary gland into the sphenoidal sinus. Shell-like calcification and plaques of calcium are present in the suprasellar region (**x**). Because of this, the possibility of craniopharyngioma instead of pituitary adenoma was considered more likely.

B, pneumoencephalogram, lateral view: This demonstrates suprasellar extension of the tumor with encroachment on the hypothalamic portion of the third ventricle (**arrow**). The optic and infundibular recesses are effaced and the third ventricle is invaginated. The indentation of the third ventricle corresponds exactly with the upper border of the shell-like calcification because the calcium is in the wall of the tumor, not within it. There is also elevation of the floor of the anterior horns of the lateral ventricles.

C, right carotid angiogram, frontal view: This shows upward displacement of the proximal portion of the anterior cerebral artery (**a**) and slight lateral displacement of the supraclinoid portion of the carotid siphon (**b**). The bifurcation of the internal carotid artery is probably high. The posterior aspect of the intracavernous portion of the internal carotid artery is slightly lateral in relation to the most anterior part of this segment due to lateral bulging of the intrasellar mass.

D, angiogram, lateral view: No significant distortion of the intracavernous segment or of the siphon is apparent in this projection. The elevation of the initial portion of the anterior cerebral artery is confirmed (**arrow**).

A right frontal craniotomy was performed with partial removal of the tumor and decompression of the optic nerves and chiasm and the hypothalamus. Postoperative radiographs revealed none of the previously noted suprasellar calcification.

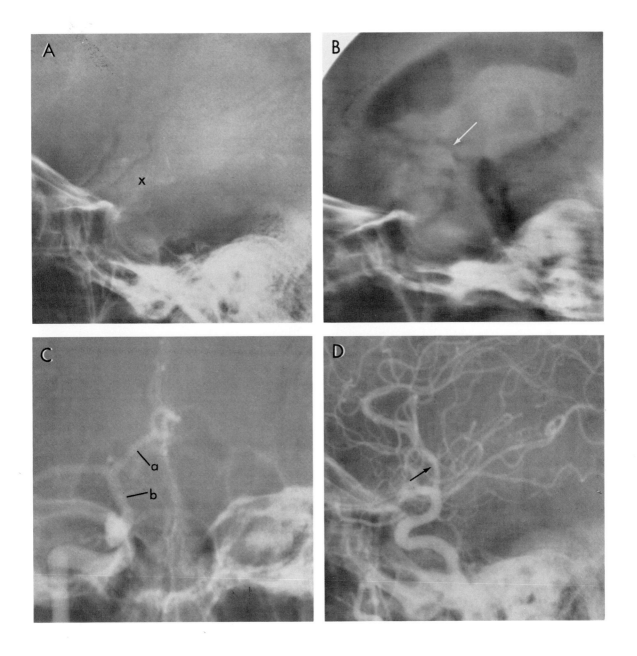

Figure 49 · Calcification in Pituitary Adenoma / 91

Figure 50.—Craniopharyngioma with suprasellar and retrosellar extension.

A 48-year-old woman had a two-year history of blurred vision and bilateral "blind spots." A pneumoencephalographic examination as well as carotid angiography had been performed elsewhere with what was said to be negative results. There had also been an intracranial exploration. At the time of our examination she had diabetes insipidus and bitemporal hemianopia with markedly decreased vision bilaterally.

A, autotomogram taken during pneumoencephalography: A large suprasellar mass (**arrows**) displaces and invaginates the third ventricle causing ventricular dilatation. It also extends posteriorly, encroaching on the cisterna interpeduncularis, and displaces the midbrain backward. The mass is unusually smooth and round, suggesting a cyst, but there is no calcification. The dorsum sellae is short and the clinoids are stubby. The pituitary fossa is shallow and the cortex of the floor is dense.

B, right carotid angiogram, frontal view: There is slight elevation of the horizontal portion of the anterior cerebral artery and there is lateral bowing of the supraclinoid portion of the carotid siphon (**arrow**). Residual air (**x**) from the pneumogram outlines the remaining patent portion of the third ventricle as a crescent over the tumor, which has collapsed the hypothalamic portion and splayed the upper portion of the ventricle.

C, vertebral angiogram, lateral view: Marked posterior displacement of the distal segment of the basilar artery (**b**) and bowing of the thalamoperforate arteries (**a**), confirming the posterior extension of the mass.

At operation a large portion of the tumor, which was partly cystic and partly solid, was removed. The patient responded poorly and died three months later.

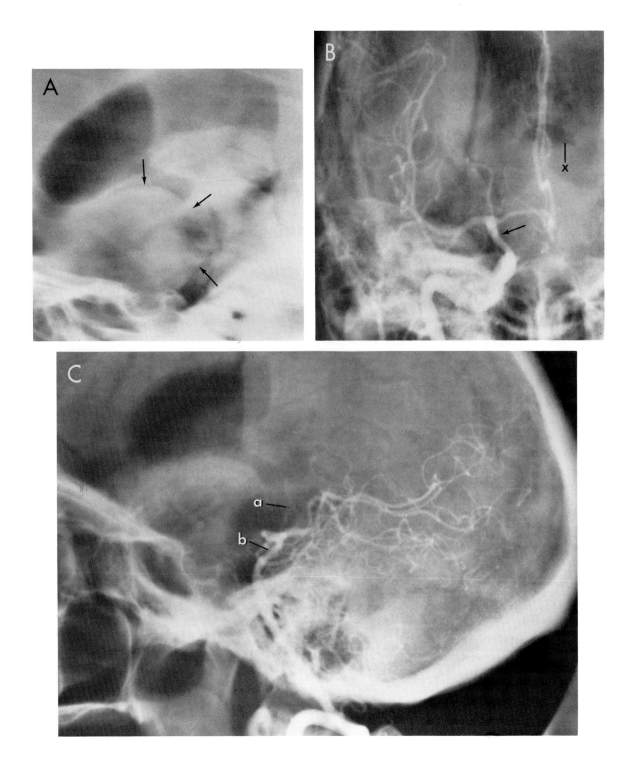

Figure 50 · Craniopharyngioma / 93

Figure 51.—Recurrent craniopharyngioma extending into lateral retrosellar region.

An 8-year-old girl was found to have impaired vision on entering school three years previously. At that time both optic discs were pale. Bitemporal hemianopia was present with more vision loss on the right than on the left. Studies elsewhere led to a diagnosis of craniopharyngioma and it was partially removed. Vision improved markedly and she did well until three months before the present examination when she again began to have blurred vision. Headache developed and she had difficulty walking. Examination again revealed a bitemporal hemianopia with marked loss of visual acuity. There were pyramidal tract signs without sensory loss.

A, polytomogram of the sellar area: This reveals a shallow fossa with a dense cortical boundary of the sellar floor and the sloping anterior wall. Numerous calcium deposits are present above the sella, some of which are curvilinear and shell-like while others appear as small plaques, probably in the wall of the cyst. Above the dorsum a more dense conglomerate collection of calcium is present.

B, pneumoencephalogram: The ventricular system is moderately dilated. The hypothalamic portion of the third ventricle does not fill but is invaginated by a mass (**arrows**) which extends well above the calcium and has a rounded anterior and superior surface. There is also a rounded edge of tumor behind the dorsum outlined by gas in the cisterna pontis (**x**), indicating significant retrosellar extension of the recurrent tumor. The aqueduct of Sylvius is seen as a thin line (**y**) extending down and back, well behind its usual position because of backward displacement of the brain stem.

C, left brachial angiography, frontal view: The basilar artery is displaced to the right (**a**). There are marked elevation and deformity of the left posterior cerebral artery (**b**) due to the greater left-sided posterior extension of the tumor. Portions of the right carotid system (**c**) are outlined by way of the right posterior communicating artery.

D, angiogram, lateral view: This shows reversal of the curve of the basilar artery (**a**), which is displaced posteriorly well away from the clivus. The left posterior cerebral artery is conspicuously elevated (**b**) as compared with the right. There are stretching of the right posterior communicating artery (**c**) and opening of the carotid siphon due to its forward displacement.

The fluid contents of the lesion were aspirated, but the recurrent tumor was in large part solid. Therefore radiation therapy was administered.

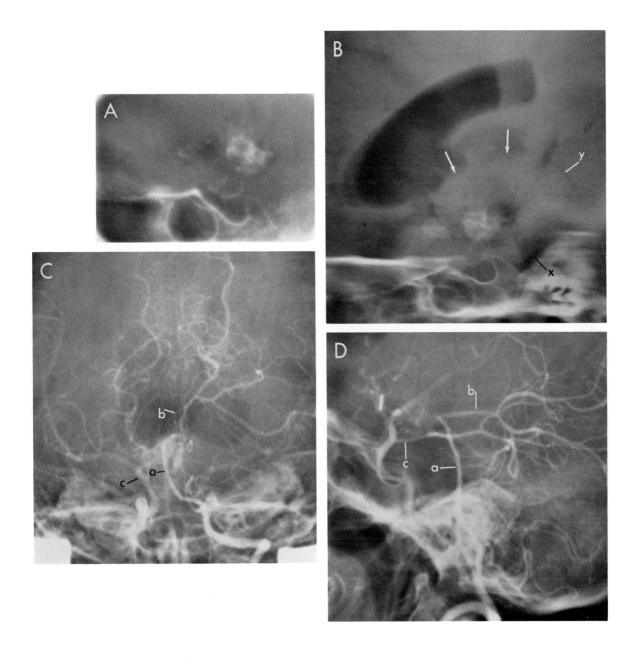

Figure 51 · Recurrent Craniopharyngioma / 95

Figure 52.—Cystic craniopharyngioma.

A 6-year-old boy complained of headaches two or three times a week. An ophthalmologist noted bitemporal field loss. Otherwise he was normal.

A, skull radiograph, lateral projection: This reveals an open type sella with a dense floor and anterior wall but with a thin dorsum. A thin line of calcium, that extends downward into the sella turcica (**arrow**), can be seen in the anterior suprasellar region.

B, pneumoencephalogram, lateral projection: There is marked suprasellar extension in a directly superior direction with invagination of the third ventricle (**arrow**). The gas projected above the anterior part of the sella is mostly lateral in position.

C, right carotid angiogram with cross-compression, frontal view: There is no evidence of elevation of the horizontal portion of the anterior cerebral artery on either side, which indicates that the tumor is extending primarily straight upward. The supraclinoid portion of the internal carotid artery is slightly displaced laterally (**arrow**), as is the proximal part of the anterior choroidal artery (**y**).

D, angiogram, lateral projection: This shows an open carotid siphon with the supraclinoid portion of the carotid artery directed straight upward (**arrow**). The bifurcation of the internal carotid is high. The left side had a similar appearance.

Surgical intervention resulted in partial removal of the tumor and satisfactory recovery. Radiation therapy was administered because the tumor was incompletely removed.

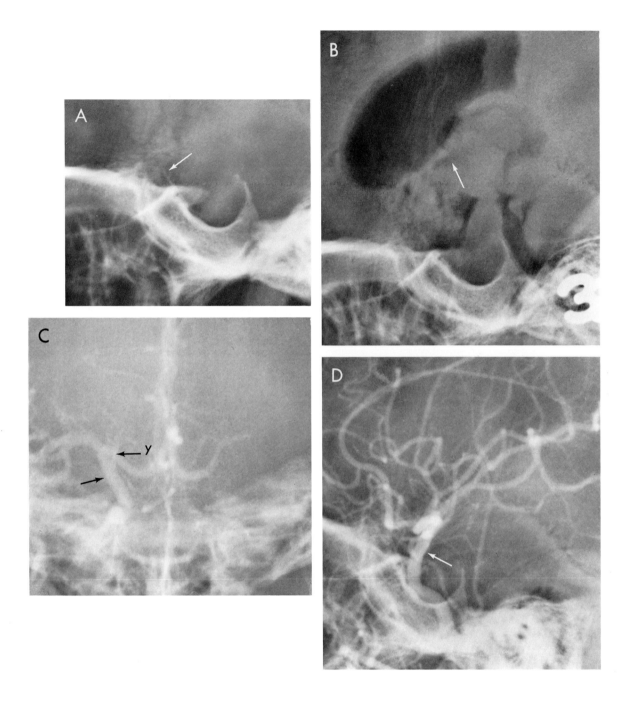

Figure 52 · Cystic Craniopharyngioma / 97

Figure 53.—Large cystic craniopharyngioma.

A 5-year-old child hospitalized with progressive vision loss was found to have bilateral papilledema. The head was moderately enlarged. No endocrinopathy was discovered.

A, right carotid angiogram, frontal view, arterial phase: Changes of hydrocephalus are evident. The anterior segment of the posterior communicating artery is normal, but the continuation of the vessel has a mild medially directed concavity (**a**), the artery being displaced laterally. The anterior choroidal artery is also displaced laterally (**b**). The lateral displacement of the lenticulostriates (**c**) is due to direct mass effect as well as hydrocephalus.

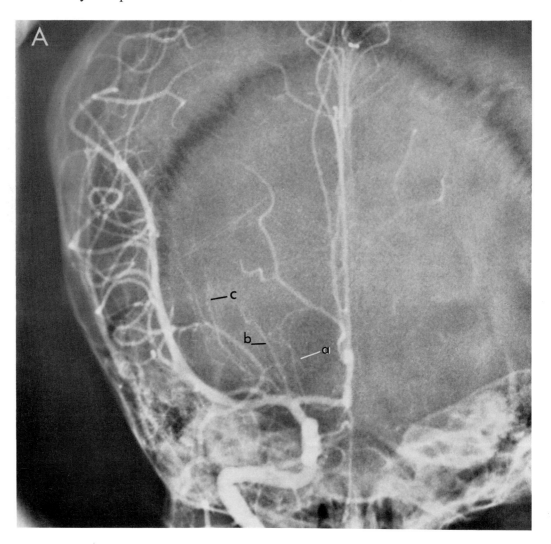

B, right carotid angiogram, lateral view, arterial phase: The posterior communicating artery and its premamillary branch are well seen (**a**). The premamillary branch is enlarged and stretched. The anterior choroidal artery also appears taut (**b**). The changes of hydrocephalus are also evident. There was flash filling of the basilar artery (**d**).

(*Continued.*)

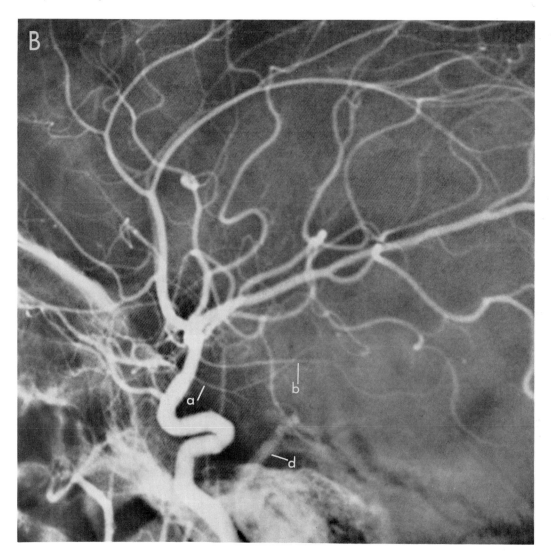

Figure 53 · Cystic Craniopharyngioma / 99

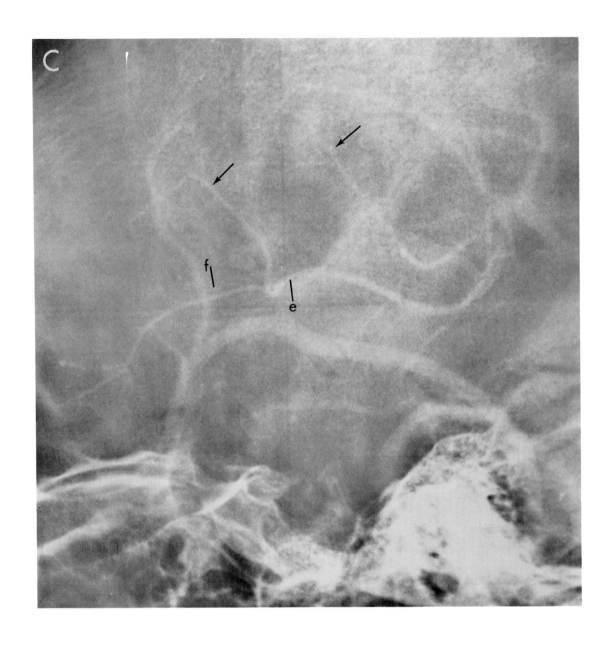

Figure 53 (cont.).—Large cystic craniopharyngioma.

C, right carotid angiogram, venous phase: This reveals a local mass effect on the internal cerebral vein (e) (upward bowing) just posterior to the foramen of Monro as demarcated by the entrance of the thalamostriate vein. In addition there is elevation of the posterior two-thirds of the septal vein (f). The lengthened subependymal veins (**arrows**) demonstrate the extent of the hydrocephalus.

D, left vertebral angiogram, frontal view, arterial phase: The tip of the basilar artery is displaced to the left (d). The flash-filled left posterior communicating artery is markedly stretched outward (g) and its normal medial convexity reversed.

(*Continued.*)

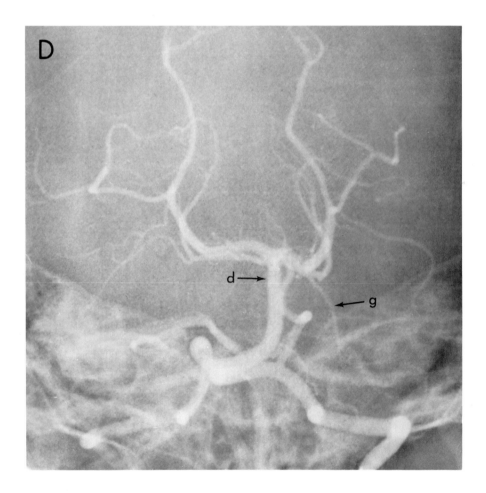

Figure 53 · Cystic Craniopharyngioma / 101

Figure 53 (cont.).—Large cystic craniopharyngioma.

E, left vertebral angiogram, lateral view: The basilar artery is displaced backward (**d**), as are its perforating thalamic branches (**d′**). The left posterior communicating artery is stretched and its premamillary branch is also quite taut. The medial and lateral posterior choroidal vessels are flattened and close together in this view secondary to the hydrocephalus. At the foramen of Monro, where the medial and lateral posterior choroidal vessels join anteriorly, there is local upward displacement of the medial vessels (**arrow**), causing an abnormally small distance between the planes of the choroid fissures of the third and lateral ventricles in this lateral projection.

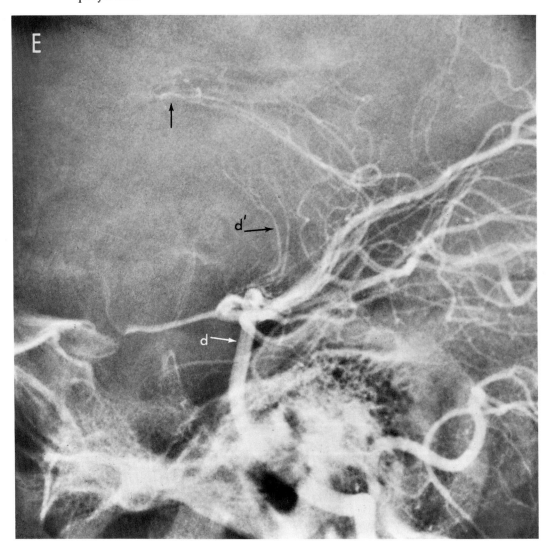

F, left vertebral angiogram, lateral view, venous phase: There is marked backward displacement of the anterior pontomesencephalic vein (**h**). The medial and lateral choroidal veins again demonstrate the local mass effect in the region of the foramen of Monro as was shown by the arteries. The precentral cerebellar vein is displaced backward (**i**) secondary to the posterior dislocation of the entire upper brain stem.

At operation a largely cystic craniopharyngioma was removed. A mild degree of diabetes insipidus developed postoperatively, but recovery was satisfactory.

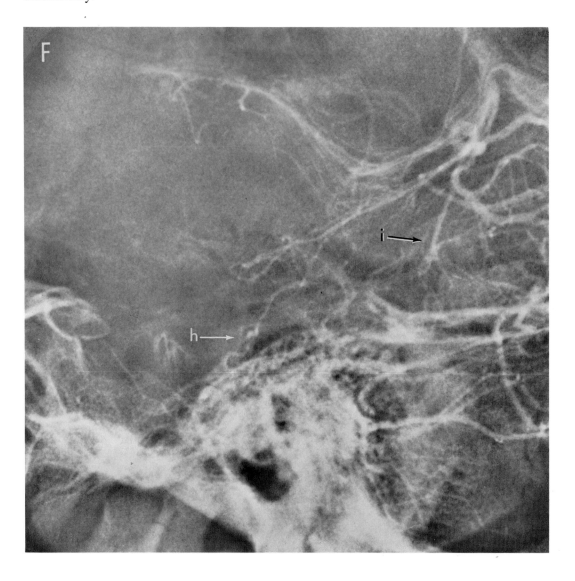

Figure 53 · Cystic Craniopharyngioma / 103

Figure 54.—Optic glioma.

A 12-year-old girl was referred from the ophthalmology service because of progressive vision loss. Both optic discs were pale, but the margins were sharp.

Pneumoencephalogram made in brow-up position, lateral projection: Air above and below the optic pathways in the suprasellar cistern outlines enlarged optic nerves (**arrows**) rostrally at the level of the anterior clinoids. The mass progressively expands backward and upward and mushrooms into a large mass effacing the anterior recesses of the third ventricle (**a**), and invaginating the hypothalamic portion of the ventricle. There is no hydrocephalus.

On a bifrontal craniotomy with exploration of the suprasellar region, the tumor was seen to involve the optic chiasm and extend into both optic nerves, which were enlarged in a funnel-shaped manner. They seemed, however, to narrow to normal size before entering the optic canals. The tumor invaded the third ventricle and hypothalamus so that only a biopsy specimen was taken. The patient received radiotherapy and was doing well when seen three years after the operation.

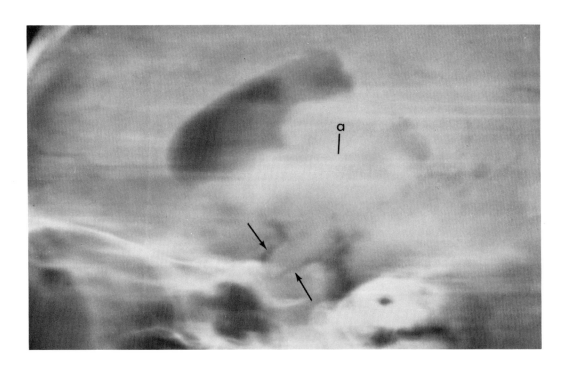

Figure 55.—Large optic glioma.

An infant was hospitalized because of failure to thrive, irritability and frequent crying and an enlarging head. There were roving eye movements and the pupils reacted poorly to light. The optic discs were very pale and the nerve head on the left was elevated.

Pneumoencephalogram, lateral projection: There is moderate dilatation of the lateral and third ventricles. A large mass (**x**) above the sella turcica has effaced the anterior recesses of the third ventricle (**arrow**) and invaginated its hypothalamic extension. The base of the brain has been lifted so that the aqueduct of Sylvius is elongated and of small caliber (**a**). The anterior part of the sella turcica has not developed normally and has a gourd shape. Note the air (**b**) rimming the inferior aspect of the optic glioma.

Operation revealed a large tumor of the optic chiasm and both optic nerves. A well-differentiated astrocytoma was diagnosed from the biopsy specimen. The patient was regaining vision when seen six months after a course of radiation therapy.

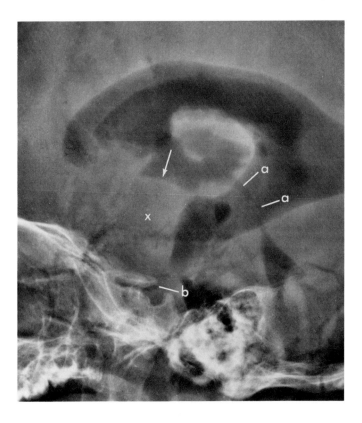

Figure 55 · Optic Glioma / 105

Figure 56.—Ectopic pinealoma presenting as a suprasellar mass.

A 14-year-old girl was seen because of blurred vision. On examination a bitemporal hemianopia was found.

A, plain radiograph of the skull, lateral projection: This demonstrates a rounded sella turcica with a thin floor suggesting an intrasellar mass.

B, pneumoencephalography, hanging-head position: A suprasellar mass (**x**) encroaches on the lumen of the hypothalamic portion of the third ventricle (**arrow**). The angles between the tumor and the anterior and posterior ventricular walls are sharp.

C, right brachial angiogram with cross-compression, frontal view, arterial phase: This demonstrates a normal appearance of the anterior cerebral arteries and no lateral displacement of the carotid siphons, although the bifurcation is slightly higher on the right than on the left. The only abnormality is slight flattening of the inward curves of the proximal portions of the anterior choroidal arteries (**arrows**) of both sides.

D, right brachial angiogram, lateral view: This shows an open carotid siphon with a straight vertical supraclinoid portion but no other abnormality.

At operation the bulk of the tumor was removed and the optic chiasm and nerves were decompressed. Histologic examination disclosed an ectopic pinealoma. Fifteen months later the patient returned complaining of weakness of the legs, particularly on the left. A myelogram demonstrated a block at T-10/T-11 and a laminectomy revealed metastatic pinealoma. Radiation therapy to the entire cerebrospinal axis was then given.

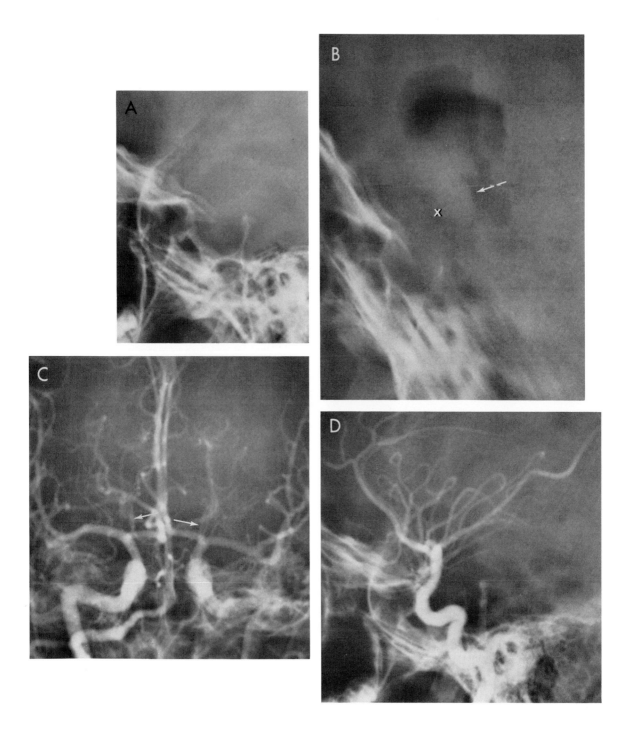

Figure 56 · Ectopic Pinealoma / 107

PART 4

Frontal Tumors

Intracerebral, Supratentorial Tumors

IN PARTS 4–9 we present the large group of intracerebral, supratentorial tumors. It is necessary, first, to outline the general manifestations of such lesions found in angiograms and pneumograms and to define a practical scheme of classification of these tumors. It is also important to appreciate the complications of tumor growth resulting from the displacement of cerebral structures in relation to the falx, tentorium and other fixed structures around which the brain is molded or herniated. It is necessary, too, to recognize the aggravation of such deformities that may result from performing various special procedures.

PNEUMOGRAPHIC AND ANGIOGRAPHIC MANIFESTATIONS

Cerebral pneumography is less commonly used than formerly as a primary procedure to diagnose supratentorial neoplasms. Cerebral angiography is almost invariably carried out as a first procedure; a pneumographic examination, performed either by lumbar pneumoencephalography or by ventriculography, may then be used to clarify the location of a tumor if the diagnosis is in question after angiography. The morbidity accompanying cerebral pneumography in patients with supratentorial brain tumors is greater than that of angiography. Also operative intervention is often necessary following a pneumographic examination because of the precipitation or aggravation of a herniation by pneumography. In general, the tumors that are more deeply situated, such as central tumors in the thalamus or basal ganglia and the corpus callosum and intraventricular masses, are more easily and clearly delineated by cerebral pneumography. The more superficially placed tumors and those neoplasms that have an inherent tumor circulation are more easily demonstrated by angiography.

PNEUMOGRAPHY

Four basic pneumographic changes may be associated with supratentorial neoplasms. These include defective filling, dilatation, deformity and displacement.

DEFECTIVE FILLING.—Lack of filling may be due to obstruction of the ventricular pathways by the tumor or to deformity at a communicating foramen or canal from angulation and compression by the tumor. By itself, it is not a reliable sign of a tumor because abnormal filling may be associated with an inflammatory process or a congenital defect. Incomplete filling of a lateral ventricle is common, although it is not now seen as often as in the past because use of the somersaulting chair allows equalization of gas in the lateral ventricles in most cases. When it is not possible to obtain equal, or nearly equal, filling of the lateral ventricles by placing the patient in the brow-up or hanging-head position, the failure of any portion of the ventricular system to fill must be explained. In some cases, filling of an obstructed ventricle may be accomplished by positioning the head with elevation of the unfilled side or by the administration of urea or Mannitol.

When defective filling is found in a patient who has ventricular dilatation, as known from prior angiography, particular attention must be directed toward accomplishing good filling. In such cases, a small local lesion such as a benign colloid cyst may obstruct one foramen of Monro. Also, when gas enters the intracranial subarachnoid space satisfactorily but there is complete failure of ventricular filling, the suspicion of a tumor in some portion of the brain, including the supratentorial areas, is greatly raised. Approximately one-half of patients who have non-filling of the ventricles on pneumoencephalography have a brain tumor. If additional information is needed after angiography, pneumoencephalography should be undertaken after the patient has been treated with dexamethasone (Decadron) for two to three days.

DILATATION OF VENTRICLES.—Like defective filling, dilatation may be associated with obstruction of some portion of the ventricular lumen by a tumor or angulation and compression of a communicating foramen or canal. In most cases of supratentorial tumors, the ventricle contralateral to the lesion undergoes greater enlargement. The ventricle on the side of the tumor is usually collapsed or compressed directly by the tumor, while the opposite ventricle does not drain properly because of compression, stretching or angulation at the foramen of Monro. Some hemispheric tumors grow through the ventricular wall, and fragments of the lesion in the cerebrospinal fluid may block the aqueduct of Sylvius, causing marked ventricular dilatation. Choroid papillomas, which may be in the hemisphere as well as in the ventricle, cause overproduction of cerebrospinal fluid with resulting hydrocephalus. In patients with tumors that produce high levels of cerebrospinal fluid protein, the large molecules are thought to block the arachnoid villi and produce dilatation through interference with fluid absorption. As with defective filling, dilatation by itself is not necessarily indicative of a tumor because it may be seen with congenital defects and inflammatory, degenerative and other cerebral abnormalities. In general, pronounced ventricular dilatation results from non-neoplastic processes, such as aqueduct stenosis, but there are exceptions, such as the marked internal hydrocephalus caused by colloid cysts.

A *pressure diverticulum* is a special type of localized ventricular dilatation usually seen with long-standing hydrocephalus. The evaginations or out-pocketings of the ventricular walls are characteristically found at specific sites which are considered to be points of greatest weakness. In the lateral ventricles, a pressure diverticulum may be found along the medial wall of the atrium in the region of the choroid fissure. The diverticulum extends to the retrothalamic region and the quadrigeminal cistern, and in some cases it herniates through the tentorial incisura into the posterior fossa. Pressure diverticula are also seen fairly frequently in the region of the lamina terminalis and the suprapineal recess of the third ventricle and at the anterior medullary velum, these diverticula occurring with tumors more central and caudad to the cerebral hemispheres.

DEFORMITY.—Ventricular deformities are usually local changes, except those produced by large tumors and herniations. The deformities characteristic of lesions in various areas classified later are changes of localizing value and are better presented under the individual tumor sites. Minor deformities caused by a tumor without accompanying changes of displacement and dilatation involve principally the lateral ventricles. In many instances, measurements found in standard text and reference books are useful in establishing the presence of an abnormality.

DISPLACEMENT.—The displacement of cerebral structures may be either minor or major. Minor displacements are related to deformities, noted above, and, as with the deformities, are better considered under individual categories of tumors.

Major displacements frequently result in herniations. A herniation is defined as a protrusion of cerebral substance through a natural opening in the skull or meninges such as the foramen magnum or the incisura of the tentorium. If it progresses, incarceration of blood vessels will occur at the hernial ring and infarction and intracerebral hemorrhages may be produced. Downward transtentorial herniation is a relatively common and very serious complication of a hemispheric tumor. The portion of the brain most often displaced through the tentorium is the hippocampus. Anterior hippocampal herniation displaces the brain stem backward and causes flattening of the corresponding cerebral peduncle. This commonly occurs with tumors of the anterior or middle fossa. Middle and posterior herniations of the hippocampus produce flattening of the midbrain, which is then displaced toward the opposite side of the incisura as well as downward. The contralateral side of the midbrain is compressed against the edge of the tentorium. Bilateral herniations are not uncommon, particularly in patients with large frontal tumors.

Uncal (anterior hippocampal) herniations are very common secondary to mass lesions of the infra-Sylvian region. The uncus is rolled over the tentorial edge and presents in the incisura. With further increase in volume of the cerebrum by a middle or anterior fossa tumor on one side, the anterior part of the hippocampus and the medial portion of the perihippocampal gyrus are displaced over the tentorial edge and forced caudad (Fig. 57). Downward herniations along the posterior portion of the incisura are most often caused by tumors behind the third ventricle. The posterior part of the perihippocampal gyrus is displaced downward, behind the brain stem.

Either an anterior or a posterior herniation may progress to severe unilateral tentorial downward herniation (complete herniation). If there is complete herniation on both sides, the process is referred to as a central herniation. Any sizable tentorial herniation compresses the brain stem and forces it against the opposite tentorial edge. There is associated compression of perimesencephalic veins causing congestion and petechial hemorrhages within the mesencephalon (Fig. 57).

There is usually defective filling of the ventricular system rostral to the fourth ventricle on pneumoencephalography and caudal to the third ventricle on ventriculography because the aqueduct is occluded. The most commonly observed changes of downward transtentorial herniation are in the subarachnoid cisterns on pneumoencephalography when the presence of a herniation is not anticipated. Anterior and middle hippocampal herniations produce a deformity or an obstruction of the cisterna interpeduncularis. This is seen in the lateral view as a soft tissue shadow sloping down and back to fuse with the outline of the brain stem, demonstrated by means of the head of the gas column in the cisterna pontis and lower part of the cisterna interpeduncularis. In some cases of supratentorial tumor the retrothalamic space, also in the lateral view, may show downward displacement on one side in comparison with the normal opposite side. Air in the quadrigeminal cistern may disclose the collicular plate tilted backward. If the aqueduct does fill, the iter is also displaced backward and lateralward with an anterior herniation.

Subfalcial herniation (midline shift) is very common with supratentorial tumors. The midline shift has been called the most important sign in neuroradiology. Such herniations vary tremendously from the slight shift seen with small tumors to incarceration of the cingulate gyrus beneath the falx. The configuration of a midline shift and its point of maximal contralateral protrusion beneath the falx, as seen in frontal views in both angiography and pneumography, are important in the localization of a hemispheric tumor. Three structures are usually involved in the shifts of pneumography: (1) the third ventricle, (2) the septum pellucidum, and (3) the callosal cistern. With a superiorly placed tumor, the septum pellucidum is usually shifted more than the third ventricle. The reverse is true when a tumor is present along the low convexity or in the infra-Sylvian region.

The shifts found on pneumography differ from those observed at angiography, described below. The shifts of pneumography are most helpful in localizing a tumor in the coronal plane, as just noted. The shifts of angiography are also useful in determining the location of a tumor in the sagittal plane as well as in the coronal plane.

The dislocations or shifts may be placed in three general categories: (1) straight, (2) angular, and (3) curved. Because the shifts of pneumography and angiography do not correlate well, the terms "square" and "round" are not usually applied to herniations observed pneumographically.

The septum pellucidum and third ventricle may be displaced contralaterally by the vectors of pressure from any hemispheric tumor, the results varying with the high, mid- or low position along the convexity. A straight shift is produced when the line of the septum pellucidum is displaced parallel to, but no longer in, the midsagittal plane. The upper portion of the third ventricle usually continues in the same plane, although the inferior portion must return to the midline because of its fixation at the base. Such a shift is produced by tumors that are near the coronal plane of the foramen of Monro and are mid- or low convexity in location, the vector of force of the new growth pressing straight laterally against the septum pellucidum. The straight shift, however, is not of as strong localizing value as the angular and curved shifts of pneumography because it may occur with a tumor in almost any portion of one hemisphere when the lesion produces generalized increased bulk of the hemisphere. For example, a straight shift can be seen with a posterior hemispheric tumor when there is compression of draining cerebral veins resulting in generalized edema. It may also be seen with an extracerebral lesion, such as a subdural hematoma which exerts widespread lateral pressure on the midline structures.

An angular shift is one in which the top of the septum pellucidum is displaced more than its base and more than the third ventricle, which usually continues in line with the septum. An angular shift is seen most often with high convexity and parasagittal tumors (Fig. 58). With high tumors the lateral angle of the lateral ventricle ipsilateral to the tumor is usually lower than the medial angle.

A curved shift is one in which the lower end of the septum is displaced more than the upper margin, the reverse of the angular shift. The third ventricle also appears to be concave toward the side of the lesion, the displacement of the upper margin of the third ventricle conforming to the maximal lateral displacement of the lower edge of the septum pellucidum. This type of shift is most often the result of a tumor of the low convexity or of the infra-Sylvian region. The bulk of such a lesion is below the transverse plane of the foramen of Monro. However, it may be either central or lateral to the temporal horn and may be in the thalamus. With central lesions, the body of the ipsilateral ventricle is narrowed by pressure from the mass displacing the lateral wall medially. When there is only mild subfalcial herniation, the ventricular roof on the involved side may be elevated rather than depressed as with the angular shift.

A tilt of the callosal space or cistern may be found with subfalcial herniation. This becomes maximal when there is herniation of the cingulate gyrus beneath the falx (Fig. 59). In many cases the pericallosal space is not well depicted in pneumograms. Characteristic angiographic findings of importance are often connected with this type of herniation, and will be illustrated subsequently. Similarly, retrosphenoidal herniations are usually best demonstrated by angiography. These are most often herniation of the base of the frontal lobe over the sphenoid ridge, but forward herniation of the temporal pole into the anterior fossa can also occur.

ANGIOGRAPHY

There are four principal changes observed on angiography that are often associated with supratentorial neoplasms. These include vascular displacement, straightening and stretching of cerebral arteries, changes in circulation time and a tumor circulation.

VASCULAR DISPLACEMENT.—As in pneumography, vascular displacement may be major or minor. Either arteries or veins may be involved, frequently both. Major displacements often involve the deep cerebral vessels and may be associated with herniations. Minor displacements are often found in the vicinity of the tumor, although there may be local major displacements as well as minor ones.

Downward transtentorial herniation can usually be diagnosed on angiography. The disturbance of cerebrospinal fluid dynamics associated with pneumography should be avoided since there may be an aggravation of the herniation.

Depending on the location of the tumor, as in pneumography, all or portions of the vascular structures bordering the tentorial ring may be displaced downward. If there is an anterior herniation of the uncus or of the anterior part of the hippocampus, the cisternal portion of the anterior choroidal artery and the posterior communicating artery are displaced downward. The choroidal artery is often displaced far medially, sometimes as far as the midline, with larger herniations. The middle and posterior thirds of the tentorial hiatus are ringed by the posterior cerebral artery, the basal vein of Rosenthal and other smaller perimesencephalic veins which may be displaced or bowed downward. In some cases the proximal portions of the superior cerebellar arteries are also depressed when the herniation is severe.

Subfalcial herniation (*midline shift*) is, as in pneumography, a highly important change of lateralizing and localizing value in the diagnosis of hemispheric tumors. Angiographic subfalcial shifts may involve only the anterior cerebral artery and not the internal cerebral vein, or it may involve both. If a tumor is more anteriorly placed, the artery may be more clearly displaced than the vein. If the tumor is more posterior the internal cerebral vein may be more significantly displaced than the anterior cerebral artery.

Because the anterior cerebral artery has a long course and throughout much of its course it is below the free edge of the falx, it is readily displaced by tumors of the anterior and the middle fossa. Even in its more posterior course, when it is beside the falx, it can be displaced downward and forward and across the midline by parasagittal and posterior tumors. The artery, coursing forward and upward, may first be affected as a *proximal shift* by deep frontal masses and tumors of the anterior portion of the middle fossa (Fig. 60). At its rostral curve, the anterior cerebral artery is still beneath the free edge of the falx and a frontal mass may displace it readily across the midline to produce a *round shift* (Fig. 60).

Tumors not in the frontal lobe but situated more posteriorly or laterally exert pressure on the anterior cerebral artery more evenly than do frontal tumors. Because of the vector of force produced by the lesion nearer the distal part of the artery, the distal segment is displaced across the midline. At the same time, the general increase in the mass of the hemisphere also exerts pressure on the forward part of the anterior cerebral artery. Thus a *square or even shift* of the anterior cerebral artery contralateral to the tumor is produced. The square shift is not as specific for localizing a tumor as the round shift because it can be produced by tumors of the parieto-occipital convexity and masses in the middle and posterior portions of the temporal lobe. In some cases there is a shift of only the *distal* portion of the anterior cerebral artery. This is produced by parasagittal or high convexity posterior tumors which displace the distal part of the anterior cerebral artery downward and beneath the falx but do not produce a transmitted force against the forward portion of the artery.

The internal cerebral vein, being beneath the free edge of the falx throughout its course, is readily displaced off the midline. The greatest shifts occur with tumors in the plane of the vein, such as those of the temporal lobe and low frontoparietal convexity. As noted above, however, frontal tumors can also displace the internal cerebral vein to some extent by increase in bulk of the hemisphere. The anterior portion of the vein is usually displaced more than the posterior part, which is more fixed.

As noted, because of the long course of the anterior cerebral artery, the configuration of its displacement is useful in the localization of a mass in the sagittal as well as the coronal plane. The proximal shift related to displacement of the proximal ascending portion, as seen in the frontal angiogram, is caused by inferior frontal and anterior middle fossa masses. A well-rounded bending or even a rounding of the upper and lower displaced corners of the ascending portion of the anterior cerebral artery in the frontal angiogram is characteristic of a frontal tumor. If, however, the entire ascending portion of the anterior cerebral artery is displaced equally up to the point where it returns to its normal position beside the falx and the corners of the displaced portions of the artery are angular, the shift will appear to be square. If only the distal portion of the anterior cerebral artery is seen to be shifted across the midline in a frontal angiogram, other evidence of the presence of a mass in the posterior part of the cerebrum and in the parasagittal or high convexity region should be sought.

Retrosphenoidal herniation is gross displacement upward or downward in relation to the lesser wing of the sphenoid bone. Downward herniation is usually caused by frontal tumors and is manifested by flattening of the middle cerebral and uncal veins and downward displacement of the carotid siphon. With larger lesions, the middle cerebral vein may be displaced well backward and the carotid siphon closed. An upward herniation, produced by mass lesions of the middle fossa, is manifested by forward and upward displacement of the same venous structures and opening of the carotid siphon.

Arterial displacements not related to herniations frequently occur as a result of superficially placed masses. With such tumors, the arterial displacement is often quite pronounced and clearly defined. Local arterial displacements with deeply placed tumors are more difficult to appreciate unless radiographs of the opposite normal side are available for comparison. Deep tumors, however, frequently cause local deformity of the subependymal veins and other deeply seated venous structures.

STRAIGHTENING AND STRETCHING OF CEREBRAL ARTERIES.—The cerebral arteries normally undulate as they follow the cerebral convolutions and sulci. In some instances a portion of an artery may lie deep in the sulcus and another portion may wander out of the sulcus, especially when it becomes elongated by atherosclerosis. Loss of the normal undulations and stretching of arteries are commonly found in the region of a tumor and sometimes in areas adjacent to the tumor due to accompanying edema.

If two adjacent gyri are affected by an increase in mass, the artery and the sulcus between them has to take a longer course. If one gyrus becomes much larger than an adjacent one, the vessel in the sulcus will be stretched in a curved manner, concave toward the tumor. When there is considerable edema in the vicinity of a tumor, several adjacent arteries may be affected. Extensive edema causes a more generalized straightening and stretching, more arteries being affected.

Stretching also occurs as a result of ventricular enlargement. In children, in whom widening of the sutures can occur, the convolutions carrying the vessels are actually stretched over the enlarged ventricles.

The deeper an artery is situated in the sulcus, the more it can become bowed if a tumor develops. The deformed sulci may be clearly outlined in the late arterial and intermediate phases of the angiogram. Veins are not straightened and stretched (or bowed) to the same degree that arteries become deformed. The veins are more superficially situated on the surface. On the other hand, the veins originating on the convexity and coursing toward the superior longitudinal sinus not infrequently have their normal rostral concavity straightened or reversed as the result of a high convexity or parasagittal tumor.

CHANGES IN CIRCULATION TIME.—Increased intracranial pressure causes a generalized lengthening or slowing of the circulation time. There may also be a local slowing of the circulation time in the presence of tumors. The arteries in the region of the mass may fill slower than elsewhere, with a corresponding slowness of filling of the veins. Such alterations occur most often with frontal and supra-Sylvian tumors. Edema contributes to increased circulation time through elevation of intracranial pressure, both general and local. The tumor itself often compresses veins so that filling of the larger veins may be through collateral vessels, thus delaying the time of appearance of contrast material in the larger surface vessels. In many cases there is a local change in circulation time with an increase in the speed of circulation through a malignant tumor.

TUMOR CIRCULATION.—Malignant tumors and meningiomas present a characteristic tumor vascularity in a very high percentage of cases. This neovascularity is a great aid in the localization and identification of such tumors. The characteristic features of intrinsic tumor circulation are presented in the next several parts of the Atlas in connection with glioblastomas and metastases of the cerebral hemispheres. In Part 13, the typical features of the tumor circulation of meningiomas are illustrated.

In some cases increase of tumor circulation is accomplished by enlargement of pre-existing arteries. In these cases many branches can be seen where the artery supplies the tumor; these may represent enlargement of previously inconspicuous vessels now feeding the new growth. In other instances new (innominate) arterial channels may develop to supply the tumor. Within the tumor a maze of new abnormal vessels (neovascularity) courses throughout the neoplasm. These new vessels are particularly prevalent in malignant tumors. At other times the most conspicuous part of the tumor circulation is in the capillary phase, so that a "tumor stain" appears to be present. A stain is most often seen in meningiomas, pituitary adenomas and other benign lesions. New or enlarged veins are found in the distal circulation to accommodate the increase in blood flow through a tumor.

CLASSIFICATION OF SUPRATENTORIAL TUMORS

Because of the difficulty in defining the several lobes of the brain on radiographs of the skull—and even in pneumographic and angiographic studies—we prefer to adhere to a classification that avoids the designation of "lobes." Instead, the divisions shown in Figure 61 are preferred. The groupings are related basically to the primary branches of the middle cerebral artery lying in the Sylvian fissure and under the frontal and parietal opercula.

It is difficult, even so, to avoid the term "frontal" to designate the most rostrally situated masses, although the term "pre-Sylvian" might be used. In Figure 61, the lateral sketch shows that the angiographic frontal region is only about one-half the size of the anatomic frontal lobe. This is due to the fact that only those masses situated rostral to the first vessel of the Sylvian triangle are considered to have a frontal location. On pneumography, it is difficult to avoid including in the frontal tumor group, lesions that deform the anterior horns; for this reason, tumors that lie rostral to the foramen of Monro in pneumograms are usually considered frontal tumors. This would include some tumors designated angiographically as anterior supra-Sylvian.

The frontal, or pre-Sylvian, area is usually divided into five subsections. Tumors may be designated as arising (1) at the frontal pole, (2) from the inferior frontal or subfrontal region, (3) from the lateral frontal area, (4) from the midfrontal and high frontal convexity, and (5) from the frontal parasagittal region.

The second group of supratentorial tumors includes those that arise in the portions of the frontal and parietal lobes that are projected above the opercular loops of the primary middle cerebral branches. These tumors also are projected above, or on a level with, the body of the lateral ventricle as seen in lateral view (Fig. 61). These tumors are further subdivided into the anterior supra-Sylvian group, which are ahead of the fissure of Rolando, and the posterior supra-Sylvian group situated behind the fissure.

Tumors of the posterior portion of the hemisphere are referred to as retro-Sylvian. These tumors are also situated around the atrium of the lateral ventricle and can be referred to as periatrial. They can also be called parieto-occipital. The retro-Sylvian tumors are further subdivided into three groups, the superior, posterior and inferior retro-Sylvian lesions.

Temporal tumors may be referred to as such, or they may be called infra-Sylvian. On angiography, in the lateral view, the tumors are observed below the loops forming the base of the Sylvian triangle. On pneumography, they are related to the temporal horn. This large group of lesions may be further divided into four subgroups: (1) superior infra-Sylvian or temporal tumors, (2) inferior temporal and subtemporal masses, (3) anterior infra-Sylvian lesions, and (4) medial or deep temporal tumors.

Some lesions are situated at the level of the Sylvian triangle, as observed in lateral views. If a transverse depiction of the hemisphere is considered, it is seen that such lesions may be lateral to the base of the Sylvian triangle, intra-Sylvian or within the Sylvian fissure, while others are medial (centro-Sylvian). Tumors may also arise within the lumen of a lateral ventricle; but because several of the intraventricular tumors are not commonly found elsewhere, they are considered separately.

It is customary also to designate the location of a tumor as specifically as possible, in the coronal plane, as seen in the frontal projection of the angiogram or pneumogram. Lesions in high and medial position may be of either parasagittal or high convexity origin. The former lie along the medial aspect of the brain and face on midline structures. The latter are situated predominantly on the convex surface of the hemisphere. Tumors situated more laterally over the greatest arcing portion of the convexity are classified as midconvexity. Tumors placed lower, but still above the temporal region, are referred to as low convexity tumors. Those below the base of the Sylvian triangle and in the middle fossa are termed infra-Sylvian, as already noted. Again, regarded laterally, the foramen of Monro is found to be near the center of the Sylvian triangle and in the oblique plane of the Sylvian fissure. In pneumograms, therefore, lesions above the foramen of Monro are chiefly supra-Sylvian, either central or lateral in location and may be high, mid- or low convexity or parasagittal.

The frontal lobe anatomically is the largest division of the brain and contains the highest percentage of brain tumors within its boundaries. Angiographically, however, it is not the largest division, only the pre-Sylvian area being considered frontal (Fig. 61). Many frontal tumors, especially those of the nondominant hemisphere, are very large when the patient is first seen. There is often a history of a change in personality, memory loss and other mental changes. In some cases there is a history of seizures, and with large lesions evidence of increased intracranial pressure may be found. Tumors extending posteriorly into the anterior supra-Sylvian region may lead to motor deficits, demonstrated on neurologic examination; those extending into the corpus callosum or corpus striatum may produce other symptoms and signs.

It is usually possible to make a diagnosis by angiography, which is more definitive than in many other areas because of the arterial surface coverage on both the medial and lateral aspects of the frontal lobe and its opercular surface. There is usually displacement of the Sylvian triangle postero-inferiorly, with crowding of the anterior branches. Deep extension into the basal ganglia can be detected by changes in the lenticulostriate arteries. Invasion of the corpus callosum can be appreciated by alterations in the pericallosal artery and corresponding deformities of the subependymal veins lying along the lateral ventricular wall. Cystic changes in large frontal tumors can often be detected from avascular areas and confirmed by sonography or computerized tomography. Pneumography is not ordinarily carried out in cases of frontal tumor unless prior angiography has shown that there are no significant herniations that might be aggravated by reduction of the intraventricular pressure.

Figure 57.—Downward transtentorial herniation.

A, an anterior and midhippocampal herniation is present on the left. The uncus and anterior part of the hippocampus (**a**) are ischemic from pressure. The brain stem is displaced toward the right. There is marked deformity on the left side with indentation of the peduncle (**b**), reversing its normal curve. On the right side the inferior surface of the hippocampus appears flattened (**c**) from pressure against the superior surface of the tentorium (removed). The left margin of the brain stem is white from infarction and edema. Elsewhere there are congestive changes and petechial hemorrhages. The patient had a left temporal lobe glioblastoma.

B, there is a complete herniation on the right which has surrounded that side of the mesencephalon. The brain stem is displaced to the left and is deformed by flattening against the tentorial edge (removed). The anterior part of the hippocampus (**arrow**) has indented and deformed the brain stem but there is swelling of the peduncle from infarction. Gross and petechial hemorrhages are evident in the midbrain produced by venous compression.

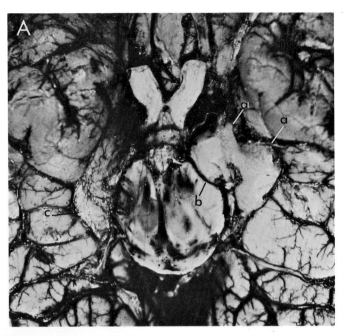

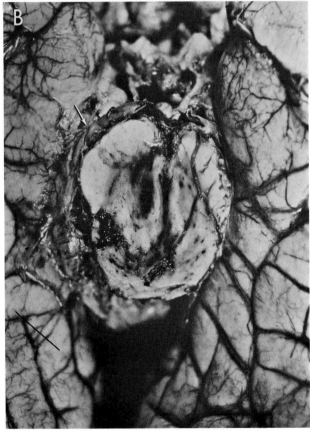

Figure 57 · Downward Transtentorial Herniation / 123

Figure 58.—Angular subfalcial herniation.

The specimen cut in coronal section illustrates how a high convexity meningioma has displaced parts of the cerebral hemisphere and produced an angular shift of the septum pellucidum (**a**) and third ventricle (**b**). There is marked contralateral dislocation of the lateral ventricles. The top of the septum pellucidum is displaced more than its inferior margin and the upper part of the third ventricle, constituting an angular shift of these normally midline structures. The left lateral ventricle is depressed and its lateral angle narrowed.

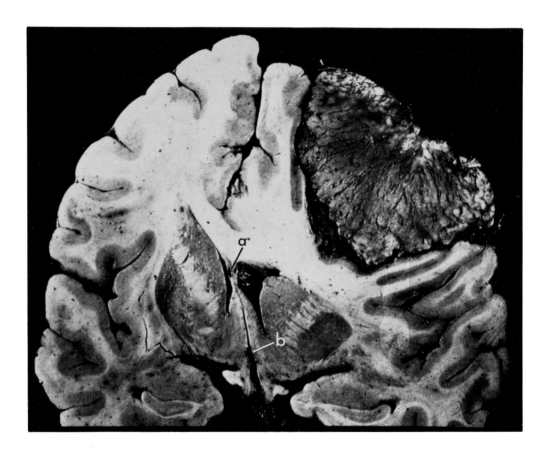

Figure 59.—Cingulate gyrus herniation.

An expanding lesion of the left cerebral hemisphere has displaced the midline and paramedian structures on the left into the right side of the cranial cavity. The cingulate gyrus (**arrows**) has become incarcerated beneath the falx (**x**) and has undergone gross swelling and infarction.

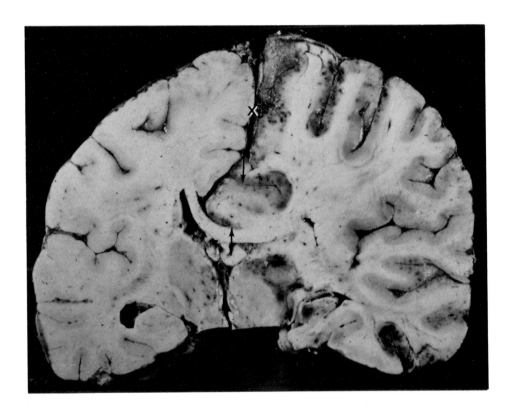

Figure 59 · Cingulate Gyrus Herniation / 125

Figure 60.—Patterns of subfalcial herniation.

A, the sites of major protrusions of the brain through openings in the skull and pachymeninges. Subfalcial herniations are manifested chiefly by shifts of the anterior cerebral artery and deep cerebral veins. The long course of the anterior cerebral artery makes it more flexible in relation to the edge of the falx than the majority of other midline structures. The variety of shifts of the anterior cerebral artery denoted on the drawing make it a sensitive indicator of the location of a tumor in the sagittal plane. The sketch also shows the sites of herniations that occur in relation to the tentorial incisura, usually with large hemispheric masses, and over the lesser sphenoid ridge with frontal or temporal masses. Herniation at the foramen magnum is dealt with elsewhere in this volume.

B, a coronal section of a pathologic specimen with a large frontal tumor illustrating a typical round shift. Because of the narrowness of the falx in the frontal region it impedes lateral movement only of the superior frontal gyrus. The large subfalcial midline plane can be freely affected by vectors from the expansion of the tumor.

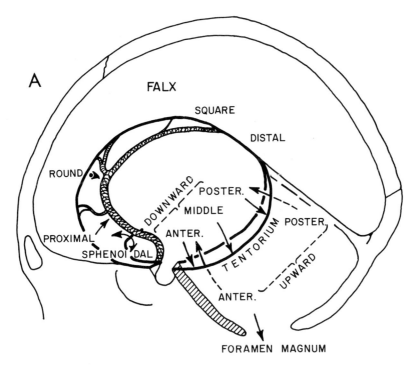

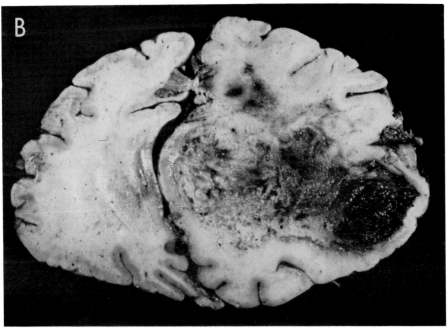

Figure 60 · Patterns of Subfalcial Herniation / 127

Figure 61.—Classification of supratentorial tumors.

A, the classification shown is based primarily on the Sylvian triangle. The base of the triangle is formed by the four or five loops of the primary branches of the middle cerebral artery under the frontal and parietal opercula. Tumors may be found anterior to, above, behind or beneath this triangular configuration.

B, lesions may also be found in the Sylvian fissure and lateral or medial to the triangle. Most of the areas designated are subdivided further as described in the text.

1, frontal; **2A,** anterior supra-Sylvian; **2B,** posterior supra-Sylvian; **3,** retro-Sylvian; **4,** infra-Sylvian; **5,** intra-Sylvian; **6,** latero-Sylvian; **7,** centro-Sylvian; **8,** intraventricular.

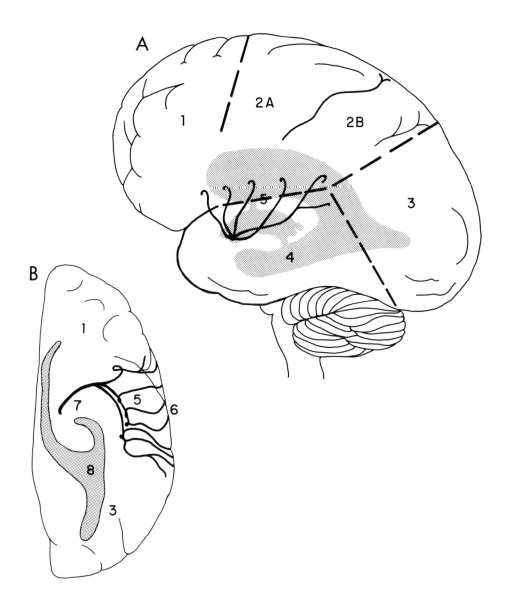

Figure 61 · Supratentorial Tumor Classification / 129

Figure 62.—Frontal pole glioblastoma.

A 54-year-old man was in good health until six months before hospitalization when he had a generalized seizure. For two months he had a change in personality and began to complain of severe headaches. Examination revealed papilledema. There was a drift of the left upper extremity with slight hyperreflexia. A Babinski reflex was found bilaterally and the jaw jerk was active. He was given high doses of dexamethasone and urea was administered on one occasion.

A, right carotid angiogram, anteroposterior projection, arterial phase: Shift of the anterior cerebral artery is evident. Its frontopolar (**a**) and anterior frontal branches (**b**) are enlarged to supply areas of neovascularity. The lenticulostriate arteries appear to be spread (**c**). The proximal insular loop of the middle cerebral artery is displaced laterally (**d**). The "U" loop of the anterior and middle cerebral arteries is greatly enlarged, and the separation of the lenticulostriate vessels suggests infiltration of the corpus striatum.

B, right carotid angiogram, lateral view, arterial phase: The carotid siphon is tightly closed. The anterior cerebral artery is displaced posteriorly and straightened. There is separation of the frontopolar (**a**), callosomarginal (**b**) and pericallosal (**c**) branches due to interposed tumor. A large area of neovascularity is apparent in the frontal pole of the brain from which an early vein (**f**) appearing in the arterial phase is seen draining into the anterior end of the superior sagittal sinus. The failure of the frontopolar branch to reach the inner table of the skull is due to an exophytic component of the tumor extending beyond the cerebral surface. Several very faintly opacified dural branches of the anterior falx artery are seen in the same region where the tumor has become parasitic upon the meninges. There is marked backward and downward displacement of the anterior part of the Sylvian triangle.

(*Continued.*)

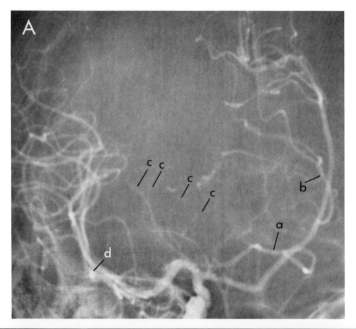

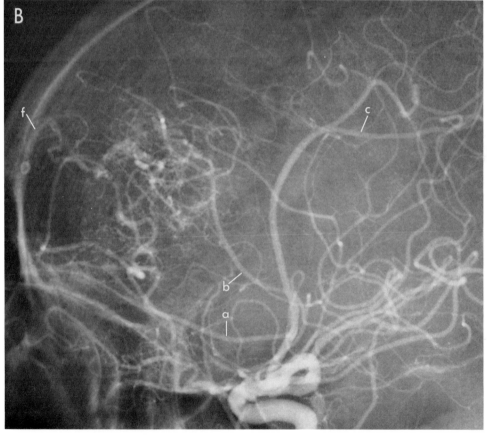

Figure 62 · Frontal Pole Glioblastoma / 131

Figure 62 (cont.).—Frontal pole glioblastoma.

C, frontal view, venous phase, same series as in **A:** The thalamostriate vein (**g**) has been largely displaced across the midline. Marked contralateral displacement of the basal vein (**h**) and internal cerebral vein (**i**) is also evident. A faint tumor stain (**x**) is evident in the mid- and medial portions of the right frontal lobe.

D, lateral view corresponding to **C:** Residual contrast material is present in the central portion of the tumor in the frontal area. There are straightening and stretching of the anterior frontal veins (**j**) and they are large. Downward transsphenoidal herniation is indicated by backward and downward displacement of the middle cerebral vein (**k**) which is draining superficially into the vein of Labbé (**l**). The uncal vein (**m**) is also displaced backward and downward. The anterior part of the internal cerebral vein and the venous angle are displaced backward so that the internal cerebral vein (**i**) is foreshortened and humped. The subependymal veins of the anterior horn are enlarged, buckled and displaced backward, acting as outflow tracts from the hypervascular tumor bed to the internal cerebral vein. Since the subependymal veins do not reach the same height as the anterior part of the pericallosal artery, extension of the tumor into the corpus callosum is suggested. **x,** tumor stain.

A right frontal lobectomy was performed, with decompression. The patient then received radiation therapy but did poorly and died five months after the first examination.

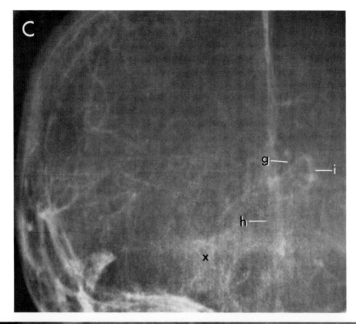

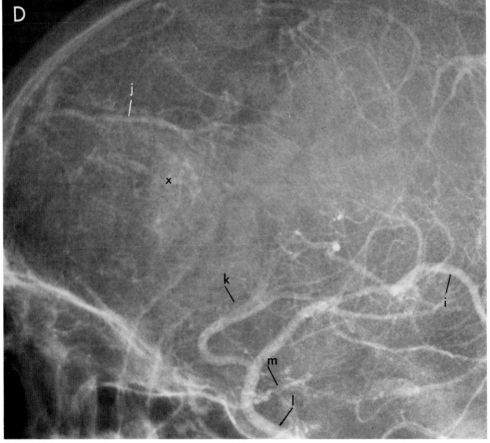

Figure 62 · Frontal Pole Glioblastoma / 133

Figure 63.—Mixed oligodendroglioma-astrocytoma of left frontal lobe with extension into basal ganglia and an exophytic component on the medial surface of the frontal pole.

A 40-year-old man had had a seizure two years previously, at which time results of a neurologic examination were within normal limits. When seen by us he complained of increasing bitemporal headache for several weeks. The only abnormality found on examination was a suggestion of papilledema.

A, left carotid angiogram, anteroposterior projection, arterial phase: The anterior cerebral artery is shifted from left to right. The vessel in the midline is an anterior falx artery (**a**) arising from the ophthalmic artery. Stretching of the frontopolar (**b**) and anterior frontal (**c**) branches of the parasagittal area is seen. The lenticulostriate arteries (**d**) are displaced medially, and the anterior insular branches of the middle cerebral artery (**e**) are displaced laterally. The tumor must have extended into the lateral basal ganglia to cause this displacement.

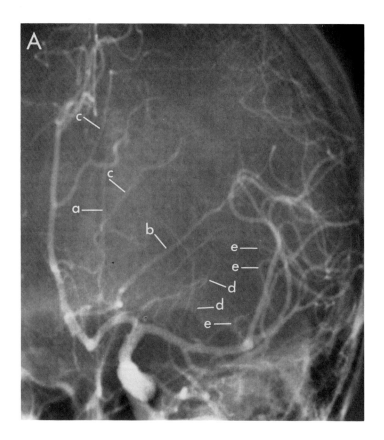

B, left carotid angiogram, lateral view, arterial phase: The first branch of the Sylvian triangle (**e**) is displaced downward and posteriorly. The orbito-frontal branch of the middle cerebral artery (**f**) becomes stretched as it approaches the convexity of the frontal pole. The frontopolar artery (**b**) and anterior frontal (**c**) branches of the callosomarginal artery are stretched and displaced away from the inner table because the tumor (**x**) is exophytic on the medial surface of the brain. The tumor is deriving some of its blood supply from the dura, as evident from the enlargement of the anterior falx artery (**a**). In addition, numerous pools of contrast material are seen within necrotic areas of the tumor supplied by the callosomarginal branches.

(Continued.)

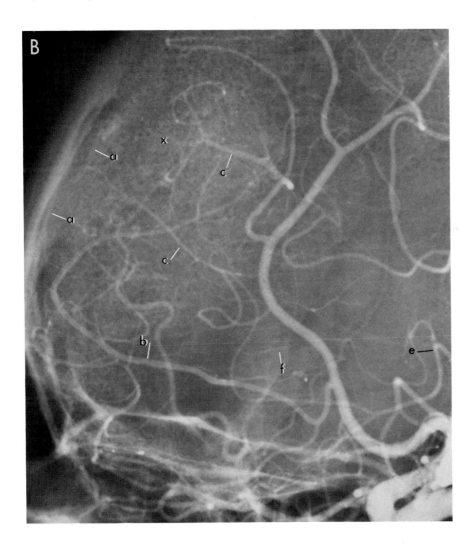

Figure 63 · Mixed Oligodendroglioma-Astrocytoma / 135

Figure 63 (cont.).—Mixed oligodendroglioma-astrocytoma of the left frontal lobe with extension into the basal ganglia and an exophytic component on the medial surface of the frontal pole.

C, left carotid angiogram, frontal view, venous phase: A faint stain is seen in the high convexity region of the frontal pole. The thalamostriate vein (**g**) is displaced downward and is enlarged as it is draining the deep portions of the tumor. The uncal vein is displaced medially (**h**).

D, lateral view made simultaneously with **C:** There is a faint stain (**x**) in the region of the frontal pole and several convexity veins surround the tumor. Transphenoidal herniation is evident from downward displacement of both the middle cerebral (**i**) and uncal veins (**h**).

Operation revealed an exophytic tumor containing a few small cystic and necrotic areas. It became rubbery in consistency and blended into normal brain in the deep regions of the frontal lobe. A partial frontal lobectomy was performed with subtotal removal of the tumor. Radiotherapy followed.

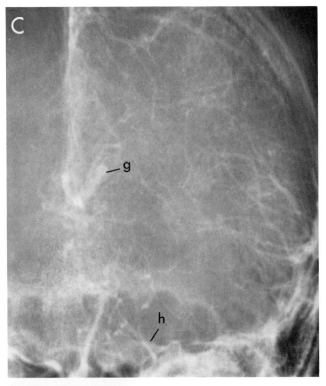

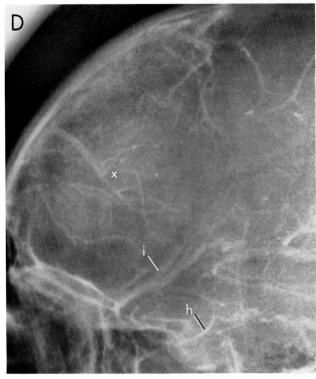

Figure 63 · Mixed Oligodendroglioma-Astrocytoma / 137

Figure 64.—Left frontotemporal glioblastoma with deep extension.

A 60-year-old man had a two-month history of right-sided focal seizures, aphasia, memory defect and headache. One week before hospitalization he became ataxic. Examination revealed bilateral papilledema, right central facial weakness, hyperreflexia on the right side and a right Babinski reflex.

A, left carotid angiogram with cross-compression, frontal view in standard anteroposterior projection, arterial phase: The supraclinoid portion of the internal carotid artery is displaced medially and downward. The ascending anterior cerebral artery exhibits a marked round shift. The lenticulostriate arteries (**a**) are displaced medially and in addition are separated as the tumor has infiltrated the medial aspects of the basal ganglia. The genu of the middle

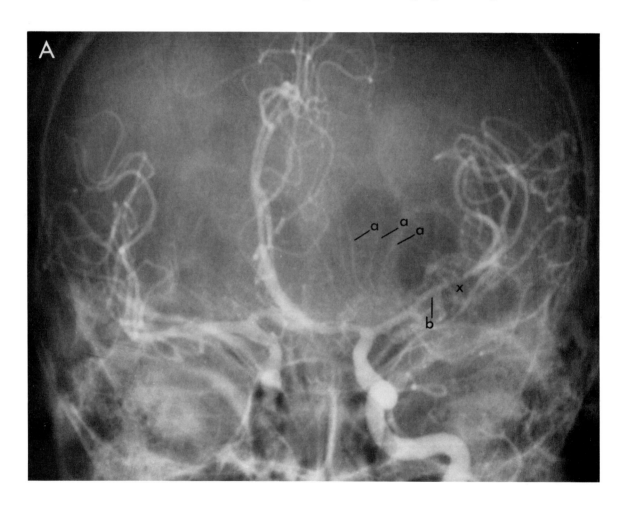

cerebral artery (**b**) is elevated and displaced medially. Areas of neovascularity (**x**) are seen in the region of the anterior aspect of the insula. This malignant lesion not only has caused separation and elevation of the loops of the middle cerebral artery in the anterior aspect of the insula but has bridged across the Sylvian fissure to extend into the temporal operculum inferiorly and into the frontal lobe adjacent to the lateral aspect of the floor of the anterior fossa. It is unusual, except for malignant gliomas, to traverse large cisterns, this property usually being reserved for benign extra-axial masses.

B, left carotid angiogram without cross-compression, lateral view, arterial phase: The siphon is opened and stretched. Displacements of the vessels seen in the frontal view are reproduced and the center of the tumor vascularity is evident (**x**).

(Continued.)

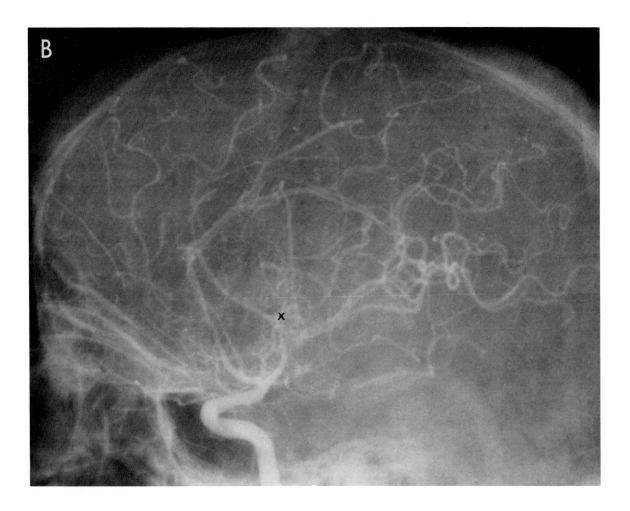

Figure 64 · **Frontotemporal Glioblastoma** / **139**

Figure 64 (cont.).—Left frontotemporal glioblastoma with deep extension.

C, left carotid angiogram with cross-compression, same frontal projection as **A,** later arterial phase: Several early veins drain the area of tumor involvement both deeply and superficially, including the basal vein (**c**), which is displaced medially, indicating impending tentorial herniation.

D, left carotid angiogram without cross-compression, lateral view, late arterial phase: The basal vein of Rosenthal (**c**) provides a course of drainage from the region of the anterior perforated substance where the tumor (**x**) has involved the basal ganglia. It is displaced downward. More superficially, the vein of Labbé (**d**) is seen to fill early.

(Continued.)

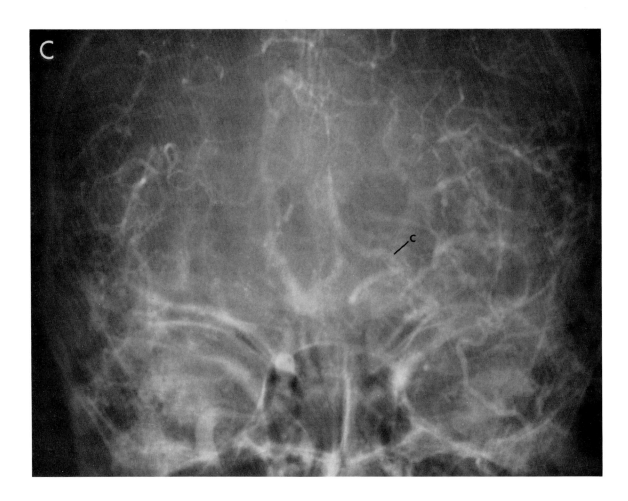

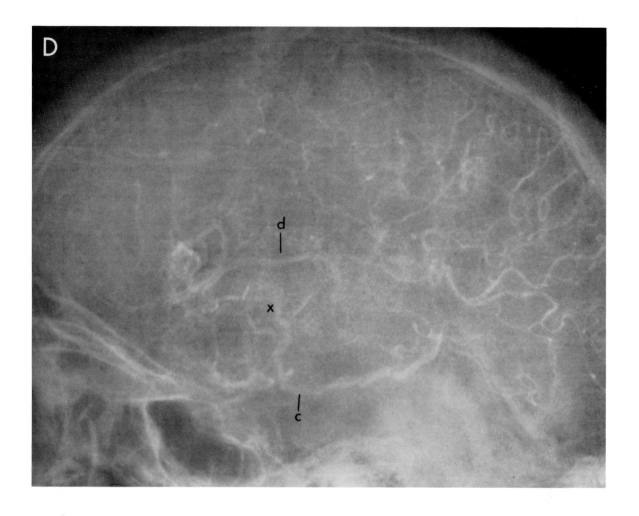

Figure 64 · Frontotemporal Glioblastoma / 141

Figure 64 (cont.).—Left frontotemporal glioblastoma with deep extension.

E, serialographic continuation from **A,** frontal view, venous phase: The internal cerebral vein (**e**) is markedly shifted from left to right to practically the same degree as the subfalcial herniation of the anterior cerebral artery.

F, lateral view corresponding to **E:** The internal cerebral vein is humped (**e**). This is secondary to the marked distortion caused by the large shift, as well as the large mass effect of the deep frontal tumor.

The patient, considered to have a glioblastoma, developed signs of downward transtentorial herniation and was judged a poor candidate for intracranial exploration. Radiation therapy was begun, but he survived only the first week of therapy.

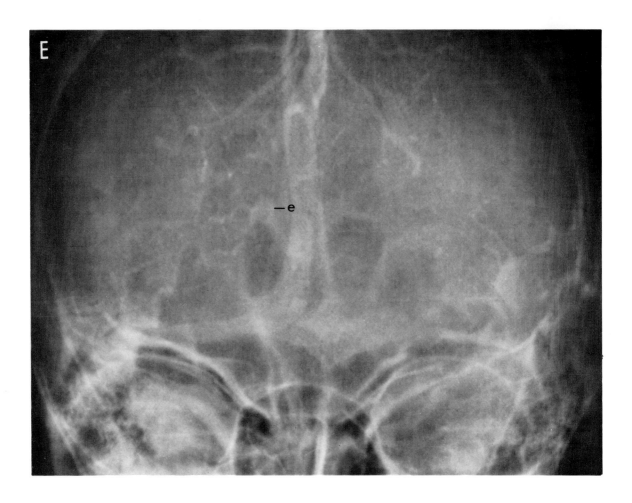

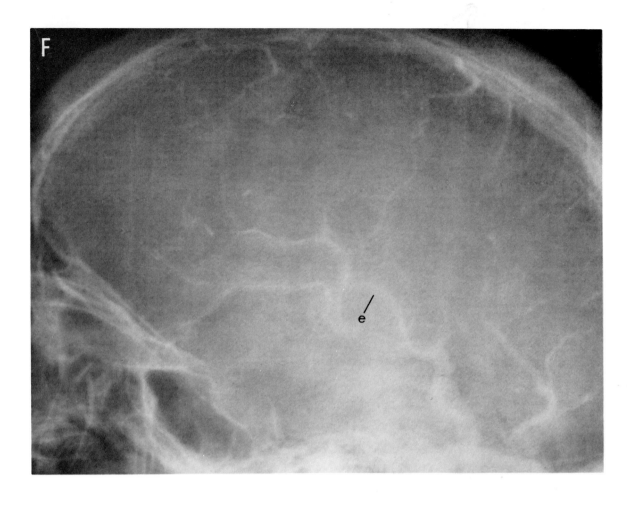

Figure 64 · Frontotemporal Glioblastoma / 143

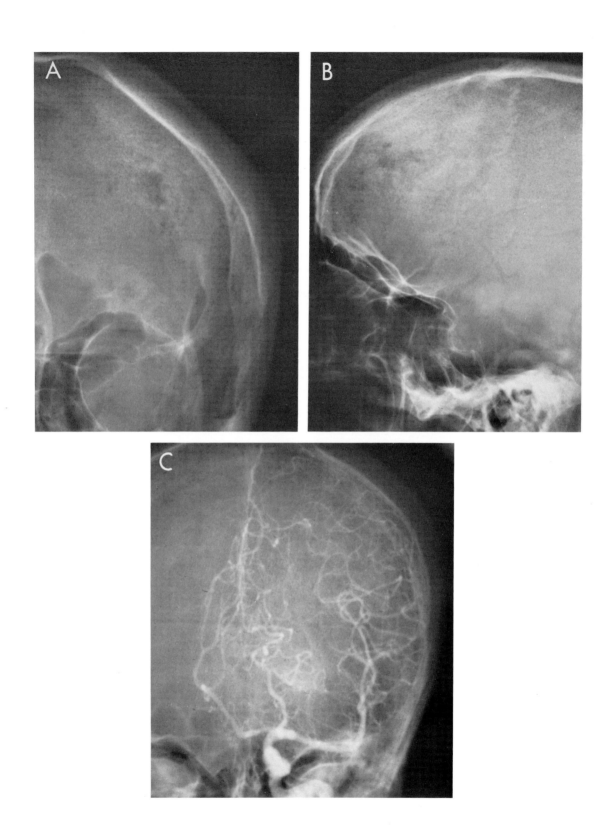

Figure 65.—Malignant lymphoma involving skull, meninges and brain.

A 51-year-old woman had a local swelling of the left forehead and was said to have suffered periods of mental confusion for several months. During the month before admission she became forgetful and complained of severe headache.

A, exposure in Caldwell projection: Sclerosis of the vertical portion of the frontal bone above the orbit is demonstrated with an irregular radiolucency below it.

B, lateral projection: This reveals changes similar to those seen in **A,** with no increased vascularity. The sella turcica exhibits atrophy due to increased intracranial pressure.

C, left carotid angiogram, frontal projection, arterial phase: The round shift of the anterior cerebral artery is characteristic of frontal lesions.

D, lateral projection corresponding to **C:** The carotid siphon is closed. The sweep of the anterior cerebral artery is blunted and the caliosomarginal artery is displaced backward with separation of branches extending into the frontal region adjacent to the bony change (**arrows**). There is striking posterior displacement of the anterior opercular branches of the middle cerebral artery with depression and crowding of the anterior aspect of the Sylvian triangle.

(*Continued.*)

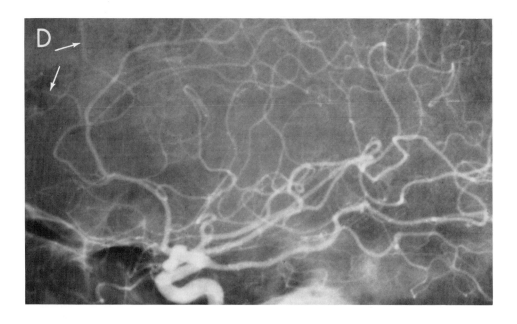

Figure 65 · Malignant Lymphoma / 145

Figure 65 (cont.).—Malignant lymphoma involving skull, meninges and brain.

E, left carotid angiogram, lateral view, intermediate phase: A faint irregularly shaped stain is evident in the anterior fossa behind the bone changes (**x**).

F, venous phase continued from **E:** A large frontal avascular area due to compression of surface veins with delayed filling is evident. The venous angle is displaced backward (**arrow**), and there is humping of the internal cerebral vein.

A craniectomy was performed with removal of the affected bone, which histologic examination disclosed to be involved by Hodgkin's disease. The adjacent meninges were infiltrated as well as the left frontal lobe, and only partial removal could be accomplished. The patient received radiation therapy and was doing well one year later, still with no evidence of generalized lymphoma.

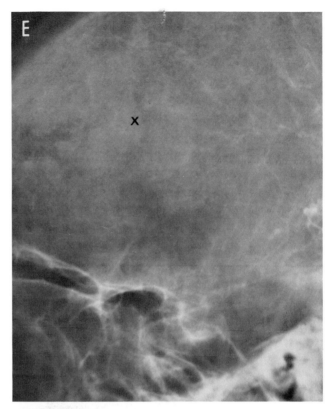

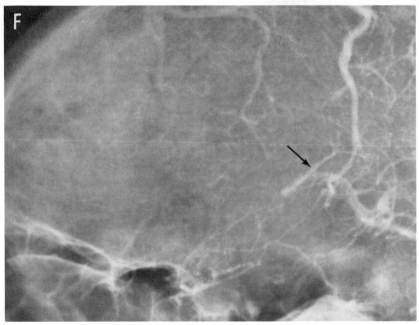

Figure 65 · Malignant Lymphoma / 147

PART 5

The Supra-Sylvian Region

Radiographic Tumor Picture

THE ANGIOGRAPHIC SUPRA-SYLVIAN group contains the largest number of tumors since it includes the posterior part of the anatomic frontal lobe. It is divided into anterior and posterior portions that conform to the posterior frontal and anterior parietal regions respectively. Localization in the coronal plane is similar to the frontal area—parasagittal and high, mid- and low convexity.

The pneumographic change most often seen is a flattening of the lateral ventricular roof. With midconvexity tumors the roof is directly compressed downward and with low convexity tumors is compressed in an upward direction. The septum pellucidum and third ventricle are displaced and angulated by the higher tumors, with the greatest angulation occurring in the most superior portion of the structures. With the deep tumors, particularly with thalamic involvement, there is significant deformity of the third ventricle.

Angiographic changes in the Sylvian triangle are classically depressions of its roof loops. Local mass effects on the surface vessels of the anterior and middle cerebral arteries help to localize the tumor in coronal plane. If these local changes are not evident, the position of the insular loops in the frontal view will help to localize the mass. If the loops are displaced medially, the mass is low convexity. If the loops are displaced laterally, the mass is high convexity, parasagittal or interhemispheric. If the loops are only depressed without side-to-side displacement, the mass is usually midconvexity. Corpus callosum involvement causes the discrepancy between the positions of the pericallosal artery and the subependymal veins described earlier. Involvement of basal ganglia causes changes in the lenticulostriate arteries similar to those described for the frontal tumors. With supra-Sylvian lesions, however, the changes involve the more peripheral medial and lateral curvatures of the arteries. Local changes of the cortical veins may be confusing in the lateral view because the medial and convexity veins are superimposed. Generally, however, the medial veins can be distinguished because of their shorter and straighter course.

Figure 66.—Anterior supra-Sylvian parasagittal glioblastoma extending into the corpus callosum.

A 67-year-old man had a four-month history of transient difficulty in balance. Three months prior to admission he noted weakness in the right upper and lower extremities. Three days before hospitalization he had a seizure followed by paresis of the right leg. Examination revealed a mild memory deficit and complete hemiparesis with a Babinski reflex on the right.

A, left carotid angiogram, frontal view, arterial phase: The anterior cerebral artery is shifted to the right. There is mild lateral displacement of the

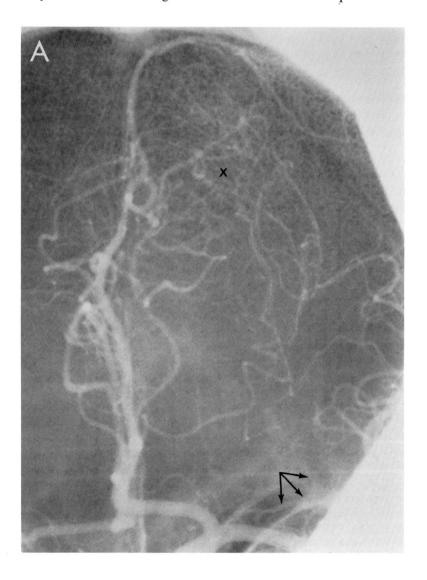

lenticulostriate vessels (**arrows**). Marked stretching and slight enlargement of the posterior frontal branch of the anterior cerebral artery is present, and numerous fine tumor vessels (**x**) occupy the parasagittal region.

B, lateral view made simultaneously with **A:** The pericallosal artery is taut and not depressed. The posterior frontal and parietal branches of the anterior cerebral artery give rise to numerous neovascular areas (**x**). The parietal branch ascending the interhemispheric area reveals encasement by tumor (**arrows**).

(Continued.)

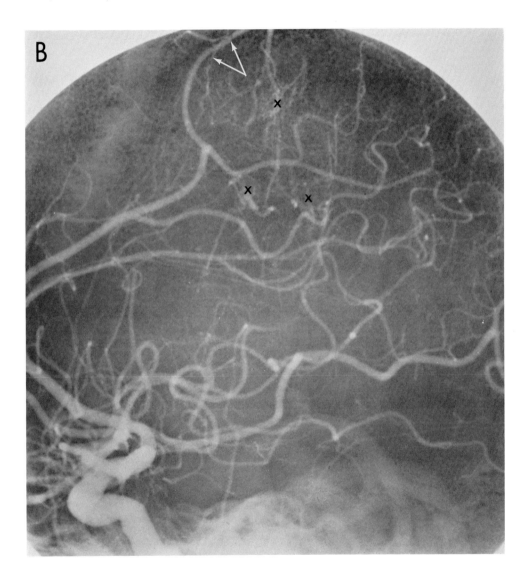

Figure 66 · Glioblastoma / 153

Figure 66 (cont.).—Anterior supra-Sylvian parasagittal glioblastoma extending into the corpus callosum.

C, lateral view, early venous phase, sequent to **B**: Local stretching and thinning of several posterior frontoparietal veins are seen (**a**). Numerous small and two large tortuous medullary veins (**b**) drain into the thalamostriate vein, which is depressed. The internal cerebral vein is also conspicuously flattened.

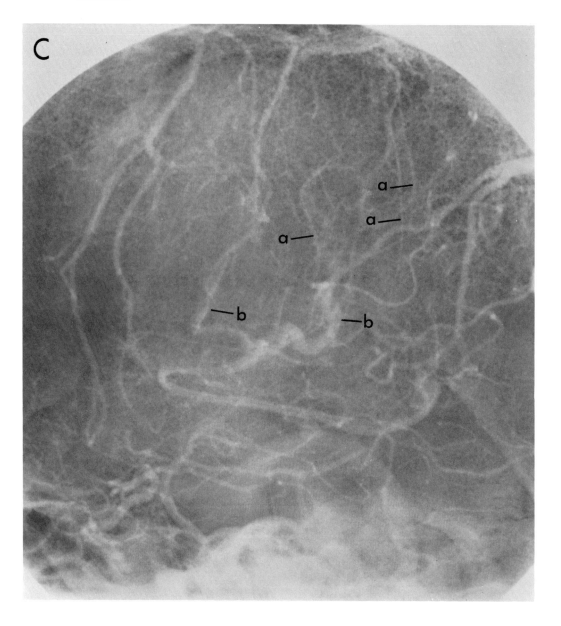

D, lateral view, late venous phase, succeeding **C:** The subependymal veins (**arrows**) outline the flattened roof of the anterior horn and body of the lateral ventricle. This depression of the ventricular roof without corresponding deformity of the pericallosal artery indicates invasion of the corpus callosum. The lack of more midline shift in **A** also suggests spread to the right hemisphere through the corpus callosum.

At craniotomy, deep involvement by the tumor was verified and a biopsy specimen was taken. The patient was discharged to a chronic care facility.

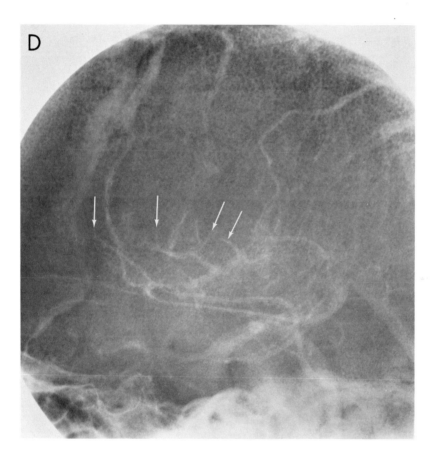

Figure 66 · Glioblastoma / 155

Figure 67.—Supra-Sylvian high convexity astrocytoma.

A 48-year-old woman had a six-year history of seizures. Recently there had been bifrontal headache. Examination revealed an outward drift of the right upper extremity and twitching of the fingers. Deep reflexes were more brisk on the right side than on the left and there was a Hoffmann sign.

A, left carotid angiogram with right carotid compression, anteroposterior projection, arterial phase: There is a shift of the anterior cerebral artery from left to right. Slight medial displacement of the anterior choroidal artery is evident (**a**). There is definite asymmetry of the Sylvian points (**b**), the left being lower than the right.

B, left carotid angiogram without cross-compression, lateral view, arterial

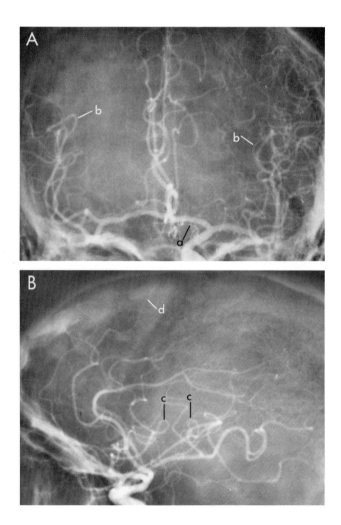

phase: The siphon is closed. There is depression of the roof of the Sylvian triangle (**c**) with straightening of a callosomarginal branch (**d**) in the midfrontal area on the interhemispheric surface.

C, frontal view, venous phase, sequent to **A:** The internal cerebral vein is not displaced. However, there is progressive displacement of the septal vein (**e**) as it courses anteriorly around the frontal horn.

D, lateral view, late venous phase: There is slight foreshortening of the internal cerebral vein. The septal vein is displaced downward (**e**), as is also the anterior caudate vein (**f**). These displacements are due to compression and forcing downward of the frontal horn of the lateral ventricle.

At operation, a hard rubbery tumor was found occupying a large portion of the frontal lobe. A subtotal removal was effected. The patient received radiotherapy.

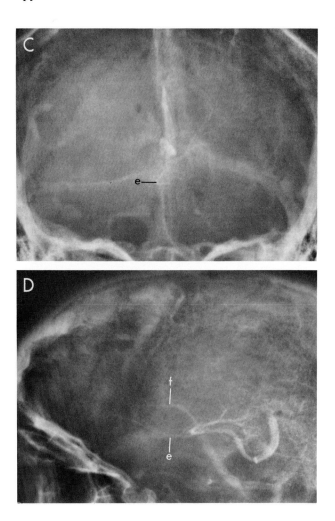

Figure 67 · Astrocytoma / 157

Figure 68.—Posterior supra-Sylvian astrocytoma.

A 59-year-old man had a three-month history of focal left upper extremity seizures as well as numbness and loss of dexterity in the left hand. Examination revealed left central facial paresis and mild weakness of the muscles of the left arm and hand. The EEG and radioactive isotope brain scan were normal.

A, right carotid angiogram with cross-compression, anteroposterior frontal view, arterial phase: There is no midline shift. There is mild but definite asymmetry of the positions of the two Sylvian points (**a**), the right being slightly lower than the left.

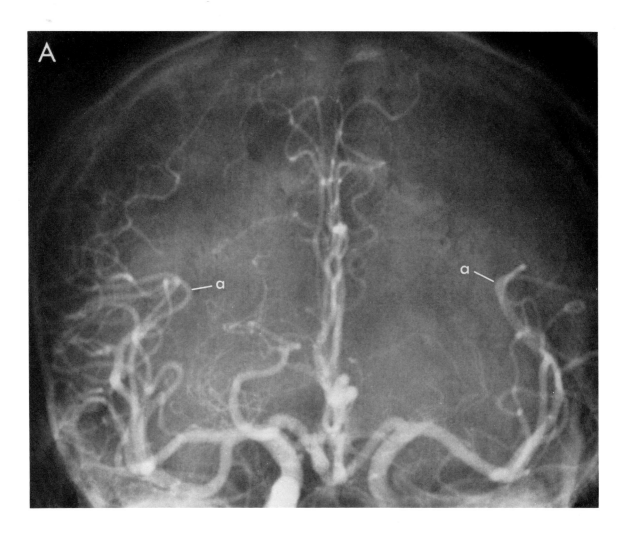

B, right carotid angiogram without cross-compression, lateral view, arterial phase: The most posterior portion of the base of the Sylvian triangle is displaced downward (**b**). As the branches of the middle cerebral artery reach the high convexity area, a mass effect is seen (**x**). A terminal branch of the large callosomarginal vessel changes abruptly to a taut arc (**c**). The increased density seen in this area of vascular change is secondary to calcification within the tumor, better shown in **F**.

(Continued.)

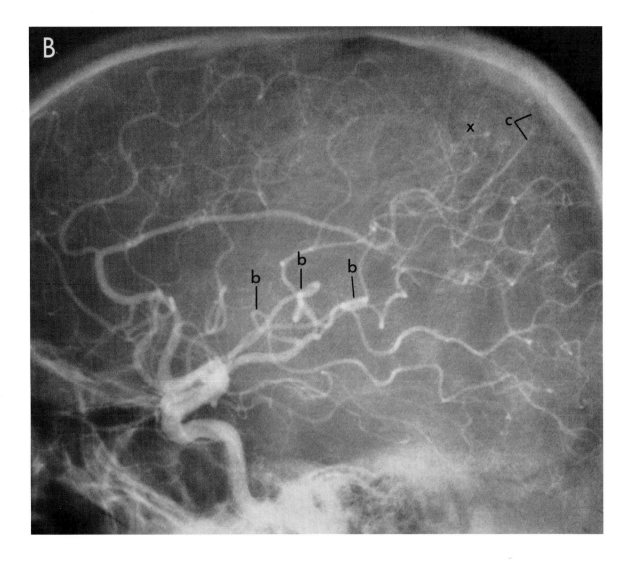

Figure 68 · Astrocytoma / 159

Figure 68 (cont.).—Posterior supra-Sylvian astrocytoma.

C, frontal view, venous phase, sequent to **A:** Note the slightly lower position of the subependymal veins on the superolateral corner of the right lateral ventricle (**d**) as compared with the left.

D, lateral view, venous phase, succeeding **B:** Very slight flattening of the posterior portion of the right lateral ventricle is outlined by the subependymal veins (**e**). Slight local mass effect (**x**) is seen in the region of the tumor calcification.

(Continued.)

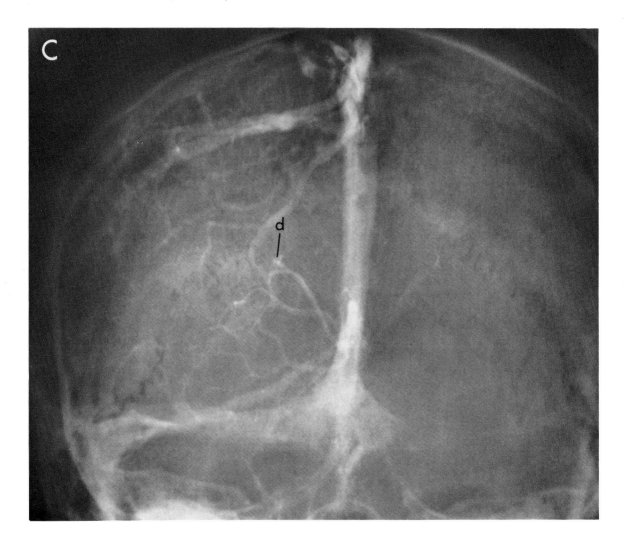

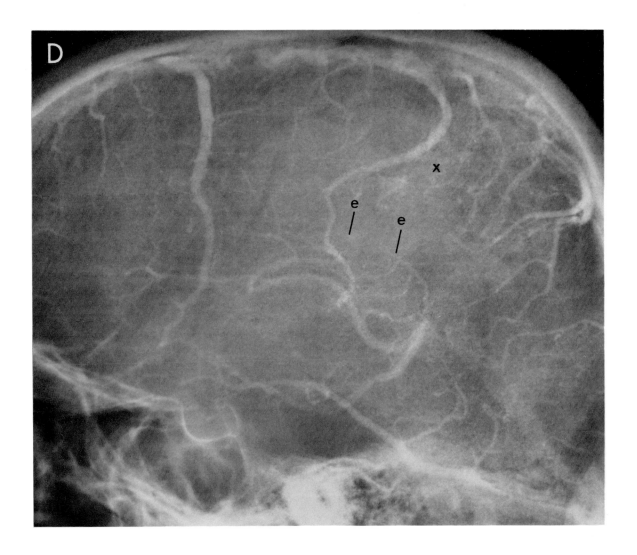

Figure 68 · Astrocytoma / 161

Figure 68 (cont.).—Posterior supra-Sylvian astrocytoma.

E, pneumoencephalogram after replacement of 30 cc of cerebrospinal fluid by gas, brow-down position, frontal tomogram through the bodies of the lateral ventricles: The pericallosal cistern (**f**) is tilted down on the right and the roof of the ventricle is lower. Calcification is faintly visible in the tumor in the high convexity region (**g**). The third ventricle, septum pellucidum and interhemispheric air (posterior to the lesion) do not appear to be displaced.

F, lateral view, corresponding to **E:** Slight downward displacement of the roof of the body of the lateral ventricle is evident.

Operation disclosed the tumor on the surface in the precentral gyrus in the arm area and extending both anteriorly and posteriorly. A small amount of tumor was removed for pathologic examination. The patient underwent radiation therapy postoperatively and was well when last seen two years later.

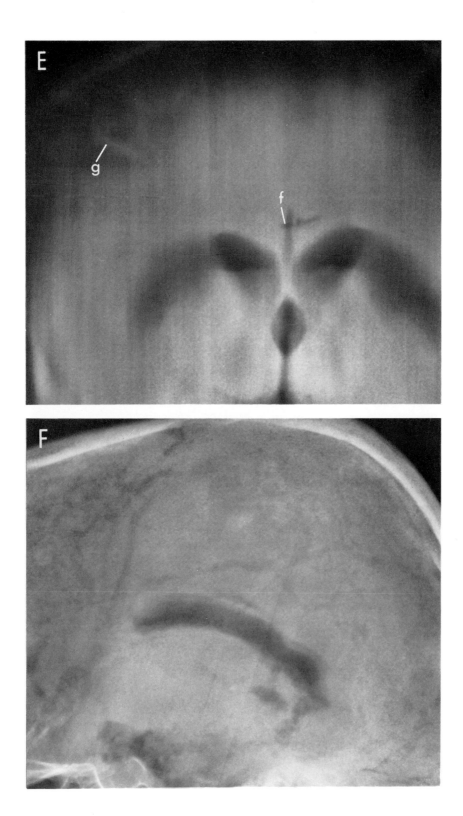

Figure 68 · Astrocytoma / 163

Figure 69.—Malignant tumor of the posterior supra-Sylvian opercular region extending into the ventricular atrium and splenium of the corpus callosum.

A 69-year-old man experienced rapid progression of expressive aphasia and loss of memory for four weeks. There was diminished sensation in the right hand. Examination revealed right hemiparesis with decrease of pain, temperature and position sense in the right upper extremity.

A, left carotid angiogram with cross-compression, frontal view, arterial phase: The anterior cerebral artery is shifted from left to right in its distal ascending portion. The lenticulostriate vessels on the left are displaced medially, straightened and separated in their posterior portions (**a**). The insular

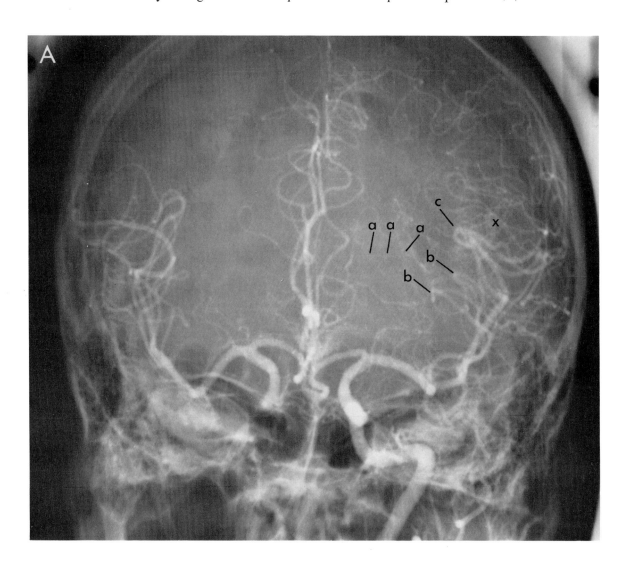

loops of the left middle cerebral artery (**b**) are displaced medially in the region of the Sylvian point (**c**). Nearby is a faint tumor stain (**x**).

B, lateral view corresponding to **A:** There are stretching and separation of the opercular and low convexity branches (**d**) of the middle cerebral artery involving mainly the posterior supra-Sylvian region. Neovascularity (**x**) is seen through the separated branches. The pericallosal artery in its distal portion (**e**) is stretched and elevated as the tumor extends medially into the splenium of the corpus callosum.

(*Continued.*)

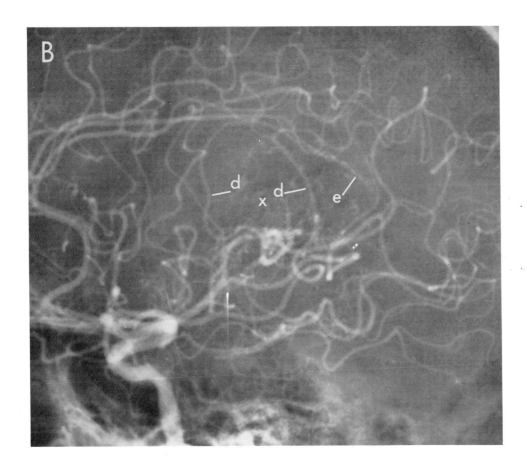

Figure 69 · **Malignant Tumor with Extension** / **165**

Figure 69 (cont.).—Malignant tumor of the posterior supra-Sylvian opercular region extending into the ventricular atrium and splenium of the corpus callosum.

C, venous phase sequent to **A:** The tumor stain (**x**) in the region of the atrium is draining via an atrial vein (**f**) into the internal cerebral vein. The internal cerebral vein is only slightly displaced to the right because of fixation by the involved splenium of the corpus callosum.

D, lateral view matching **C:** Tortuous neovascularity drains into the atrial vein (**f**). There is widening of the curve of the vein of Galen and distal internal cerebral vein (**g**), indicating involvement of the corpus callosum in the splenial region. A low convexity posterior frontal cortical vein, tributary to the middle cerebral vein, is deformed by the tumor (**y**).

Because of the deep parietal location in the dominant hemisphere, and in the absence of increased intracranial pressure, neurosurgical decompression was thought inadvisable and radiotherapy was given. The patient did poorly and died seven months after the first admission.

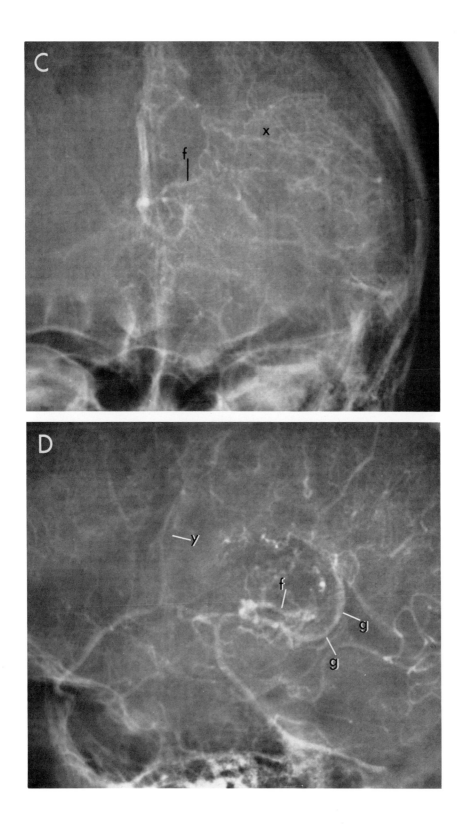

Figure 69 · Malignant Tumor with Extension / 167

Figure 70.—Posterior supra-Sylvian astrocytoma with extension into the basal ganglia.

A 46-year-old woman had a one-year history of progressive headache associated with blurred vision. On examination her affect was flat. There was a slightly decreased left arm swing, and increased reflexes were noted on the left. (See Figs. 10 and 15 for this patient's routine roentgenograms).

A, carotid angiogram, frontal projection, arterial phase: The posterior portion of the pericallosal artery is being shifted from right to left. A local mass effect has displaced the anterior choroidal artery (**a**) and posterior communicating artery (**b**) downward and laterally. Tumor extension into the anterior portion of the tentorial hiatus is greater on the right side than on

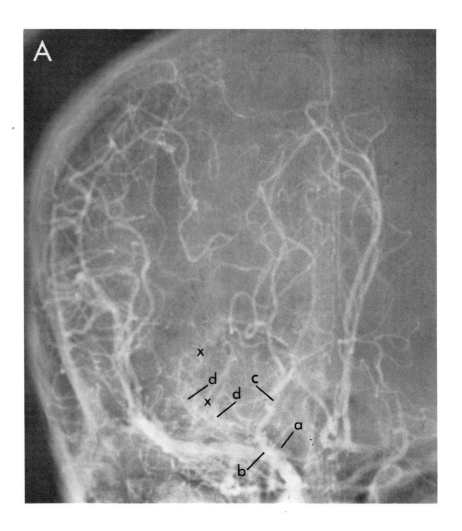

the left as demonstrated by the lower position of the right posterior cerebral artery (**c**). The lenticulostriate arteries (**d**) are displaced laterally and a small tumor stain (**x**) arises from these vessels.

B, lateral view corresponding to **A:** The Sylvian triangle is depressed, and major arteries coursing over the medial surfaces show the mass effects of herniation and separation (**arrows**).

(Continued.)

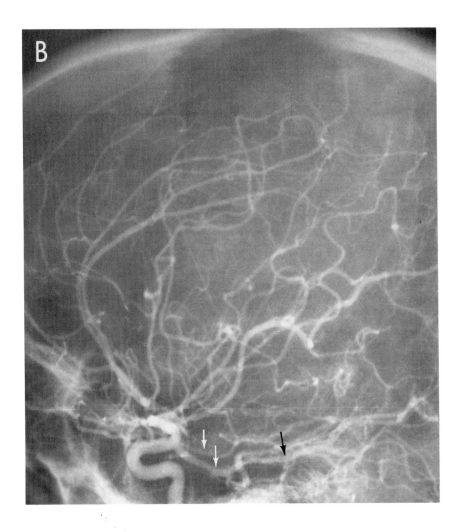

Figure 70 · Astrocytoma / 169

Figure 70.—Posterior supra-Sylvian astrocytoma with extension into the basal ganglia.

C, late arterial phase succeeding **A:** Early filling of a convexity vein (**e**) and the internal cerebral vein (**f**) is clearly seen.

D, lateral projection conforming to **C:** The large vein (**e**) on the convexity and the internal cerebral vein (**f**) seen in **C** are again delineated.

(*Continued.*)

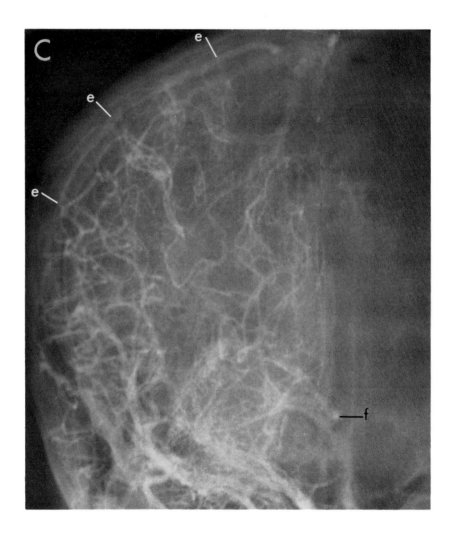

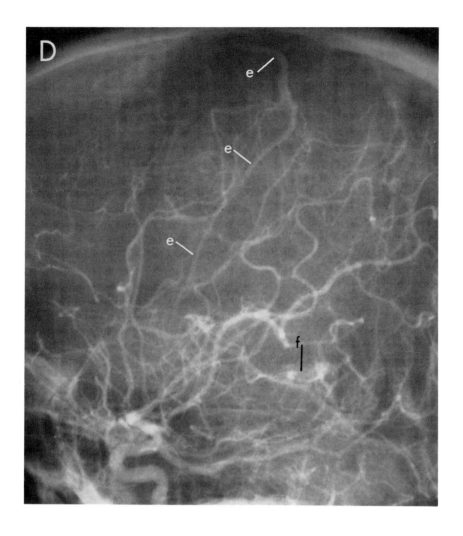

Figure 70 · Astrocytoma / 171

Figure 70 (cont.).—Posterior supra-Sylvian astrocytoma with extension into the basal ganglia.

E, right carotid angiogram, frontal view, venous phase: Hydrocephalus is demonstrated by the course of the thalamostriate vein. There is local deformity of the two tributaries of the thalamostriate vein, particularly superiorly (**g**). The septal vein (**h**) is shifted toward the side of injection.

F, lateral venous phase, matching **E**: A local mass effect narrows the septal vein (**h**) just prior to its junction with the thalamostriate vein. These findings attest to the deep extension of the glioma which at the plane of the foramen of Monro has crossed to the opposite side and obstructed the ventricular

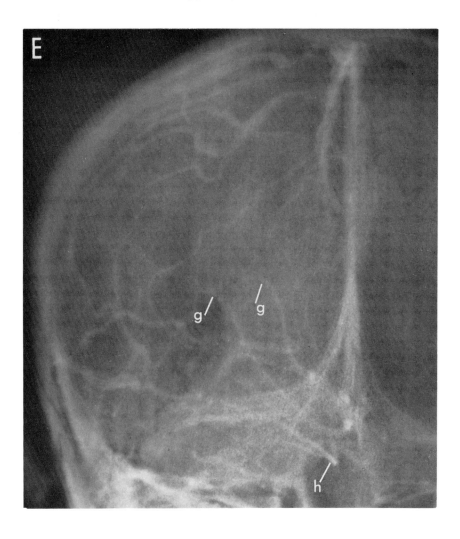

system. A mass effect deforms the convexity veins (**i**). Deformity of the two tributaries of the thalamostriate veins is again seen (**g**).

The day before a scheduled operation the patient became lethargic and because of the transtentorial herniation observed in the angiograms was taken promptly to the operating room. An extensive subcortical glioma was found extending deeply into the basal ganglia and into the motor area. A subtotal excision of the tumor was performed and internal decompression effected. The patient then received radiotherapy and chemotherapy.

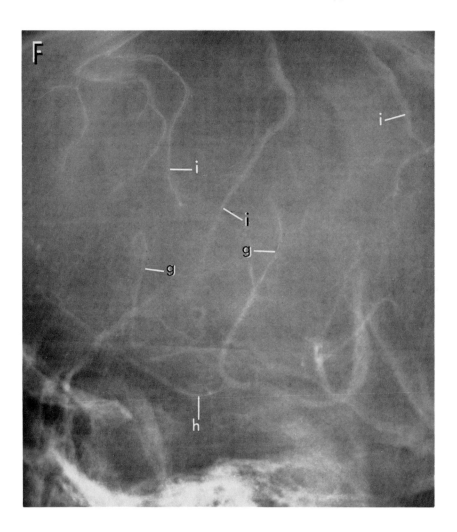

Figure 70 · Astrocytoma / 173

PART 6

The Retro-Sylvian Area

The Angiographic Picture of Tumors

RETRO-SYLVIAN MASSES are, by definition, behind the angiographic Sylvian point (see Fig. 61) and are posterior parietal, occipital or posterior temporal in location. The deeper lesions within the thalamus, splenium of the corpus callosum and other paraventricular areas are dealt with separately in Part 8. Some of the difficulty encountered in diagnosing the precise location of these lesions develops because filling of the posterior cerebral artery is not constantly accomplished by carotid angiography. Lesions involving the medial and inferior aspects of the hemisphere in the retro-Sylvian area will not produce an appreciable local mass effect on the small terminal anterior cerebral artery branches or the more laterally located posterior parietal, angular or posterior temporal branches of the middle cerebral artery. In the diagnosis of extracerebral or exophytic masses it is easy to see displacement away from the falx medially in the frontal views or the occipital pole forward in the lateral views whenever the posterior cerebral artery is filled. The more laterally located masses, even with the posterior cerebral artery delineated, are not seen in profile in the standard views and may require oblique projections, base projections or other tailored views because of the curvature of the skull posteriorly. Opacification of the vertebral-basilar system is usually required in addition to carotid angiography, and this is being done more routinely through retrograde femoral catheterization.

Appreciation of venous changes of the retro-Sylvian group of lesions is difficult because of the normal paucity of veins in the occipital pole in the region 5-6 cm superior to the torcula. Changes in the cortical veins are otherwise similar to those elsewhere. It should be remembered that in the occipital pole, as in the frontal pole, the veins course horizontally in order to maintain a more or less perpendicular orientation to the superior sagittal sinus. In immediate proximity to the sinus the veins normally turn in a countercurrent direction to the sinus.

There are two interesting aspects of the distant effects of these masses. One is the relative lack of shift of the anterior cerebral artery from the midline. Because of the protection of the wide falx posteriorly, and because the lesions are at such a distance from the flexible portions of both the internal cerebral vein and the anterior cerebral artery, there appears to be a relative lack of shift. A distal step of the artery is the most characteristic finding. Second, larger lesions can cause a paradoxical frontal component of anterior cerebral artery shift. This develops because very large tumors can produce forward trans-sphenoidal herniation of the temporal pole; the herniation is in the plane of the anterior portion of the anterior cerebral artery.

Figure 71.—Posterior retro-Sylvian tumor.

A 54-year-old man had difficulty in seeing to the right for three months. More recently he realized that he had difficulty in concentrating. He was found to have early papilledema, right central facial paresis, right homonymous hemianopia and difficulty in reading and calculating. He was mildly anemic. An abnormal density was seen in the left lung on a chest radiograph. Bronchoscopy provided no evidence of a lesion.

A, right brachial angiogram, anteroposterior projection with vertebral angulation, arterial phase: There is good filling of the left posterior cerebral artery, which is larger than the right. The internal occipital (**a**) and posterior inferior temporal (**b**) branches give off many tumor vessels. Even in the early arterial phase a number of draining veins were demonstrated.

B, right brachial angiogram, lateral view, arterial phase: The vascular tumor is shown well with early draining veins (**c**) denoting a malignant neoplasm.

At craniotomy, a highly vascular tumor was removed from the left occipital region. Pathologic examination revealed a tumor of squamous cell type, consistent with bronchogenic origin. Steroid therapy was begun, and 4000 rads were administered to the lung and the occipital area. The patient did well for six months, then had recurring headache and mental confusion. A radioactive isotope brain scan disclosed recurrence of the left occipital lesion and another metastasis in the left frontal region. He died one year after operation.

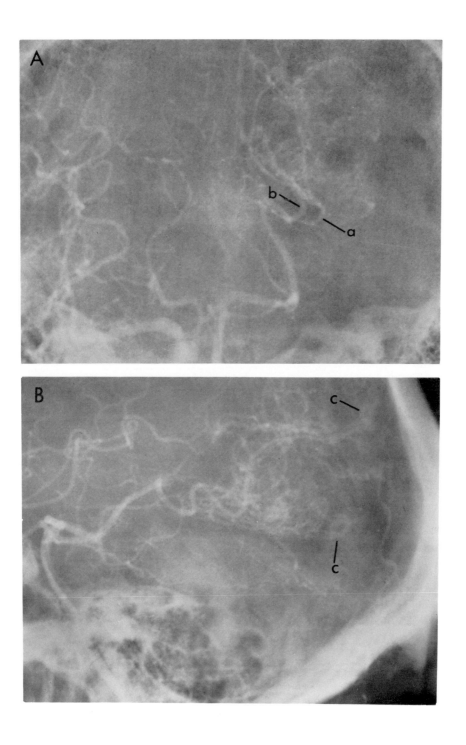

Figure 71 · Posterior Retro-Sylvian Tumor / 179

Figure 72.—Inferior retro-Sylvian tumor.

A 60-year-old man had increasingly frequent severe headaches for three months. He had memory loss for recent events and pathologic euphoria. Left homonymous hemianopia was found on examination. Changes of Paget's disease were seen in the skull radiographs.

A, right carotid angiogram, frontal projection, arterial phase: A distal shift of the anterior cerebral artery is present. The angiographic Sylvian point is displaced slightly medially (**a**). Stretching of the angular (**b**) and posterior temporal branches (**c**) of the middle cerebral artery is evident, and there is a faint tumor stain (**x**) near the termination of these vessels.

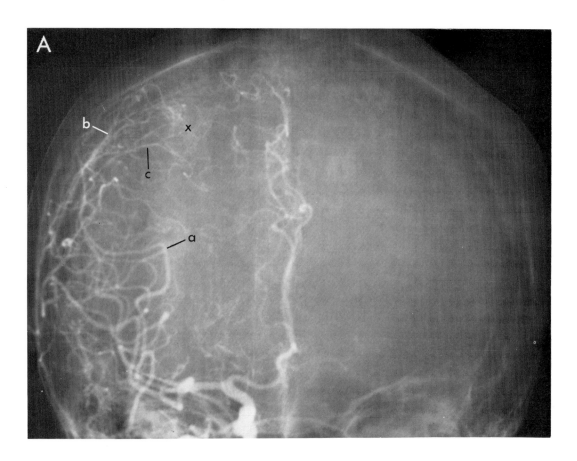

B, lateral view of arterial phase matching **A:** The Sylvian triangle is displaced forward and upward. There is crowding of the angular branches (**b**) and separation and stretching of the posterior temporal branches (**c**).

(Continued.)

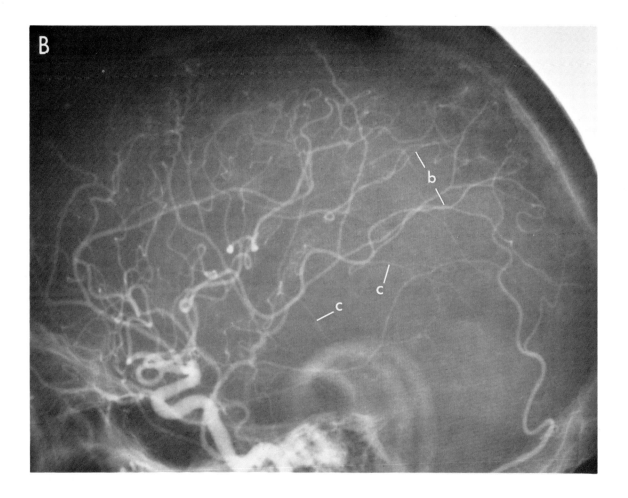

Figure 72 · Superior Retro-Sylvian Tumor / 181

Figure 72 (cont.).—Superior retro-Sylvian tumor.

C, early venous phase sequent to **B:** Compression of the sulci in which several posterior parietal veins (**d**) are running is disclosed, with upward displacement secondary to the posterior mass. The distal portion of the basal vein of Rosenthal has lost its downward convexity (**e**).

D, lateral view, late venous phase, succeeding **C:** Marked separation and stretching of the temporo-occipital tributaries of the vein of Labbé (**f**) is evident. The posterior portion of the vein of Labbé is displaced forward and downward.

The patient died about five weeks after hospitalization.

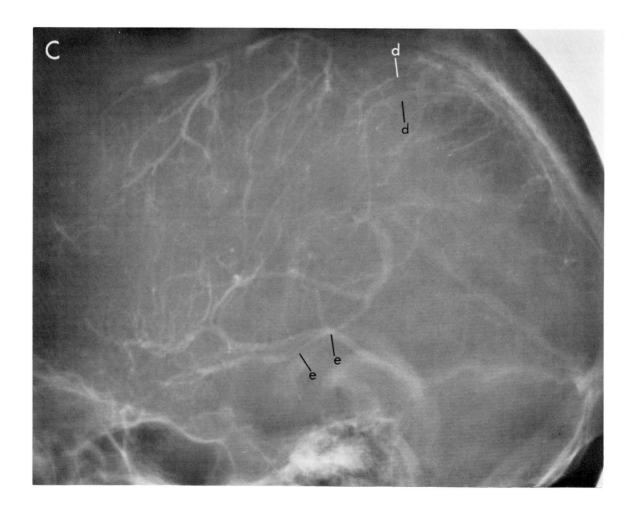

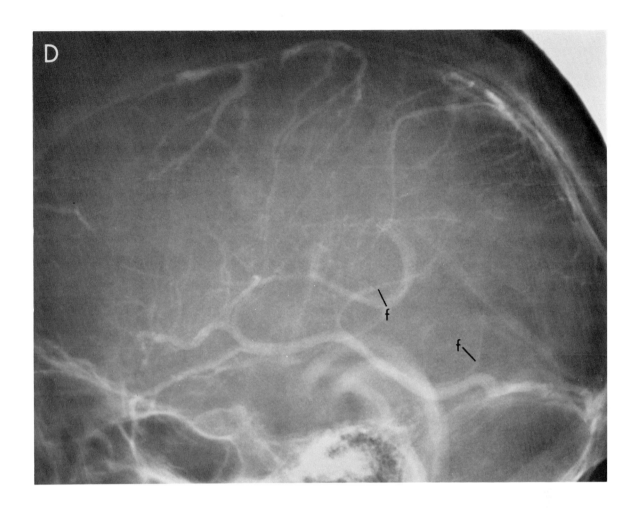

Figure 72 · Inferior Retro-Sylvian Tumor / 183

Figure 73.—Superior retro-Sylvian metastatic carcinoma extending from para-sagittal and midconvexity region.

A 70-year-old man had sudden onset of left-sided weakness about three weeks previously. The weakness progressed, and he began to complain of headache, mostly on the right. On examination, left hemiparesis was present.

A, right carotid angiogram, frontal projection, arterial phase: A slight distal shift of the anterior cerebral artery is revealed. The angiographic Sylvian point (**a**) is displaced downward. An area of neovascularity is seen in the high convexity area (**x**) being fed by a branch of the anterior cerebral artery, as well as the angular artery from the middle cerebral group.

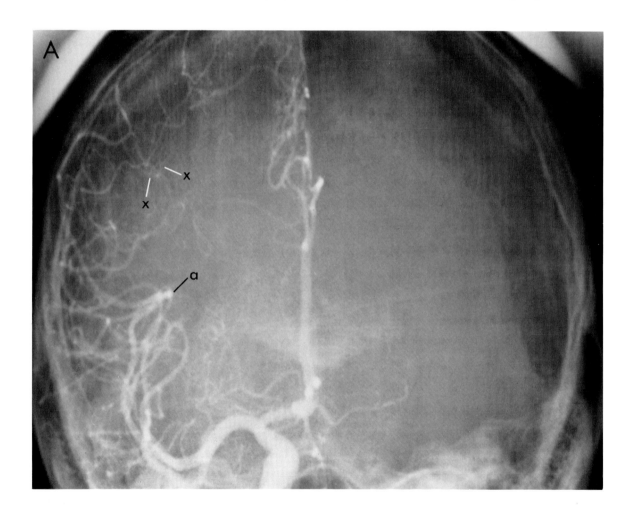

B, lateral view corresponding to **A:** The area of neovascularity is seen in the superior retro-Sylvian region (**y**). The mass effect extends well forward so that there is stretching of callosomarginal branches (**b**). The Sylvian triangle is displaced forward and downward.

(Continued.)

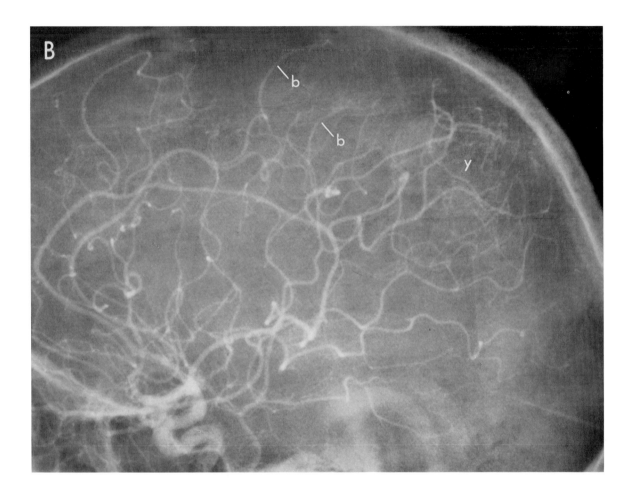

Figure 73 · Metastatic Carcinoma / 185

Figure 73 (cont.).—Superior retro-Sylvian metastatic carcinoma extending from parasagittal to midconvexity region.

C, right carotid angiogram, frontal view, venous phase: The internal cerebral vein is shifted to the left (**c**). Small, ill-defined, rather straight venous channels are perceptible in the region of the tumor stain in the high convexity area (**x**).

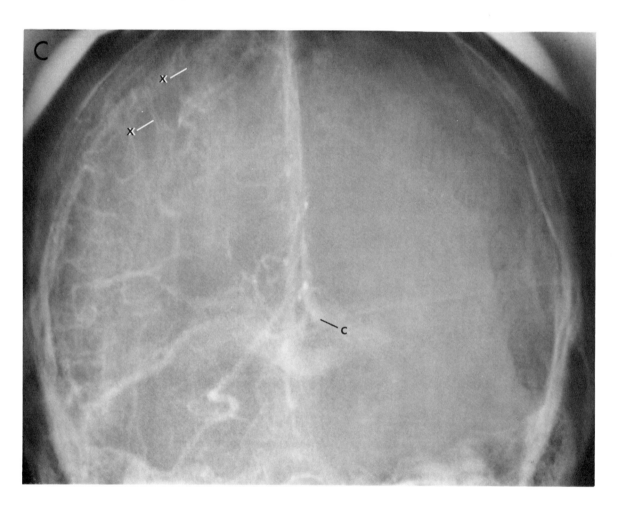

D, lateral projection matching **C:** Areas of tumor staining in the posterior parietal region extend anteriorly into the supra-Sylvian region where there is local deformity of high convexity cortical veins (**d**). Some short abnormal venous channels leading from the region of staining to the cortical veins can be appreciated. The posterior part of the internal cerebral vein is displaced downward, and subependymal tributaries (**e**) of the internal cerebral vein have a similar deformity.

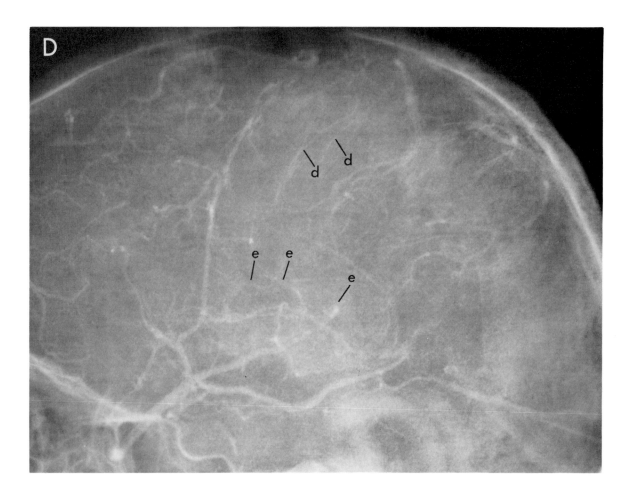

Figure 73 · Metastatic Carcinoma / 187

Figure 74.—Large retro-Sylvian glioma.

A 55-year-old man was hospitalized because of blurred vision, headache and weakness on the left side. He had papilledema, left hyperreflexia and a Babinski reflex, a left sensory deficit with astereognosis, and left homonymous hemianopia.

A, right carotid angiogram, anteroposterior projection, arterial phase: The anterior cerebral artery is shifted throughout its course beneath the falx (square shift). The distal internal carotid artery is straightened and the posterior communicating artery is displaced medially (**a**). There is downward and medial displacement of the angiographic Sylvian point (**b**).

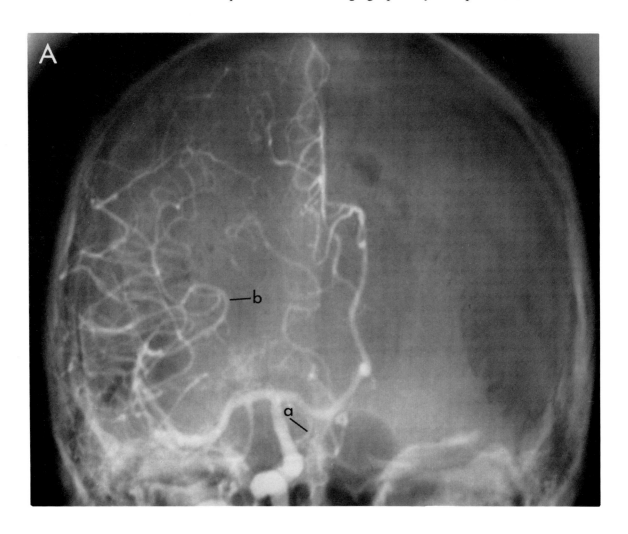

B, lateral view corresponding to **A:** There are crowding and straightening of the vessels in the parietal and occipital regions. The Sylvian triangle is compressed and telescoped forward. A mass effect is apparent in the posterior temporal region as well, where there are straightened vessels (**c**).

(Continued.)

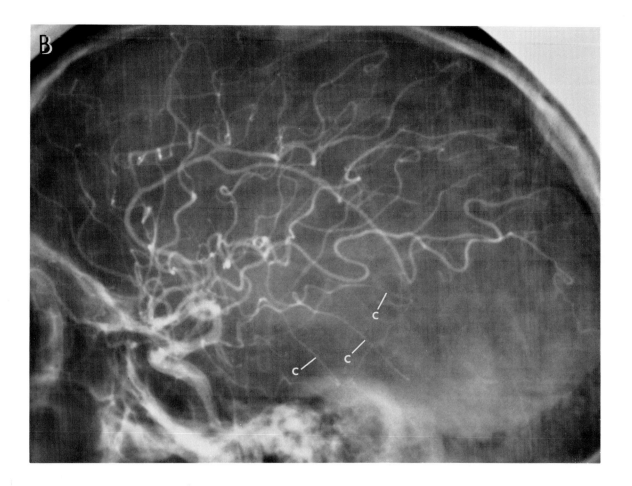

Figure 74 · Glioma / 189

Figure 74 (cont.).—Large retro-Sylvian glioma.

C, right carotid angiogram, frontal view, venous phase: The internal cerebral vein is conspicuously shifted to the left, its distal part (**d**) shifted more than the frontal portion. The basal vein of Rosenthal (**e**) is markedly displaced medially.

D, lateral view matching **C:** The posterior one-third of the cranial cavity is relatively avascular from slowing of the circulation around the tumor. Straightening and forward displacement of the parietal convexity cortical veins (**f**) are seen. The internal cerebral vein (**d**) is flattened, and the basal vein of Rosenthal (**e**) is also displaced far downward in its distal two-thirds, indicating posterior hippocampal herniation.

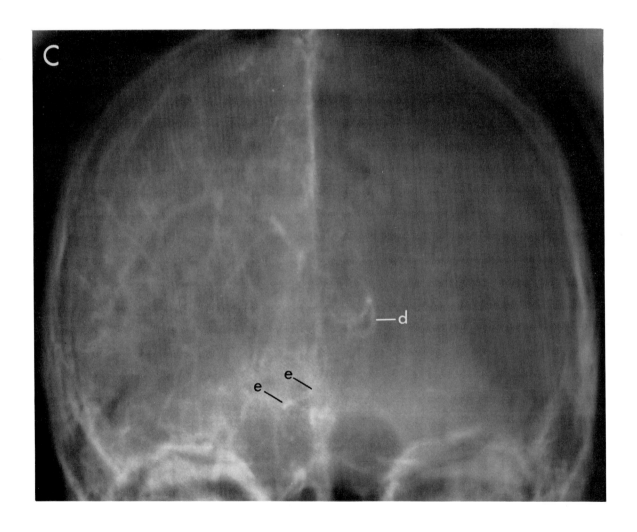

Surgical treatment was refused. The patient received radiation and steroid therapy and did remarkably well in the follow-up of two years without any signs of increased intracranial pressure. There was complete reversal of neurologic signs. Angiography two years after the first study showed diminution in size of the mass by at least one-half.

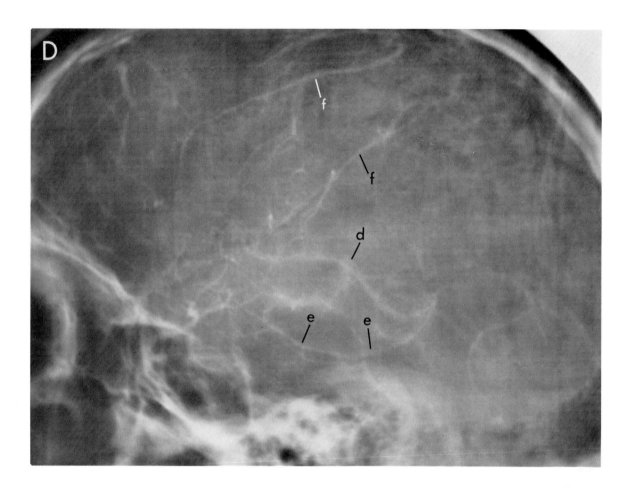

Figure 74 · Glioma / 191

Figure 75.—Retro-Sylvian cystic astrocytoma.

A 7-month-old baby girl was hospitalized because of a rapidly enlarging head and swelling in the left parietal area. Examination confirmed the enlarged head size and swelling and disclosed prominent scalp veins. Downward deviation of the eyes was observed intermittently. The neurologic examination revealed no other abnormality. (See Fig. 20 for this patient's routine roentgenogram.)

A, left carotid angiogram, frontal view, arterial phase: The terminal branches of the middle cerebral artery are displaced laterally by the mass, indicating its intracerebral position. There is significant subfalcial herniation of the anterior cerebral artery (**a**) with the form of a distal shift. The areas of neovascularity are primarily at the periphery of the mass (**x**). This observation correlates well with the pathologic finding of a vascular wall around this cystic tumor.

B, left carotid angiogram, lateral view, arterial phase: Stretching of the posterior parietal (**b**), angular (**c**) and posterior temporal (**d**) branches of the middle cerebral artery around the large mass is evident. Several areas of neovascularity are scattered throughout the tumor. There is marked upward and forward displacement of the anterior Sylvian vessels.

Operation disclosed the tumor on the surface in the retro-Sylvian region. Gross total removal was accomplished with dissection of the tumor from the atrial portion of the left lateral ventricle, which it had invaginated.

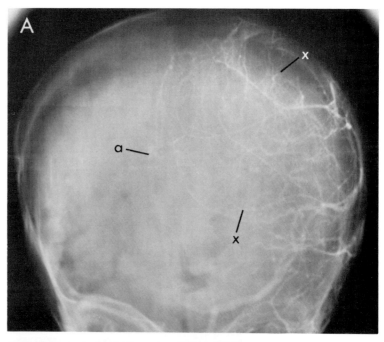

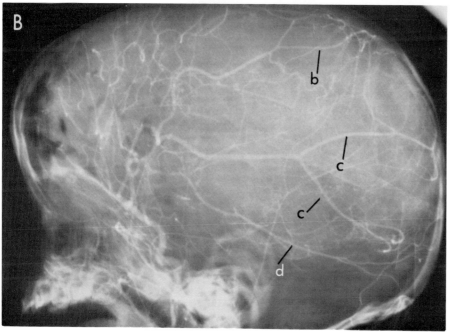

Figure 75 · Cystic Astrocytoma / 193

Figure 76.—Retro-Sylvian intracerebral ependymoma, mostly extraventricular.

A 5-year-old girl had a generalized convulsion 2½ months before hospitalization. Pneumoencephalography was performed elsewhere at that time. Nausea developed with frequent vomiting, and she became lethargic. Papilledema was found on admission together with left homonymous hemianopia and clumsiness of the left hand.

A, lateral view of the skull: A few specks of calcium (**arrow**) are present in the parieto-occipital region which, in the frontal projection, were seen to be deeply situated.

B, posteroanterior projection, brow-down, from the pneumoencephalogram obtained 2½ months before our study: Asymmetry is present in the atrial regions, with depression of the atrium on the right side. The position of the calcifications (**arrow**) in relation to the ventricle is demonstrated.

C, lateral pneumogram corresponding to **B:** An indentation of the right ventricular roof is obvious at the junction of the body and atrium, with forward and downward displacement of the ventricle (**arrow**).

D, right brachial angiogram, frontal view, arterial phase: Stretching and separation of the parieto-occipital and calcarine branches of the posterior cerebral artery are evident (**a**). There is a distal shift.

(Continued.)

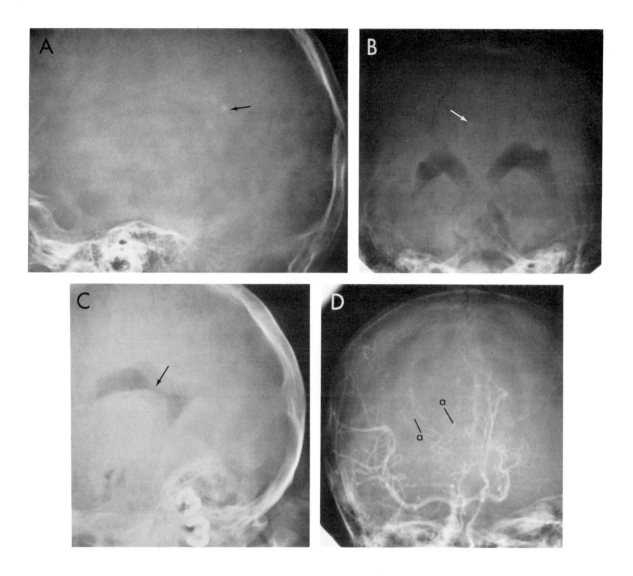

Figure 76 · Ependymoma / 195

Figure 76 (cont.).—Retro-Sylvian intracerebral ependymoma, mostly extraventricular.

E, lateral view conforming to **D:** Elevation of the posterior branches of the middle cerebral artery is present, and there is forward displacement of the angiographic Sylvian point (**b**).

F, lateral brachial angiogram, venous phase, sequent to **E:** There is pronounced downward displacement of the internal cerebral vein (**c**).

It is interesting to note how much the tumor increased in 2½ months. The diagnosis of supratentorial ependymoma was made at the time of the first examination because of the deformity of the ventricles and the calcification, but the family refused treatment. At operation following angiography, a large intracerebral tumor with intraventricular extension was removed and radiation therapy given. At the time of discharge the child was asymptomatic and the hemianopia had disappeared.

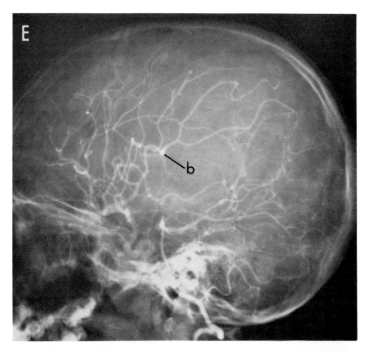

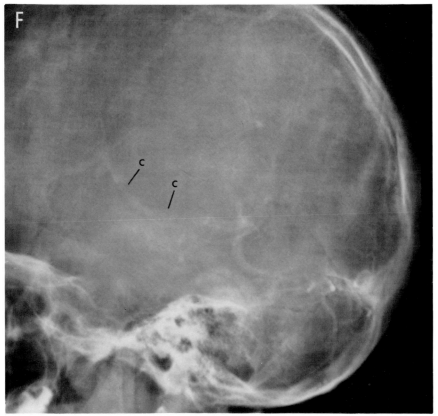

Figure 76 · Ependymoma / 197

PART 7

The Infra-Sylvian Region

Tumor Characteristics

THE INFRA-SYLVIAN INTRACEREBRAL TUMORS are temporal lobe neoplasms. Next to the frontal region, the temporal lobe is the most common site of origin of cerebral hemispheric tumors. The patients frequently present a history of psychomotor seizures. The temporal lobe is also often the site of the long-standing glioma which replaces cerebral tissue rather than displacing it; atrophic changes may be associated and therefore a relative lack of distant mass effect.

There is a practical need for very precise localization of infra-Sylvian lesions because surgical resectability is limited to the more anterior portions of the temporal lobe. As these lesions extend deeply toward the thalamus, diagnosis is aided by delineation of the posterior circulation, particularly the demonstration of changes in the posterior choroidal vessels. Evidence of local mass effects on atrial and temporal horn veins is particularly helpful, as well as the classic separation of the internal cerebral vein and the basal vein of Rosenthal. Pneumography often reveals deformity of the third ventricle when there is deep extension.

Extracerebral lesions, particularly those arising from the floor of the middle fossa, cause sharp elevation of the anterior choroidal artery. A nearly similar change may be found, however, when there is a local mass effect in the region of the uncus or fusiform gyrus of the temporal lobe. It is imperative, when studying a possible extracerebral lesion, to see the relationship of the anterior temporal branch of the middle cerebral artery to the greater wing of the sphenoid bone. It is also important to identify the posterior temporal branches of the posterior cerebral artery and determine how they relate to the undersurface of the temporal lobe and the floor of the middle cranial fossa.

Figure 77.—Anterior infra-Sylvian astrocytoma.

For three years a 40-year-old man had had grand mal and psychomotor seizures that became increasingly difficult to control with anticonvulsant medication. There were no neurologic deficits. Early in his illness an electro-encephalogram showed bilateral slowing without the presence of a slow wave focus in the temporal area, which was later evoked by nasopharyngeal leads.

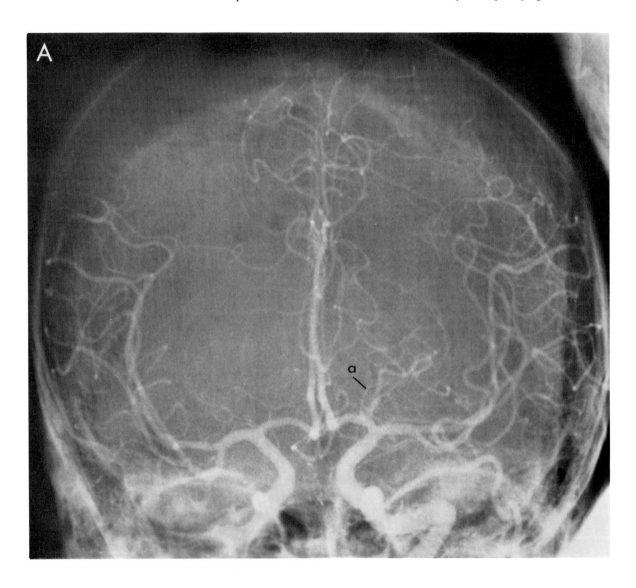

A, left carotid angiogram, with cross-compression, standard frontal view, arterial phase: A slight proximal shift of the anterior cerebral artery from left to right is present. There is mild asymmetry of the genu portions of the middle cerebral arteries, the left being slightly elevated. The middle cerebral vessels are otherwise symmetrical. A definite asymmetry of the two anterior choroidal arteries is demonstrated, with the left being straightened (**a**) as it passes around the uncus.

B, left carotid angiogram without cross-compression, lateral view, arterial phase: The anterior choroidal artery (**a**) is elevated, as faintly seen beneath a large middle cerebral vessel within the Sylvian fissure. The posterior temporal branch of the posterior cerebral artery is filled from the carotid circulation and is unremarkable. A stretched vessel is seen coursing around the upper surface of the temporal tip (**b**).

(Continued.)

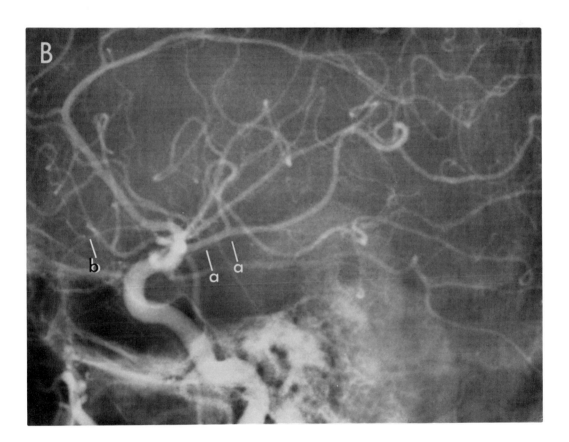

Figure 77 · Astrocytoma / 203

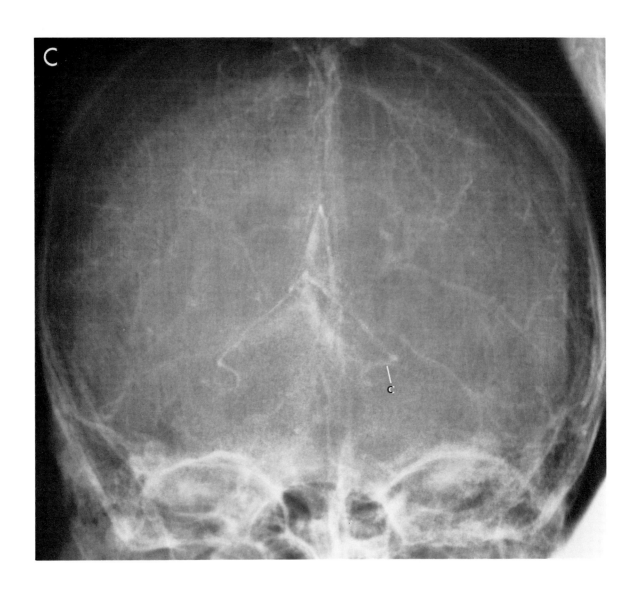

Figure 77 (cont.).—Anterior infra-Sylvian astrocytoma.

C, venous phase sequent to **A:** A slight shift of the internal cerebral vein is present. Asymmetry of the two veins of Rosenthal is demonstrated, with the proximal portion of the left basal vein (**c**) being slightly elevated and displaced medially.

D, lateral venogram succeeding **B:** Two stretched veins (**d**) course over the lateral surface of the temporal lobe and drain into the transverse sinus.

(*Continued.*)

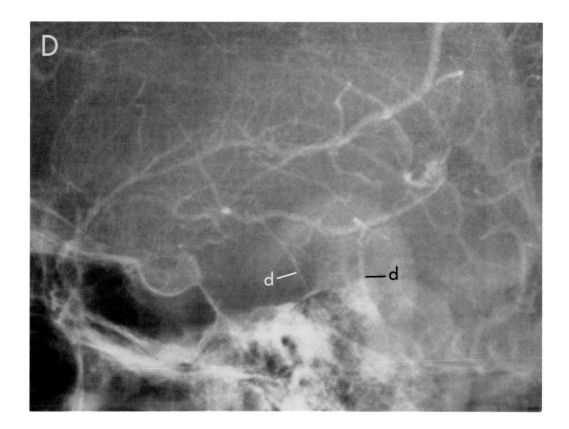

Figure 77 · Astrocytoma / 205

Figure 77 (cont.).—Anterior infra-Sylvian astrocytoma.

E, pneumoencephalogram, temporal horn series made in brow-up position following a forward somersault, reverse Towne projection: A local deformity (**x**) of the lateral aspect of the left temporal horn is shown. There is medial displacement of the temporal tip.

F, lateral view matching **E:** Truncation of the tip of the left temporal horn is evident (**x**).

At operation an infiltrating tumor was found in the anterior part of the left temporal lobe and a left temporal lobectomy was performed. Following operation the patient had a great reduction in the number and severity of psychomotor seizures. There was apparent improvement in his mental ability. Radioactive cobalt therapy was given with a dose of 5000 rads in five weeks to the area of involvement.

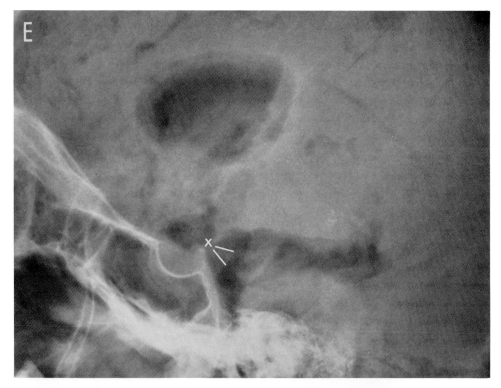

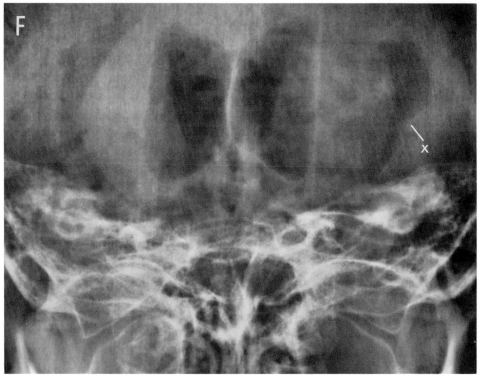

Figure 77 · Astrocytoma / 207

Figure 78.—Inferior infra-Sylvian cystic astrocytoma.

A 33-year-old man had difficulty reading, in that he could not put into words what he had read, for five months. Three weeks prior to admission he had a generalized convulsion and complained of frontal headache. On examination his recent memory was poor. Superior right quadrantonopia was present. He had visual agnosia, severe dyslexia and dyscalculia, and dysnomia. Electroencephalography revealed a prominent slow wave focus in the left midtemporal area.

A, left carotid angiogram, standard frontal view, arterial phase: A slight proximal shift of the anterior cerebral artery is evident. The angiographic Sylvian point is displaced medially and is also slightly elevated. There is medial displacement of the posterior mesencephalic portion of the posterior cerebral artery (**a**) as well as stretching of two temporal branches (**b**) arising from this structure. The anterior choroidal artery is within normal limits.

B, left carotid angiogram, lateral view, arterial phase: Upward displacement of the posterior half of the base of the Sylvian triangle is revealed. Draping of the posterior temporal branches is evident (**c**). Stretching of the temporal and occipital branches of the posterior cerebral artery is also shown (**d**).

(*Continued.*)

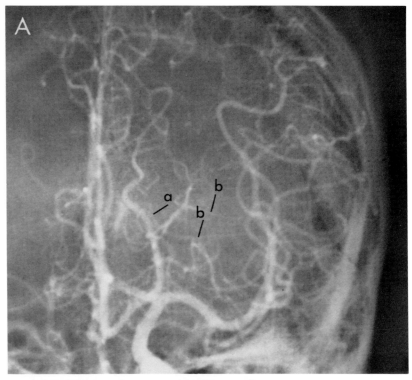

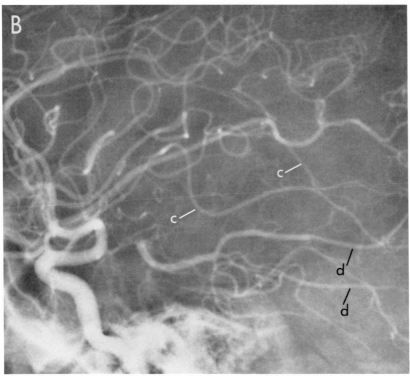

Figure 78 · Astrocytoma / 209

Figure 78 (cont.).—Inferior infra-Sylvian cystic astrocytoma.

C, left carotid angiogram, frontal view, venous phase: The internal cerebral vein is displaced left to right (**e**). A prominent vein of the temporal horn is markedly displaced medially (**f**). This vein enters the basal vein of Rosenthal (**g**), which is also medially displaced.

D, venous phase, lateral view, matching **C:** Striking upward displacement of the vein of the temporal horn is seen (**f**). Slight upward displacement of the proximal part of the basal vein of Rosenthal (**g**) is also demonstrated. The internal cerebral vein is somewhat anomalous, with the septal vein entering the internal cerebral vein far posteriorly (**h**).

The patient underwent a left temporal craniotomy with aspiration of a cyst containing nearly 20 cc of dark yellow proteinacious fluid. He did well for a few months, with reduction of the headache and visual field defect, while receiving a course of radiation therapy. However, within five months he again had severe headache, papilledema developed, and another operation (with removal of solid tumor to effect an internal decompression) was required.

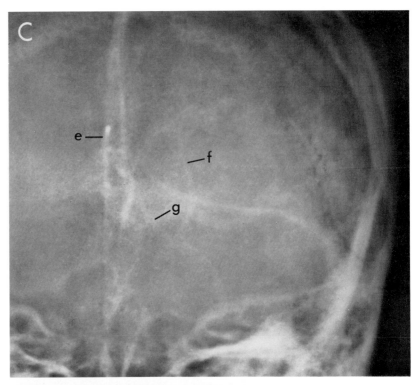

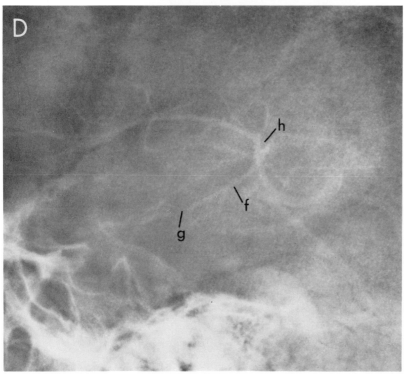

Figure 78 · Astrocytoma / 211

Figure 79.—Oligodendroglioma of the right temporal lobe.

A 12-year-old girl began to have psychomotor seizures four years prior to admission. For two years there were grand mal seizures. On examination she was slow in calculating and had a poor memory for recent events. Other results of the neurologic examination were within normal limits.

A, routine lateral exposure: An area of calcification is revealed in the plane of the dorsum sella (**x**), which is positioned laterally within the temporal lobe. The sella turcica is abnormal, with thinning of the anterior cortical margin of the dorsum and atrophy of the cortex of the sellar floor. Both the anterior and the posterior clinoid process are atrophic from intracranial hypertension.

B, right carotid angiogram, lateral view, arterial phase: Stretching and upward displacement of the anterior choroidal artery (**a**) occur as it enters the choroid fissure of the temporal horn. In addition, the main group of middle cerebral vessels within the anterior half of the Sylvian fissure is elevated.

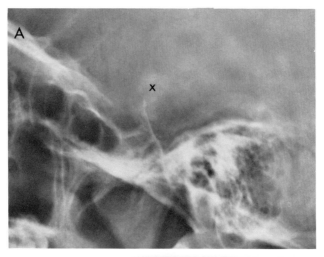

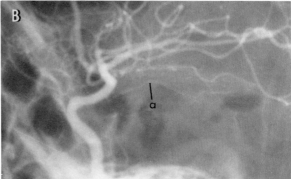

Air is seen in the subarachnoid space from the previous pneumoencephalogram.

C, pneumoencephalogram, brow-up temporal horn view after a forward somersault, reverse Towne projection: The temporal horn on the right is dilated with poor definition of its lateral recess throughout the entire length of the visible portion of the temporal horn (**arrows**). The right temporal horn is elevated. The third ventricle (**y**) is displaced slightly to the left, but this is difficult to appreciate here because of rotation.

D, lateral view, made with the patient in the same position as in **C:** The elevated and dilated right temporal horn is seen (**arrows**), with loss of the normal outline of the supracornual recesses.

At operation a grayish gelatinous tumor, which was quite hard and gritty in parts, was found. Subtotal removal of the tumor was accomplished by resecting the anterior portion of the temporal lobe. For the subsequent three years seizures have been controlled and mental status has improved.

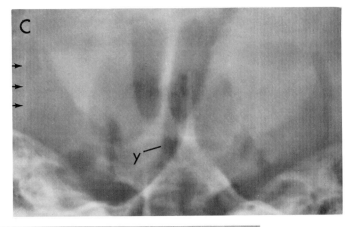

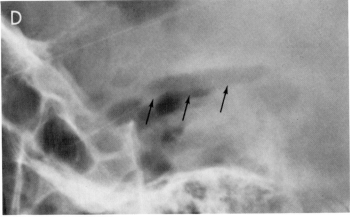

Figure 79 · **Oligodendroglioma** / **213**

Figure 80.—Infra-Sylvian glioblastoma.

A 43-year-old man began to complain of recurring headache 2½ years before admission. About 6 months later, he had his first seizure. Seizures recurred with increasing frequency and were accompanied by an auditory aura characterized as a repetitive whirring noise. When hospitalized he had a slight reduction of swing of the left arm and low-grade papilledema. An electroencephalogram revealed a slow wave focus in the right temporal region. A radioactive isotope brain scan showed no abnormality. Spinal puncture revealed normal pressure but a total protein level of 65 mg per 100 cc.

A, right brachial angiogram, standard frontal projection, arterial phase: Slight medial displacement of the angiographic Sylvian point (**arrow**) is present as well as displacement of one of the midinsular loops (**a**).

B, right brachial angiogram, lateral view, arterial phase: No local mass effect is apparent except for straightening of one thin posterior temporal branch of the middle cerebral artery (**b**) crossing the middle and inferior temporal gyri.

(Continued.)

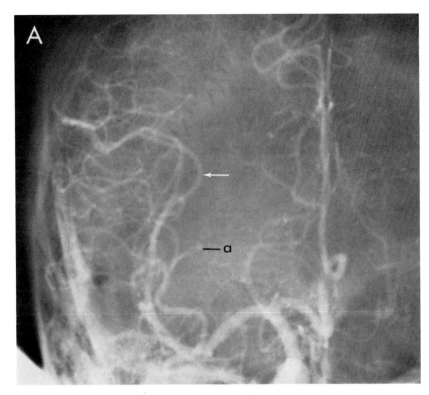

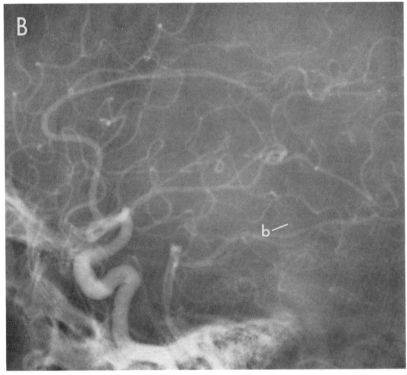

Figure 80 · Glioblastoma / 215

Figure 80 (cont.).—Infra-Sylvian glioblastoma.

C, lateral view, venous phase, sequent to **B:** There is slight separation of two large cortical veins draining the convex surface of the temporal lobe (**c**).

The seizures were controlled with anticonvulsant medication, and the papilledema receded under treatment with dexamethasone. Intracranial exploration was not advised and the patient was discharged. Ten months later the seizures had broken through the anticonvulsant medication to return at frequent intervals. He complained of blurred vision and weakness of the left arm. On examination, well-developed papilledema and left hemiparesis were found.

D, right brachial angiogram, standard frontal projection, arterial phase, on re-admission: A straight shift of the anterior cerebral artery to the left of the midline is revealed. The middle cerebral branches are elevated and stretched, especially the distal branches, and the angiographic Sylvian point is farther medial than before (compare with **A**). The genu of the middle cerebral artery is also medial in position (**d**) and its curve is flattened.

(*Continued.*)

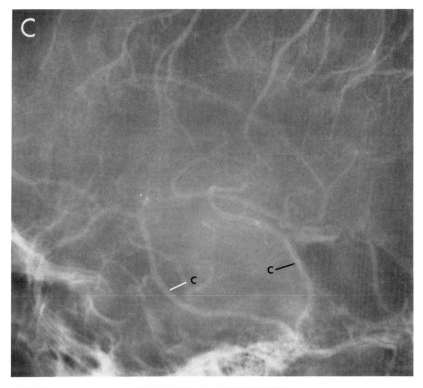

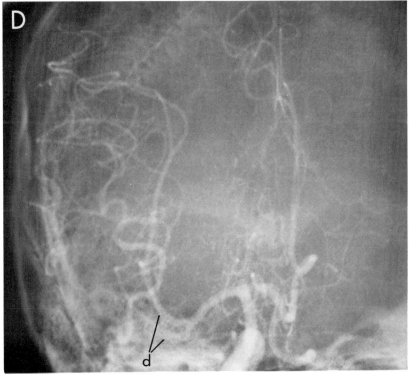

Figure 80 · Glioblastoma / 217

Figure 80 (cont.).—Infra-Sylvian glioblastoma.

E, lateral view conforming to **D:** A temporal mass effect is disclosed, with elevation and forward crowding of the middle cerebral branches producing disruption of the Sylvian triangle. An early draining view is evident (**e**), denoting the malignant nature of the tumor. The proximal segments of the posterior cerebral artery are now stretched and displaced downward (**f**), indicating downward transtentorial herniation.

F, lateral view, venous phase sequent to **E:** There is now marked separation of the cortical veins on the surface of the temporal lobe (**g**). The internal cerebral vein is elevated, straightened and stretched (compare with **C**).

At operation a large glioma was found filling most of the right temporal lobe. A large cyst was present, which was evacuated, and a large part of the glioblastoma was excised by temporal lobectomy, effecting a generous decompression. The patient was receiving radiation therapy when last seen.

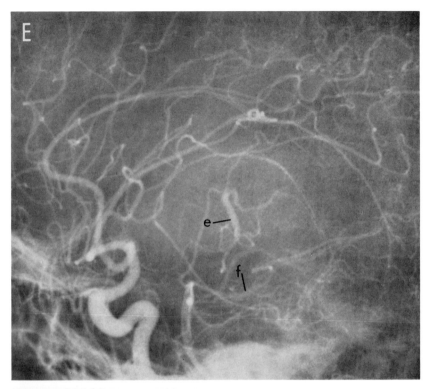

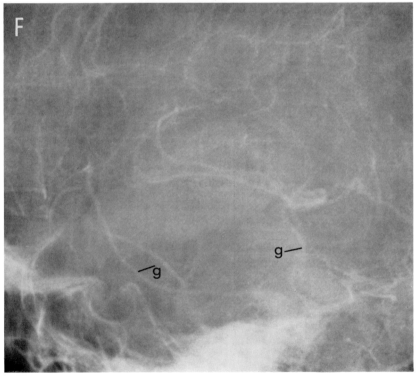

Figure 80 · Glioblastoma / 219

Figure 81.—Large infra-Sylvian glioblastoma with extension into the corpus striatum and thalamus.

A 40-year-old woman had an eight-year history of odd falling attacks, subtle personality changes and memory loss. Three weeks before hospitalization she began to experience severe headache and difficulty with speech. On examination she was found to be obtunded, dysphasic and to have right hemiparesis.

A, left carotid angiogram, frontal view, arterial phase: A square shift of the anterior cerebral artery is present. The anterior choroidal artery is displaced almost to the midline (**a**), indicating anterior hippocampal herniation at the tentorial incisura. The lenticulostriate arteries are straightened and displaced away from the insular vessels, indicating deep extension of the tumor (**b**). A striking mass effect is present in the infra-Sylvian region (**x**) with marked elevation and medial displacement of all of the middle cerebral branches. There is no longer a genu of the middle cerebral artery.

B, lateral projection matching **A:** There is complete disruption of the Sylvian triangle with elevation of all of the middle cerebral branches, which are tightly crowded. The anterior choroidal artery is elevated (**c**).

(Continued.)

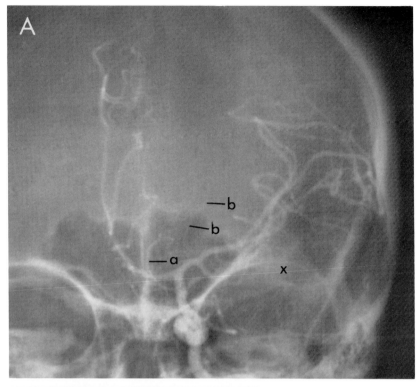

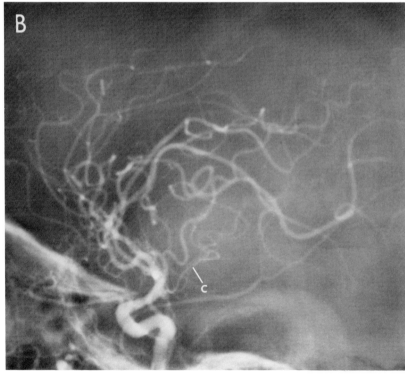

Figure 81 · Glioblastoma / 221

Figure 81 (cont.).—Large infra-Sylvian glioblastoma with extension into the corpus striatum and thalamus.

C, lateral view, slightly later arterial phase succeeding **B:** The mass effect extends into the region of the posterior temporal and angular gyri. The draping temporal convexity branches are separated, and one large branch (**d**) shows areas of definite encasement of the artery with delayed flow.

D, left carotid angiogram, frontal view, venous phase: There is pronounced displacement of the internal cerebral vein (**e**) to the right of the midline. The thalamostriate vein has a markedly arcuate course (**f**) and the width of the ventricle is narrowed, indicating deep extension with thalamic involvement.

Intracranial exploration disclosed a diffusely swollen, soft left temporal lobe which contained a grayish spongy tumor. Internal decompression was attempted. The postoperative course was downhill and the patient died on the sixth postoperative day.

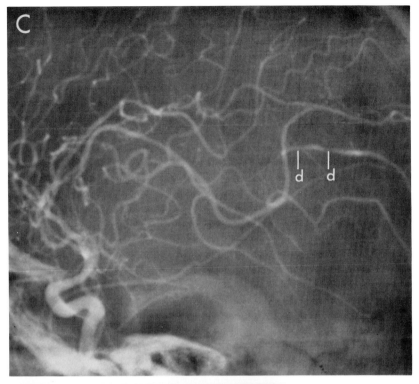

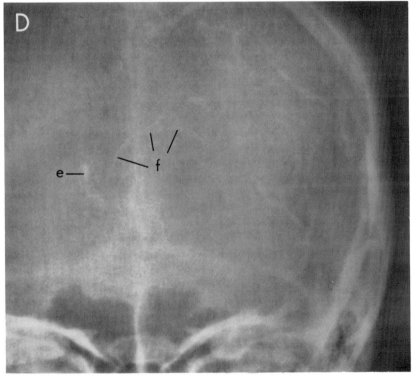

Figure 81 · Glioblastoma / 223

Figure 82.—Infra-Sylvian metastatic carcinoma.

A 54-year-old man had had a right upper lobectomy for a solitary pulmonary nodule, proved to be a bronchogenic carcinoma, two years previously. He did well until one month before this study, when retro-orbital pain developed. The pain persisted and he had difficulty in expression and periods of mental confusion. Examination revealed left hemiparesis and papilledema.

A, right carotid angiogram, standard frontal view, arterial phase: A square shift of the anterior cerebral artery is evident. The carotid bifurcation is high, with conspicuous elevation and medial displacement of the entire middle cerebral group of vessels. The anterior choroidal artery is displaced medially (**a**). There is marked stretching of the middle cerebral branches draping over the temporal tip and anterior part of the temporal lobe (**b**).

B, lateral view corresponding to **A:** This reveals an opening of the carotid siphon and marked straightening of the proximal segment of the middle cerebral artery. The anterior temporal branches passing over the temporal tip are in close apposition to the greater wing of the sphenoid bone (**c**). The anterior choroidal artery is depressed and markedly straightened (**a**). Smaller convexity middle cerebral branches also exhibit draping (**d**).

(*Continued.*)

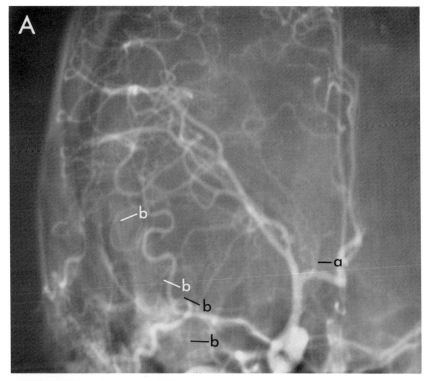

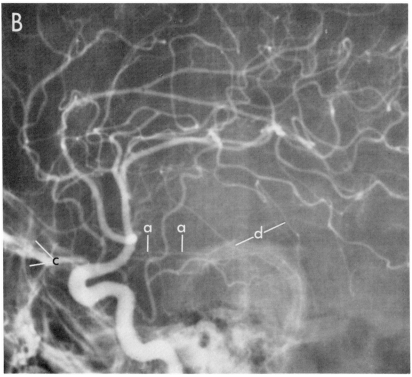

Figure 82 · Metastatic Carcinoma / 225

Figure 82 (cont.).—Infra-Sylvian metastatic carcinoma.

C, right carotid angiogram, frontal view, venous phase: The internal cerebral vein is displaced to the left of the midline. The basal vein of Rosenthal is displaced medially (**e**).

D, right carotid angiogram, lateral view, venous phase: The basal vein is conspicuously elevated (**e**) in its anterior portions. Drainage of the Sylvian fissure is into the basal vein of Rosenthal and into a large lateral vein of Labbé. The vein of Labbé is also elevated in its anterior portions but returns to normal position posteriorly.

No definite evidence of a left hemispheric lesion was found by further angiography, radioactive isotope scanning, electroencephalography or other tests, although the possibility of a hidden left focus was suggested by the lack of greater midline shift. As a result, the patient underwent intracranial exploration and a right temporal lobectomy was carried out with resection 6 cm from the temporal tip. The removed tissue was yellowish green and very soft and contained areas of mucinous degeneration. He did well briefly and was given radiation therapy. Three months later, however, there was definite evidence of a second lesion on the left side and the course was progressively downhill.

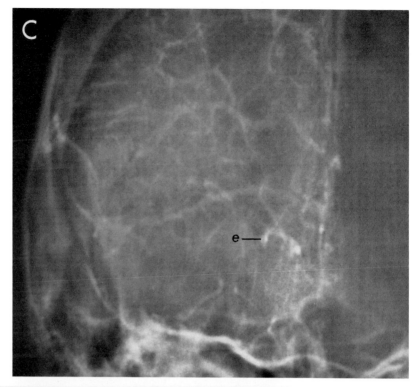

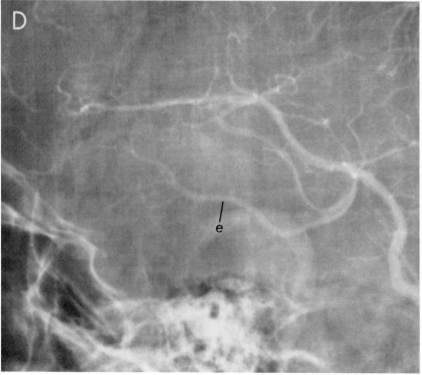

Figure 82 · Metastatic Carcinoma / 227

Figure 83.—Posterior infra-Sylvian hematoma with extension into the lateral ventricle.

A 55-year-old man suffered a subarachnoid hemorrhage and right hemiparesis four weeks previously. When seen he had marked receptive and expressive aphasia.

A, left carotid angiogram, frontal view, arterial phase: The anterior cerebral artery is shifted 8 mm to the right of the midline. The anterior choroidal artery is normal proximally but is definitely bowed medially, with a reversal of its curve, in the portion lying within the choroid fissure of the temporal horn (**a**). The angiographic Sylvian point (**x**) is displaced medially,

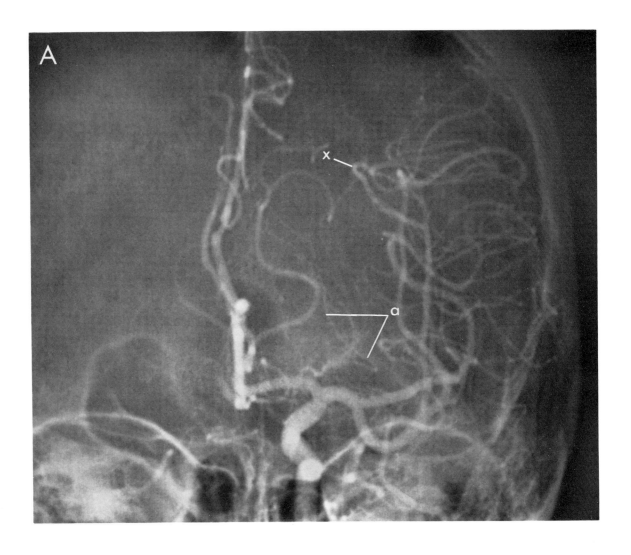

with a lesser degree of displacement of the insular loops of the middle cerebral artery branches more anteriorly.

B, left carotid angiogram, lateral view, arterial phase: Pronounced elevation of the Sylvian triangle is disclosed. Draping of the temporal vessels is seen (**c**), with frank stretching and separation in the region of the posterior part of the temporal lobe. The anterior choroidal artery (**d**) is stretched as it reaches the atrium of the lateral ventricle. The findings of this marked local mass effect correlates well with the rupture of a hematoma into the temporal horn.

(Continued.)

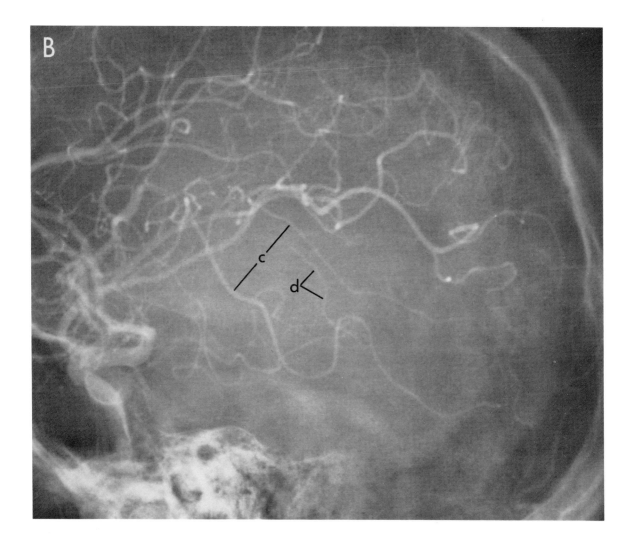

Figure 83 · Hematoma / 229

Figure 83 (cont.).—Posterior infra-Sylvian hematoma with extension into the lateral ventricle.

C, left carotid angiogram, frontal view, venous phase: The internal cerebral vein is displaced to the right, and significant hippocampal transtentorial herniation is outlined by the medially displaced basal vein of Rosenthal (**e**).

D, lateral view matching **C:** Local separation and stretching of the cortical veins (**f**) are apparent in the mid- and posterior temporal regions.

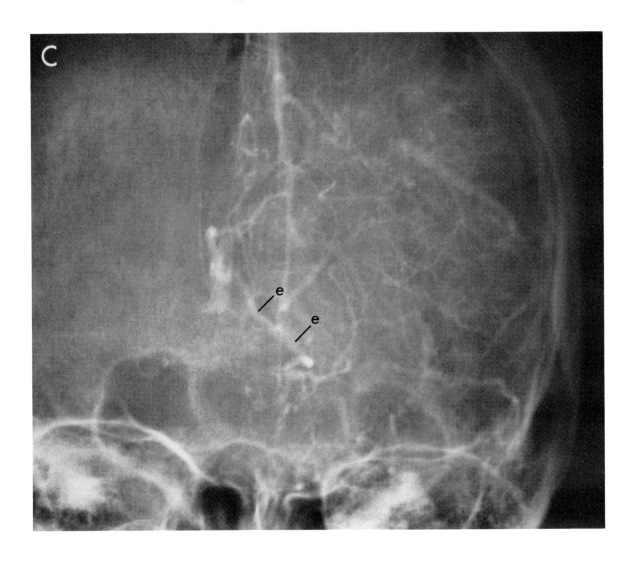

On left temporal craniotomy, evacuation of an intracerebral hematoma was accomplished. It extended from the junction of the anterior and middle thirds of the temporal lobe into its most posterior portion. Rupture into the temporal horn was verified. The hemiparesis cleared almost completely, but speech deficit was only moderately improved.

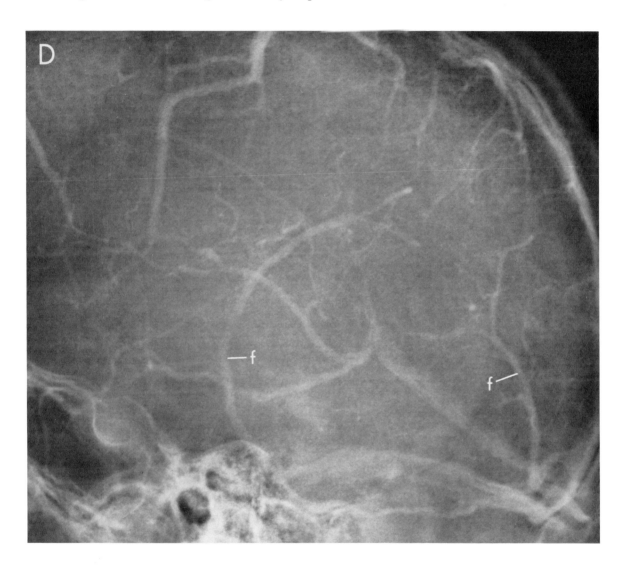

Figure 83 · Hematoma / 231

PART 8

Intra-Sylvian and
Latero-Sylvian Tumors

General Characteristics

INTRA-SYLVIAN TUMORS are distinctly uncommon. A lesion seen to be purely within the lips of the Sylvian fissure will more often than not prove to be a meningioma. If there is evidence of a local mass effect only on the bordering structures of the Sylvian fissure (middle cerebral artery and veins on the opercula) and circular sulcus (insular portion of the middle cerebral arteries and insular veins), it must be assumed that the mass is purely extra-axial. The separation of the temporal, frontal and parietal opercula is best analyzed by tracing the temporal and frontoparietal convexity branches back along their intra-Sylvian course on the lateral view. It should also be possible to demonstrate separation on the frontal view. It is not uncommon, however, for a glioma of the adjacent frontoparietal or temporal operculum to extend into the Sylvian fissure. Therefore it is necessary to look for evidence of tumor beyond the opercula either in the frontoparietal and temporal convexity laterally or in the insula, external capsule and deeper structures medially.

Latero-Sylvian tumors are, in many instances, meningiomas; they are discussed fully in Part 13. Gliomas of the opercula, however, are also latero-Sylvian, but they usually have expanded into the supra-Sylvian or infra-Sylvian region by the time they are diagnosed. In addition, other intracerebral tumors arising in the neighborhood of the Sylvian fissure may grow in an exophytic manner and be predominantly latero-Sylvian. One must keep in mind the fact that lesions that are so far lateral and have no true intracerebral features may not be neoplastic but may be subdural hematomas or abscesses.

Figure 84.—Intra-Sylvian meningioma.

A 53-year-old man had a one-year history of headache and dragging of his right foot when he was tired. Recently the headache had become more intense and he complained of blurred vision. Neurologic examination revealed left central facial paresis, decreased left arm swing and reduced strength in the left arm and leg with hyperreflexia. There was blurring of the margins of the optic discs on ophthalmoscopic examination.

A, routine exposure of the skull, Caldwell projection: A broad vascular groove is present in the squamous portion of the right temporal bone (**a**). The cortical boundaries of the lesser wings of the sphenoid bone and of the planum sphenoidale are indicative of chronic increased intracranial pressure. The calcified pineal (**b**) is projected through the left frontal sinus and is displaced well to the left of the midline.

B, lateral view: There is marked atrophy of the anterior wall of the dorsum sellae with loss of cortex along the sellar floor extending to the planum sphenoidale. The broad vascular groove noted in **A** is again well demonstrated (**a**). A small area of hyperostosis is present adjacent to the point where the groove shows evidence of branching and where it becomes smaller (**c**).

(Continued.)

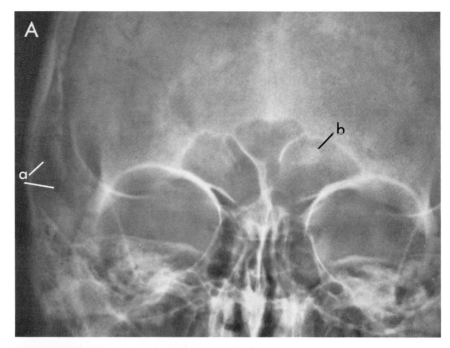

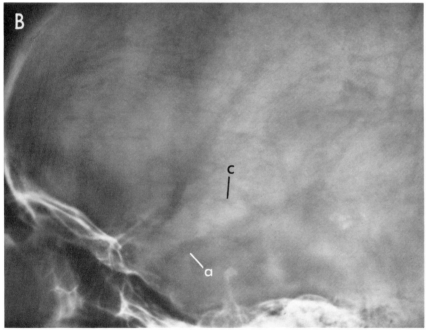

Figure 84 · Meningioma / 237

Figure 84 (cont.).—Intra-Sylvian meningioma.

C, carotid angiogram, frontal view, arterial phase: The middle cerebral arterial tree is medially displaced to a striking degree in the depths of the Sylvian fissure. The opercular branches are separated and stretched (**d**) by the large tumor within the lips of the Sylvian fissure. Small areas of tumor stain are evident (**x**). The anterior middle cerebral branches (**e**) extending laterally out of the fissure do not course all of the way to the inner table of the skull at several points because of the dural attachment of the tumor in this area. In addition to the deformities and displacements of the middle cerebral vessels, the supraclinoid segment of the internal carotid artery (**f**) is displaced almost to the midline, and a proximal shift of the anterior cerebral artery is present.

D, lateral view, corresponding to **C:** The carotid siphon (**f**) appears to be tightly closed. The insular loop forming the base of the Sylvian triangle is elevated, and there is obvious separation of the anterior and posterior groups. The frontal opercular branches (**g**) are elevated well above the temporal branches (**h**), which is a feature of tumor in an intra-Sylvian location.

Intracranial exploration revealed a large low convexity meningioma, and subtotal intracapsular removal was accomplished. The patient did very well for nine years, when a recurrence required a second operation.

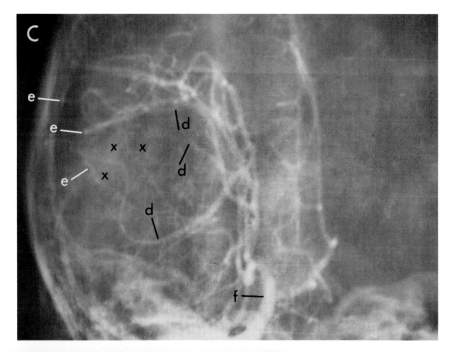

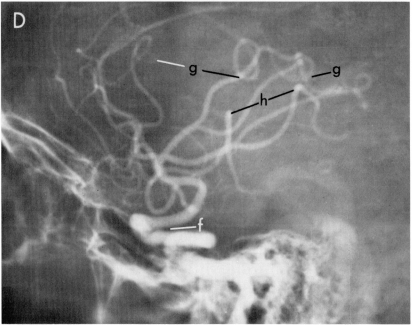

Figure 84 · Meningioma / 239

Figure 85.—Intra-Sylvian cystic glioma extending into the supra-Sylvian convexity.

A 39-year-old man experienced parasthesias of the right arm for one year. For several weeks before hospitalization he complained of headache of increasing severity, weakness of the right arm and blurred vision. Examination revealed only mild right hemiparesis with hyperreflexia and papilledema. The electroencephalogram revealed a large midtemporal focus on the left side.

A, left carotid angiogram, frontal projection, arterial phase: The anterior cerebral artery is displaced to the right. There is also medial displacement of the anterior choroidal artery (**a**). The adjacent lenticulostriate vessels (**b**) are crowded and medially displaced. The middle cerebral vessels within the Sylvian fissure exhibit marked medial displacement, and measurement of the angiographic Sylvian point (**x**) was greatly increased above normal. A small area of neovascularity (**y**) is demonstrated near the angiographic Sylvian point.

B, lateral view matching **A:** Stretching and separation of the middle cerebral branches (**c**) are evident on the low convexity of the supra-Sylvian region. The insular loops are depressed in the midportion of the Sylvian triangle and they also appear to be separated in this area. One area of neovascularity is visible in the low convexity and two in the opercular area (**arrows**).

(*Continued.*)

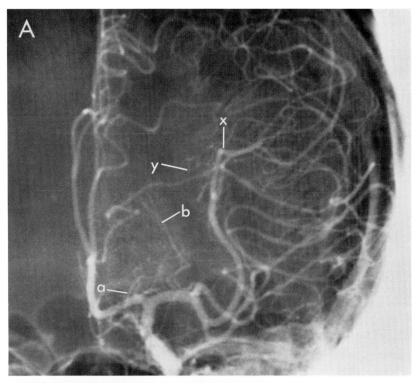

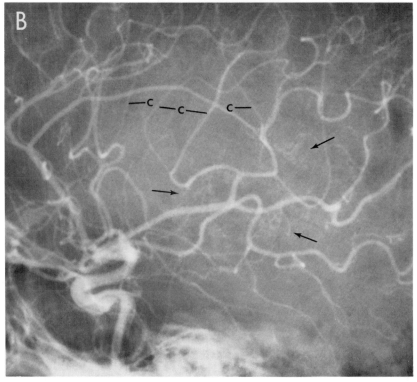

Figure 85 · Glioma / 241

Figure 85 (cont.).—Intra-Sylvian cystic glioma extending into the supra-Sylvian convexity.

C, left carotid angiogram, venous phase sequent to **A:** The internal cerebral vein (**d**) is displaced to the right. Incisural hippocampal herniation is evident from medial displacement of the basal vein of Rosenthal (**e**). Marked separation of the deep and superficial middle cerebral veins is shown outlining the intra-Sylvian component of the tumor (**f**).

D, lateral view matching **C:** Only slight straightening of the middle cerebral veins is evident (**g**) because most of the displacements are taking place in a transverse plane. There is some elongation of the subependymal veins (**h**) draining into the internal cerebral vein because of the subfalcial herniation of the left lateral ventricle.

At operation, a cyst was evacuated, effecting a decompression. Radiation therapy was then administered.

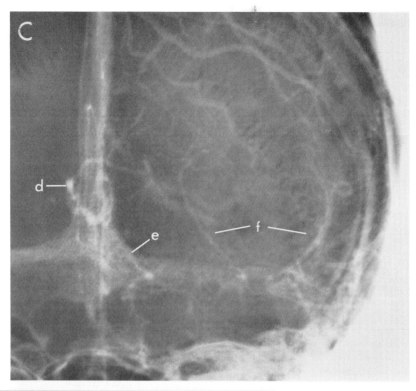

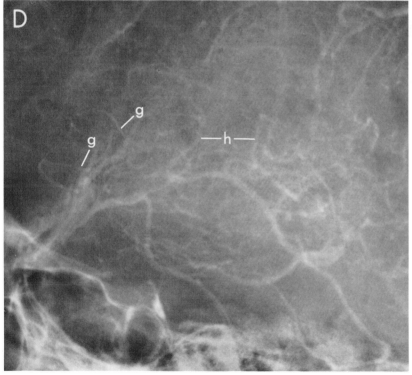

Figure 85 · Glioma / 243

Figure 86.—Oligodendroglioma of the frontal operculum extending into the insula.

A 38-year-old woman had Jacksonian seizures beginning in the left side of the face, then involving the entire left side. They began nine years before hospitalization and originally were infrequent. For the past two years the seizures were frequent and uncontrolled and she underwent a personality change with periods of severe depression. Examination revealed left facial weakness and decreased swing with posturing of the left arm. Deep reflexes on the left were exaggerated throughout.

A, right carotid angiogram, frontal projection, arterial phase: The horizontal portion of the right anterior cerebral artery is hypoplastic; the ascending portion (**a**) is faintly outlined and displaced to the left. The transverse portion of the middle cerebral artery appears to be straightened and stretched. The ascending frontal branch is displaced medially, as are other anterior branches that are ascending the insular surface (**b**).

B, right carotid angiogram, lateral view, arterial phase: There is marked separation of the first two branches forming the anterior portion of the Sylvian triangle (**arrows**). A local mass effect extends into the convexity of the anterior supra-Sylvian area.

At operation the tumor was found presenting superficially in the middle and inferior frontal gyri. At a depth of 3 cm a cyst was encountered and 40 cc of yellowish fluid evacuated. The tumor lying more superficially was removed; removal of the deeper portions extending into the Sylvian fissure was not feasible. Radiation therapy was administered. Three years later the seizures were controlled by anticonvulsant medication and the left hemiparesis had cleared.

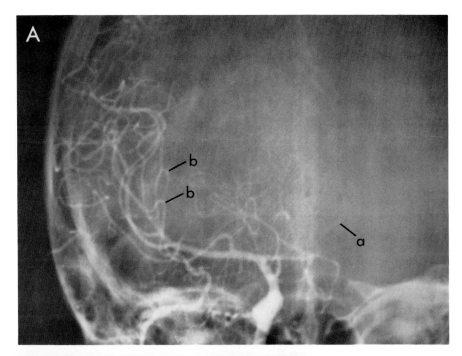

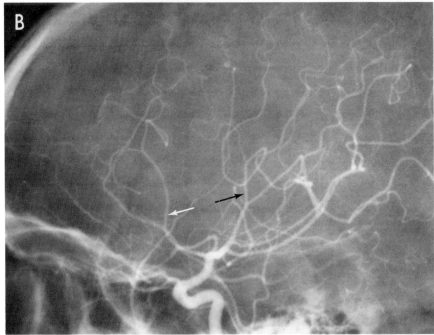

Figure 86 · Oligodendroglioma / 245

Figure 87.—Posterior temporal glioma with intra-Sylvian extension.

A 51-year-old woman suffered an episode of unconsciousness 2½ months previously. Following this she had left-sided headaches which became severe. The day before hospitalization she became lethargic and vomited. Neurologic examination revealed head tremor, shuffling gait, drift of the right arm and extinction phenomena in the right arm and leg. Right homonymous hemianopia was demonstrated.

A, left carotid angiogram, frontal view, arterial phase: A square shift of the anterior cerebral artery to the right of the midline is revealed; the shift is slightly greater in its distal portion. The Sylvian vessels are displaced markedly toward the midline, and the posterior branches show evidence of separation (**arrows**).

B, left carotid angiogram, lateral view, arterial phase: The posterior portion of the Sylvian triangle is elevated, with separation of the posterior temporal (**a**) and angular (**b**) branches of the middle cerebral artery. The center of the tumor is located in the temporal operculum. Thus the proximal portion of the posterior temporal artery within the Sylvian fissure (**c**) is elevated due to the tumor. The distal portion of the artery on the convexity of the temporal lobe is depressed (**a**).

A left temporoparietal craniotomy was performed and a large portion of the tumor presenting on the cortex removed. An internal decompression was accomplished by removing a large portion of the central part of the tumor. The patient died the next day. The tumor proved to be a glioblastoma.

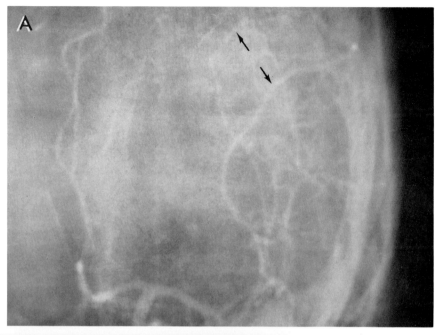

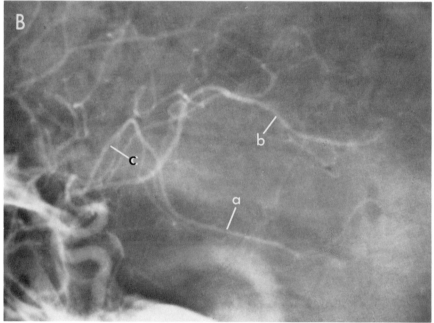

Figure 87 · Glioma / 247

PART 9

Centro-Sylvian Tumors

Tumor Characteristics

THIS DISCUSSION concerns deep tumors, usually alongside the lateral and third ventricles. The lesions may invade a ventricle, and it may be difficult to differentiate such a neoplasm from an intraventricular tumor extending outward. The tissue types, and therefore the growth characteristics, of the intraventricular group set them apart from the lesions of the corpus striatum, thalamus, corpus callosum and centrum semiovale.

The patient may present a thalamic syndrome, or a much more bizarre clinical picture when the tumor is in the corpus callosum or basal ganglia. Tumors of the latter structures often evoke behavioral changes or Parkinson-like movements. Because of their proximity to the foramen of Monro, foraminal obstruction and consequent increased intracranial pressure are not unusual.

Angiographically, the thalamic tumors cause backward displacement of the posterior choroidal arteries, elevation of the internal cerebral vein (humping) and depression of the basal vein of Rosenthal. If a tumor extends laterally, the distal portions of the anterior choroidal artery within the choroid fissure of the temporal horn are pushed outward and the middle cerebral arterial branches along the insula and distal portion of the Sylvian fissure are displaced laterally.

Corpus callosum tumors elevate the pericallosal arteries and depress the subependymal and internal cerebral veins. In the splenial portion of the corpus callosum, the splenial artery from the posterior cerebral artery often contributes a significant vascular supply to the tumor. The tumors alongside the lateral ventricles in the corpus striatum are often infiltrative gliomas and may not become greatly expanded masses. When they obstruct the foramen of Monro, they add to their own mass effect. Angiographically, the lesions displace the lenticulostriate vessels laterally and the ganglionic arteries often enlarge as they supply the lesion. Local, and often striking, deformities of the subependymal veins coursing from the superolateral corner of the lateral ventricle to the internal cerebral vein are seen. Normally, the internal cerebral vein progressively enlarges as each tributary enters on its course to the vein of Galen. Subtle changes of contour of it or its tributaries may be extremely significant.

Pneumography, by either ventriculography or pneumoencephalography or a combination of the two, has long been the definitive method of diagnosis of centro-Sylvian lesions. In many instances ventriculography is required because a thalamic tumor may compress together the side walls of the third ventricle and impair entrance of gas from below. Striatal tumors often block the foramen of Monro so that it is necessary to tap both lateral ventricles for good visualization.

The classic finding with thalamic lesions is the triad of (1) elevation of one lateral ventricular floor, (2) contralateral displacement of the third ventricle, usually a curved shift, with narrowing to a slitlike passage, and (3) outward displacement of the ipsilateral temporal horn. With corpus callosum tumors the roofs of both lateral ventricles are locally deformed as well as generally depressed. One ventricle is almost always affected more than the other, as seen in frontal view, where the slope of the roof is reduced and the ventricular angles are narrowed. Extension of the lesion into the septum pellucidum is very common; this is usually best appreciated in frontal view where the shadow of the septum is widened, often in an asymmetrical manner.

Figure 88.—Thalamic glioma.

A 66-year-old man had mental deterioration for three months. On examination he was disoriented as to place and time and showed a gross deficit in recent and remote memory. Extinction to touch was found consistently on the left. Position and vibratory senses were decreased in the left hand. The cerebrospinal fluid was normal except for a protein content of 57 mg per 100 cc.

A, right carotid angiogram with left-sided compression, frontal view, arterial phase: A slight shift of the anterior cerebral artery, right to left, is evident. There is mild lateral displacement of both lenticulostriate groups (**arrows**) and the insular loops of both middle cerebral branches, presumably secondary to hydrocephalus.

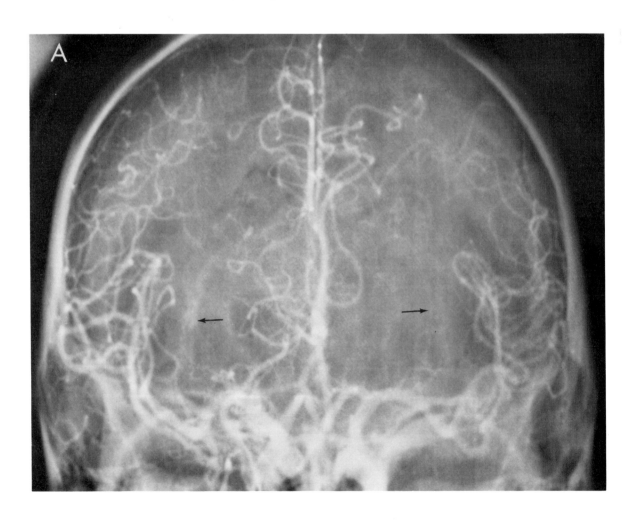

B, right carotid angiogram, lateral view, arterial phase: The pericallosal sweep is widened because of hydrocephalus. The lateral posterior choroidal artery is displaced backward (**a**), and an area of neovascularity (**b**) is seen anterior to the choroidal branches.

(Continued.)

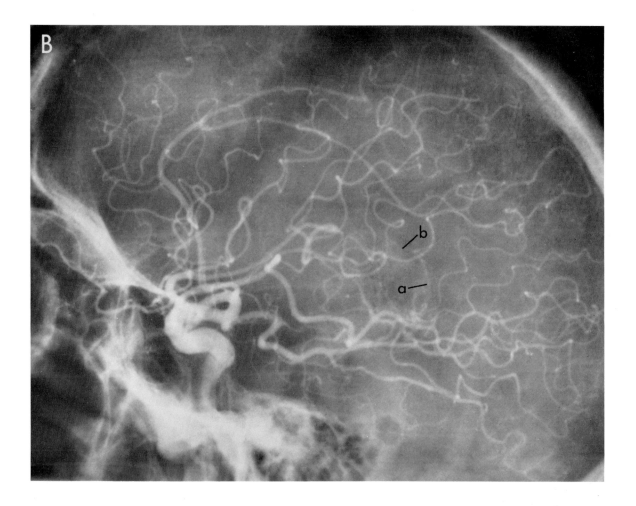

Figure 88 · Thalamic Glioma / 253

Figure 88 (cont.).—Thalamic glioma.

C, right carotid angiogram, frontal view, venous phase: The thalamo-striate veins outline greatly enlarged ventricles (**c**). Both internal cerebral veins are filled and are displaced right to left (**d**). The right internal cerebral vein is higher than the left. The posterior portions of the internal cerebral veins (**e**) are displaced to a greater extent than the anterior portions. Farther posteriorly the veins come to the midline, where they join to form the vein of Galen (**f**). A local mass effect elevates the right atrial vein medially and laterally (**g**).

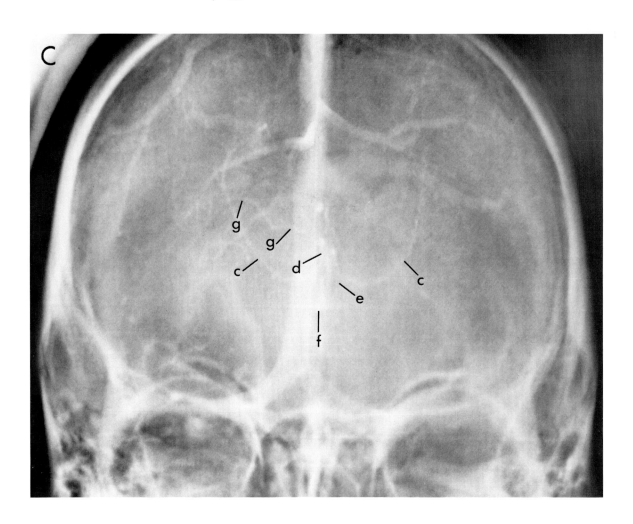

D, right carotid angiogram with cross-compression, lateral view, venous phase: The subependymal tributaries (**h**) to the internal cerebral veins outline the enlarged ventricles. One internal cerebral vein is higher than the other; both are displaced upward by the thalamic tumor.

(Continued.)

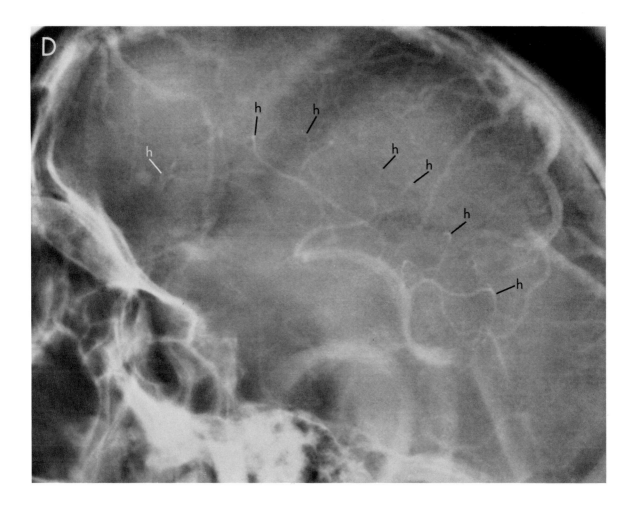

Figure 88 · Thalamic Glioma / 255

Figure 88 (cont.).—Thalamic glioma.

E, pneumoencephalogram, lateral view, filling position, autotomogram: A portion of the posterior part of the third ventricle in front of the supra-pineal recess is not clearly outlined because of compression of its side wall by the thalamic tumor. Both the third ventricle and the aqueduct appear out of focus in comparison with the fourth ventricle, because of displacement from the midline.

F, pneumoencephalogram, posteroanterior view, filling position: The third ventricle and aqueduct are displaced to the left by the tumor, which makes a concave impression upon the right side of the third ventricle. The more caudal portions of the brain stem are also tilted, as evident from the

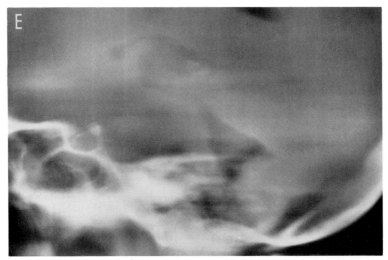

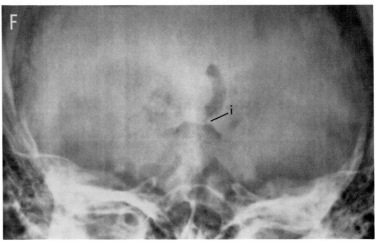

downward displacement of the left side of the superior medullary velum of the fourth ventricular roof (**i**).

G, pneumoencephalogram, posteroanterior view, brow-down position: Extension of the thalamic mass into the right atrium (**j**) is demonstrated. The relative lack of distortion of the perimesencephalic cisterns is due to the fact that only the infratentorial portions of the cisterns are filled. Compression of the right retropulvinar cistern (**k**) is evident, however.

H, pneumoencephalogram, lateral view, erect position: The thalamic mass expands and elevates the floor of the body of the lateral ventricle (**arrows**). The second lobular density seen above the tumor impression represents normal choroid.

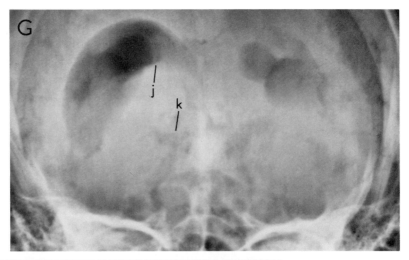

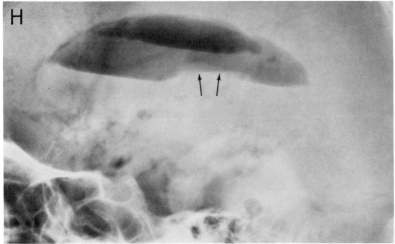

Figure 88 · Thalamic Glioma / 257

Figure 89.—Thalamic tumor with temporal extension.

A 60-year-old man had a left mastectomy and postoperative radiotherapy for a carcinoma three years previously. For a year he had had progressive left-sided motor and sensory impairment which had become worse in the past month. Examination revealed left hemiparesis and hyperreflexia, pronounced left-sided sensory deficit and left homonymous hemianopia.

A, right brachial angiogram, modified Towne projection, arterial phase: There is slight distal shift of the anterior cerebral artery. The right posterior cerebral artery (**a**) is displaced medially and its lateral posterior choroidal branch (**b**) is displaced laterally. The angiographic Sylvian point on the right is elevated as compared with the left.

B, right brachial angiogram, lateral view, arterial phase: The posterior portion of the base of the Sylvian triangle is elevated. Some straightening of the posterior temporal branches (**c**) is evident. One posterior cerebral artery and one posterior communicating vessel are depressed. The lateral posterior choroidal branch is elongated and displaced backward (**b**).

(*Continued.*)

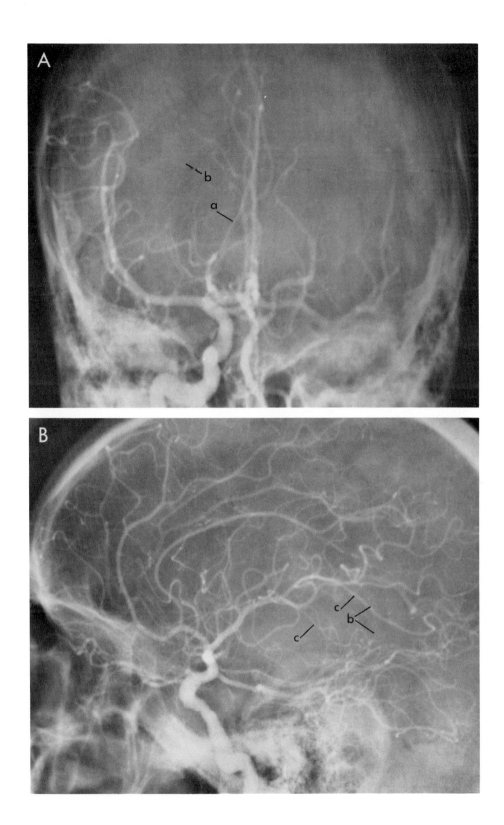

Figure 89 · Thalamic Tumor / 259

Figure 89 (cont.).—Thalamic tumor with temporal extension.

C, brachial angiogram, frontal view, venous phase: The internal cerebral vein is shifted to the left. The thalamostriate vein (**d**) is displaced upward and medially.

D, brachial angiogram, lateral view, venous phase: The basal vein of Rosenthal (**e**) and a temporal horn vein (**f**) which is superimposed on it are slightly depressed. A subependymal vein running forward along the body of the lateral ventricle from the atrial region is elevated (**g**).

The patient received radiation therapy and regained considerable strength of his left arm and leg. Eight months later he was able to walk with a cane.

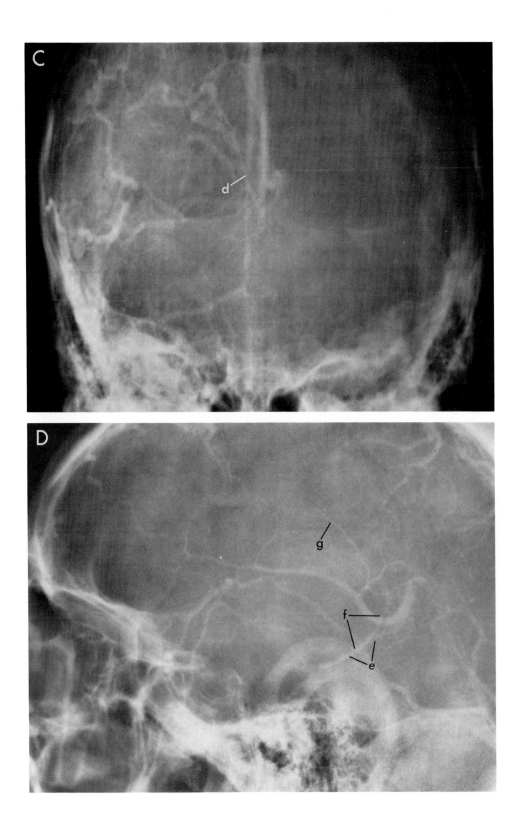

Figure 89 · Thalamic Tumor / 261

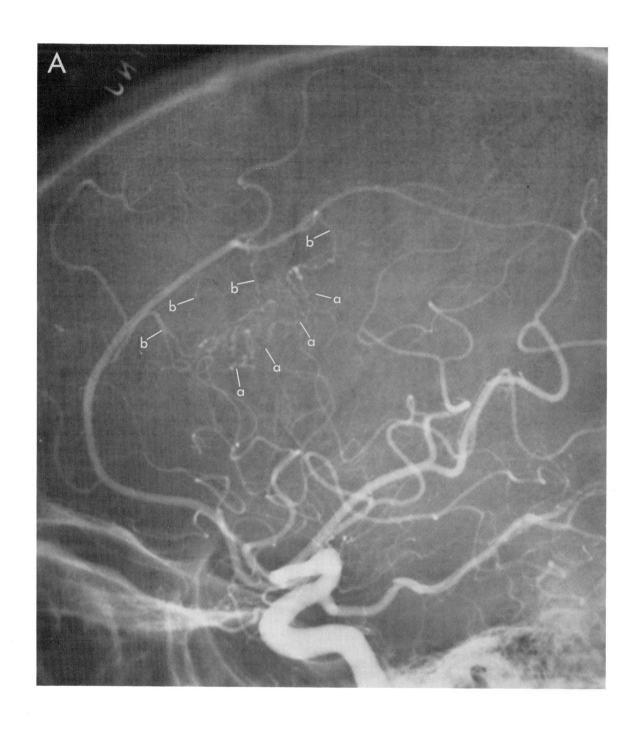

Figure 90.—Corpus callosum glioblastoma.

A 54-year-old woman manifested peculiar behavior for six days preceding hospitalization. She was disoriented as to place and showed impairment in calculations and recent memory. Results of the neurologic examination were otherwise essentially uninformative. The plain skull radiographs were normal. A brain scan showed an uptake in the deep left frontal region with possible extension to the opposite side.

A, left carotid angiogram, lateral view, arterial phase: There is elevation of the pericallosal artery, but the Sylvian triangle is only minimally disrupted. Many fine vessels project between the Sylvian triangle and the pericallosal artery (**a**). The area of neovascularity is supplied by enlarged branches of the pericallosal artery extending downward (**b**). Normally, such branches directed down toward the corpus callosum are not demonstrated.

B, left carotid angiogram, frontal projection, arterial phase: There is bowing of the midportion of the anterior cerebral artery. The Sylvian vessels are normal in appearance. The parasagittal tumor vessels (**a**) and feeding arteries (**b**) are evident on both sides of the midline.

(Continued.)

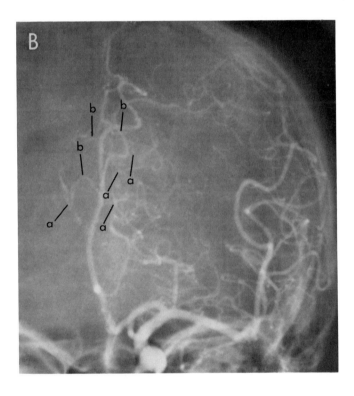

Figure 90 · Corpus Callosum Glioblastoma / 263

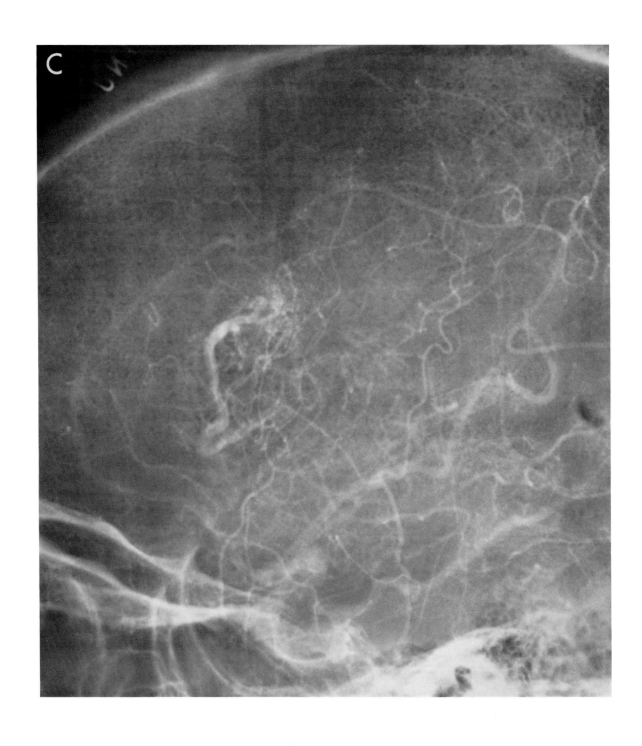

Figure 90 (cont.).—Corpus callosum glioblastoma.

C, left carotid angiogram, lateral view 2½ seconds after beginning of the injection: There is early filling of a deep vein arising from the area of hypervascularity.

D, left carotid angiogram, lateral view 4 seconds after start of the injection: The early vein is draining deeply into the anterior caudate vein (**c**) and internal cerebral vein (**d**). The venous angle (**e**) between the thalamostriate vein and the internal cerebral vein is closed, indicating downward displacement of the thalamostriate vein.

(Continued.)

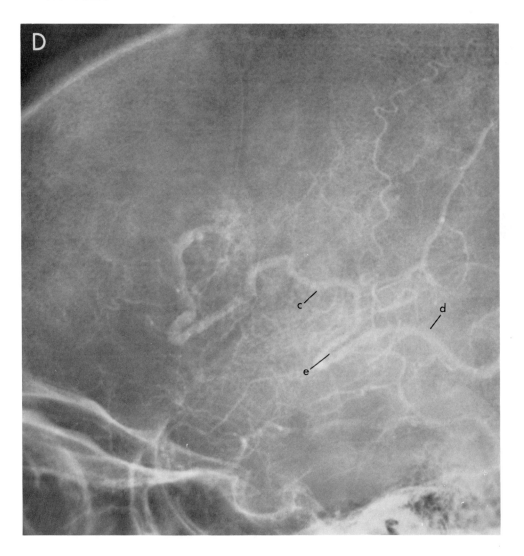

Figure 90 · Corpus Callosum Glioblastoma / 265

Figure 90 (cont.).—Corpus callosum glioblastoma.

E, left carotid angiogram, lateral view 6 seconds after start of the injection: The large draining veins have now disappeared and the septal vein (**f**) is well outlined. The septal vein is moderately depressed as well as the anterior aspect of the internal cerebral vein (**d**) in the region of the foramen of Monro, which is displaced slightly backward. The depression of the ventricular cast as outlined by the subependymal veins (**g**) is greatest in the regions of the frontal horn and body of the left lateral ventricle.

The patient deteriorated rapidly and died before completion of a course of radiation therapy.

Comment: The findings are those of a centrally placed malignant tumor, with circulation typical of malignant neoplasms. The elevation of the pericallosal artery and depression of the thalamostriate and internal cerebral veins suggest that the tumor either arose in or was invading the corpus callosum.

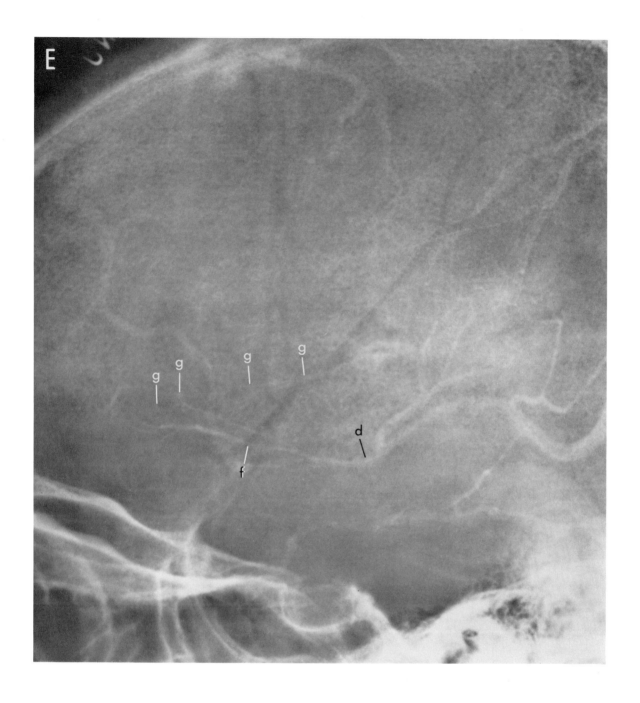

Figure 90 · Corpus Callosum Glioblastoma / 267

Figure 91.—Glioblastoma of corpus callosum.

A 59-year-old man had a three-week history of forgetfulness with increasing depression and lethargy. One week before hospitalization he became unsteady on his feet and for two days vomited intermittently and complained of diffuse headache. On examination, he was slow and apathetic. There was early papilledema. Diffuse weakness and truncal ataxia were present.

A, right brachial angiogram, frontal view, arterial phase: There is a very slight shift of the anterior cerebral artery toward the side of injection. No tumor stain is seen. The lenticulostriate and middle cerebral vessels are normal.

B, right brachial angiogram, lateral view, arterial phase: The middle and posterior cerebral vessels are normal. There are elevation and widening of the sweep of the anterior cerebral artery (**a**), but no tumor vessels are seen.

C, right brachial angiogram, frontal view, venous phase: The internal cerebral vein is displaced very slightly to the right (**b**). The thalamostriate vein (**c**) outlines a slightly widened lateral ventricle but does not extend upward in keeping with the markedly increased sweep of the anterior cerebral artery.

(*Continued.*)

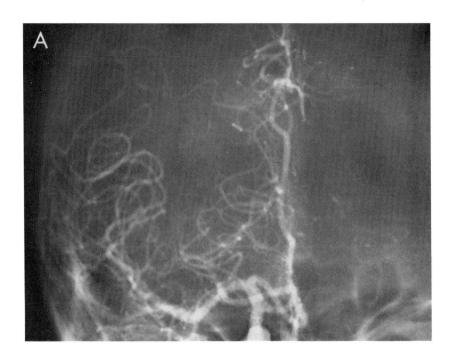

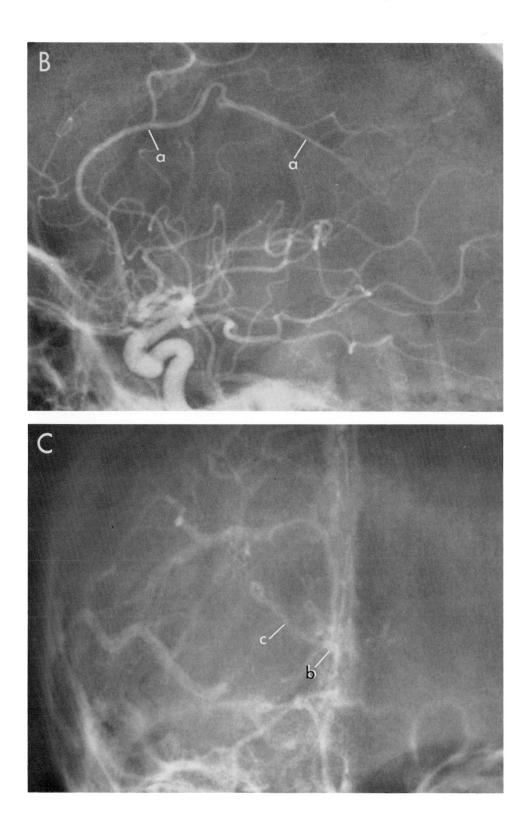

Figure 91 · Corpus Callosum Glioblastoma / 269

Figure 91 (cont.).—Glioblastoma of corpus callosum.

D, right brachial angiogram, lateral view, venous phase: The internal cerebral vein (**b**) is displaced downward and conspicuously flattened. The thalamostriate vein (**c**), with its large posterior thalamic tributary (**d**), outlines a ventricle which is much smaller than suggested by the wide sweep of the anterior cerebral artery. The compression and downward displacement of the internal cerebral vein connote involvement of the septum pellucidum.

E, combined ventriculogram-pneumoencephalogram, posteroanterior projection after injection of 20 cc of gas, upright position: The upper portions of the lateral and third ventricles are filled. The septum pellucidum is displaced to the right. The roof of the left lateral ventricle is flattened, and the roof on each side has an irregular nodular contour (**e**). An abnormal collection of subarachnoid gas (**f**) partially outlines the superior surface of the mass on the left.

The patient was given radiation therapy to a dosage of 5000 rads in a five-week period, but he died four months after he was first seen.

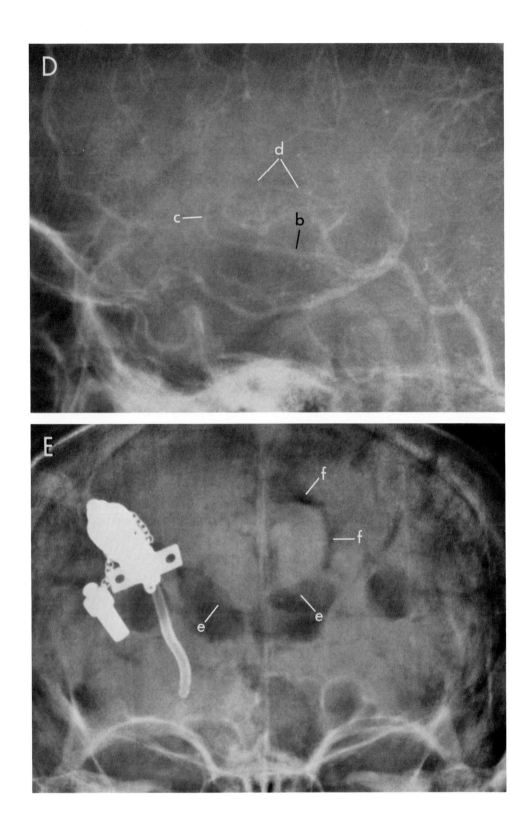

Figure 91 · Corpus Callosum Glioblastoma / 271

PART 10

Intraventricular Tumors

Characteristics and Demonstration

PATIENTS WITH INTRAVENTRICULAR MASSES often present a stuttering progressive course. The reason for this is the benign or well-differentiated nature of many tumors. Because of the slow growth, the ventricle is able to enlarge and accommodate the lesion so that it is not perpetually obstructed.

In the lateral ventricles, the more benign lesions such as meningiomas, cholesteatomas and choroid plexus papillomas, are found in the region of the atrium. The more invasive lesions are usually found farther forward in the ventricular lumen; they include the septal oligodendrogliomas and the astrocytomas. In addition to epidermoidomas, other congenital tumors may be found in the lateral ventricles, such as a ganglioglioma associated with tuberous sclerosis. Some of the choroid papillomas may be aggressive and some of the meningiomas sarcomatous.

Angiographic delineation of the lesion is important for two reasons. One is for primary diagnosis, and the second is to give the surgeon a vascular roadmap for his extensive dissection into the ventricle. Pneumoencephalography and ventriculography are the definitive methods of completely outlining intraventricular masses.

The angiographic characteristics of intraventricular lesions, when present, are related to the choroidal vessels. Therefore both the anterior choroidal artery from the carotid system and the posterior choroidal vessels of the vertebral-basilar system must be opacified, often bilaterally. The lenticulostriate vessels may also provide blood supply to an intraventricular lesion. Good localizing findings may be obtained from the venous phase of the angiogram, by which local deformity and enlargement of the ventricles can be diagnosed by the appearance of the subependymal veins and the course of the internal cerebral veins. The internal cerebral veins coursing in the third ventricular roof undergo characteristic deformities anteriorly with a colloid cyst and posteriorly with a typical pineal tumor. The choroidal veins give a good outline of the posterior portions of the third ventricle but do not reach forward beyond the foramen of Monro.

Although the pinealomas and teratomas of the posterior third ventricular area are usually thought of as extra-axial, they do invaginate and locally invade the ventricle. This is particularly true of teratomas, which may even extend forward into the anterior third ventricle. The posterior third ventricular tumors may be manifested clinically in a variety of ways, with precocious puberty, Parinaud's syndrome or only with symptoms and signs of obstructive hydrocephalus.

The course of the posterior portion of the internal cerebral vein is just above the pineal gland; it is often locally elevated in spite of the hydrocephalus which develops. However, some posterior third ventricular tumors may displace the posterior portion of the internal cerebral vein forward. One reason is that the lesions may be horseshoe-shaped and extend around the internal cerebral vein. In other cases a pinealoma may grow predominantly backward into the quadrigeminal cistern, gaining a position behind or above the great vein of Galen and its internal cerebral tributary. In still other instances the tumor is a glioma which has grown into the pineal region from behind. In addition to a local deformity of the internal cerebral vein, the medial choroidal (and sometimes the lateral choroidal) vessels exhibit mass effects secondary to a tumor in the posterior third ventricular region. When the lesion is vascular the choroidal vessels are significant contributors of the blood supply. The geniculate arteries supply the large pineal tumors, and the perforating thalamic vessels may be enlarged, straightened and displaced forward with the large tumors.

Because of the propensity of pineal lesions to grow infratentorially and particularly into the medullary precentral recess of the quadrigeminal cistern and to displace the brain stem forward, vertebral angiography may be very helpful in diagnosis. The precentral cerebellar vein is usually displaced downward and backward. The midbrain is outlined by the lateral mesencephalic and the anterior pontomesencephalic veins, which are pushed forward by the enlarging tumor. Tumors of the fourth ventricle are relatively common and many are of tissue types frequently seen in the lateral ventricles. Fourth ventricular tumors are presented in Part 11 along with intra-axial posterior fossa neoplasms.

Figure 92.—Oligodendroglioma of the septum pellucidum.

A 38-year-old man had experienced headache about once a month (lasting from one-half to two days and associated with nausea, vomiting and dizziness) since childhood. During the month before hospitalization the symptoms increased in severity and frequency, occurring almost daily. The neurologic examination revealed no abnormality. At lumbar puncture the opening pressure was 260 mm H_2O and the closing pressure was 135 mm H_2O. Cerebrospinal fluid protein content was normal.

A, routine skull radiograph, Caldwell projection: A quadrilateral mass (**x**) of fairly homogeneous calcification is projected through the upper part of the left frontal sinus. The greatest portion of the calcification is left parasagittal, but a small part extends across the midline to the right.

B, lateral view: The calcification is projected above the sella turcica and in the coronal plane of the dorsum sellae. It has a coarsely lobulated configuration in this projection. There is demineralization only of the base of the anterior wall of the dorsum sellae to suggest increased intracranial pressure.

(*Continued.*)

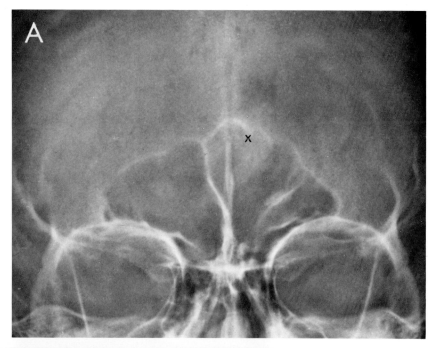

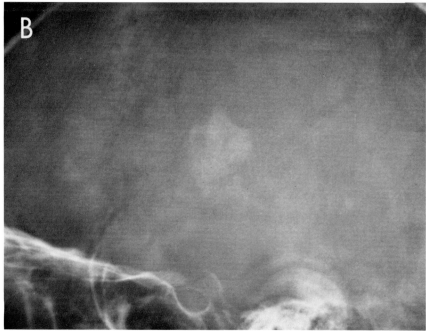

Figure 92 · Oligodendroglioma / 277

Figure 92 (cont.).—Oligodendroglioma of the septum pellucidum.

C, left carotid angiogram, standard frontal projection, arterial phase: There is a slight tilt toward the right of both anterior cerebral arteries, the right being filled spontaneously. The lenticulostriate vessels (**a**) are displaced laterally. No abnormal branches are seen in the region of the calcified mass.

D, left carotid angiogram, lateral view, exposed simultaneously with **C:** There is widening of the arc of the pericallosal arteries. No other definite abnormality is demonstrated.

E, venogram, frontal view, sequent to **C:** The thalamostriate vein (**b**) is stretched beneath the ependyma of an enlarged left lateral ventricle in the plane of the tumor. An anomalous medial tributary of the septal vein (**c**) extends vertically, apparently in a displaced septum pellucidum. The internal cerebral vein gradually returns to the midline posteriorly (**d**).

(Continued.)

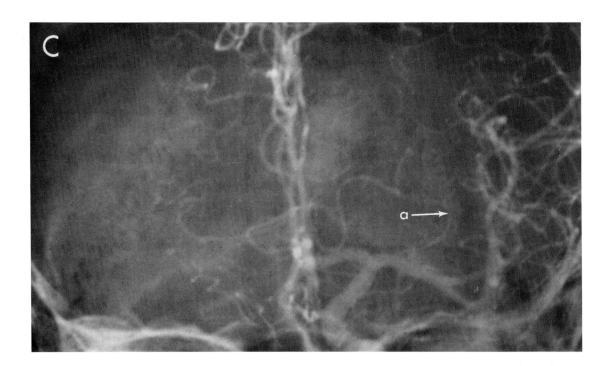

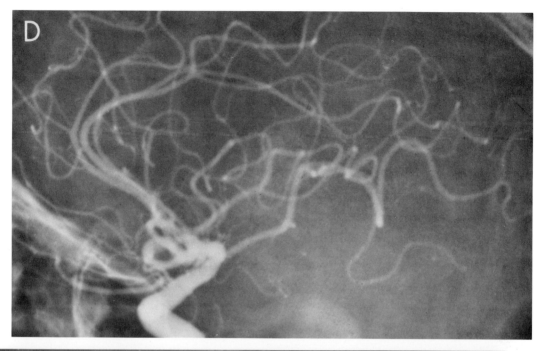

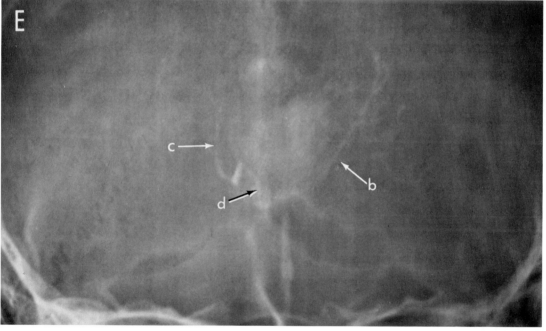

Figure 92 · Oligodendroglioma / 279

Figure 92 (cont.).—Oligodendroglioma of the septum pellucidum.

F, venogram, lateral view, succeeding **D:** The subependymal veins (**e**) form an enlarged ventricular cast. At the level of the calcified tumor the subependymal veins are even more stretched, and the thalamostriate vein (**b**) is locally narrowed at the foramen of Monro.

G, ventriculogram after displacement of fluid by gas on the left side only, posteroanterior projection, brow-up position: The calcified tumor (**x**) lies in the ventricular lumen and is surrounded by gas on all except its medial side. The anterior part of the dilated left lateral ventricle has herniated beneath the falx into the right side of the cranial cavity.

H, ventriculogram, lateral view, matching **G:** Most of the left ventricular gas is anterior to the tumor, and the rostral margin of the lesion is sharply outlined because of its direct contact with the air. A small amount of gas is present along the floor of the ventricular body beneath the mass (**x**). Some air is trapped in the left temporal horn, but no gas entered the third ventricle because of obstruction of the foramen of Monro by the neoplasm.

A diagnosis of oligodendroglioma was made because of the intraventricular position of the tumor based on the septum pellucidum and because it was largely calcified. At operation, gross total removal of the neoplasm was accomplished; the lateral ventricles were left in free communication through the resultant defect in the septum pellucidum. Two years after operation the patient was asymptomatic.

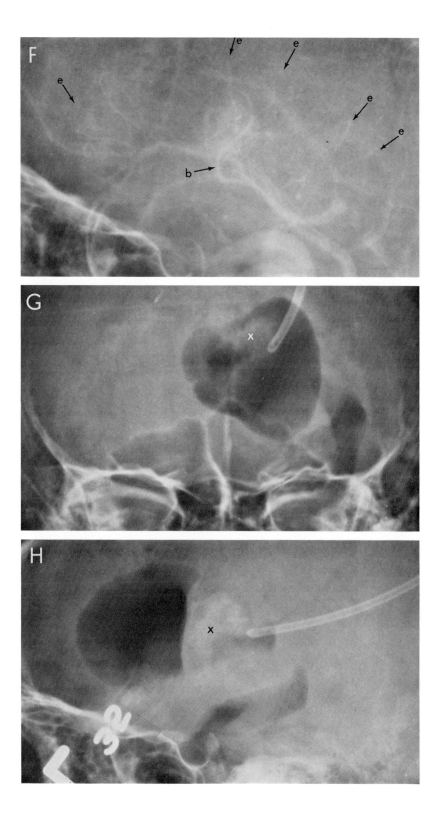

Figure 92 · Oligodendroglioma / 281

Figure 93.—Intraventricular oligodendroglioma.

A 57-year-old woman had a history of an organic mental syndrome for two to three months. She was disoriented, confused and had an ataxic gait that was thought to be hysterical. The gait was described as a listing to the right with moderately short, quick forward steps. Occasionally she took numerous short steps backward in an uncontrollable manner, then fell softly to the floor. The neurologic examination was otherwise uninformative. Cerebrospinal fluid protein content was 77 mg per 100 cc. There was a prominent slow wave focus bifrontally on electroencephalography. The radionuclide brain scan revealed a large frontal collection deeply situated and larger on the right than on the left.

A, right brachial angiogram, frontal projection, arterial phase: The anterior cerebral artery is in the midline. There is slight lateral displacement of the lenticulostriate arteries (**a**) and of the insular loops of the middle cerebral group (**b**).

B, right brachial angiogram, lateral projection, arterial phase: The pericallosal artery is elevated and takes a locally irregular course just behind the plane of the coronal suture. Several unusual branches extend down from the pericallosal artery (**c**). There is downward displacement of the most anterior insular loop of the middle cerebral group.

C, venogram, frontal view, sequent to **A:** The internal cerebral vein, like the anterior cerebral artery, is not shifted from the midline. Its subependymal tributaries (**d**) outline an enlarged right lateral ventricle.

(*Continued.*)

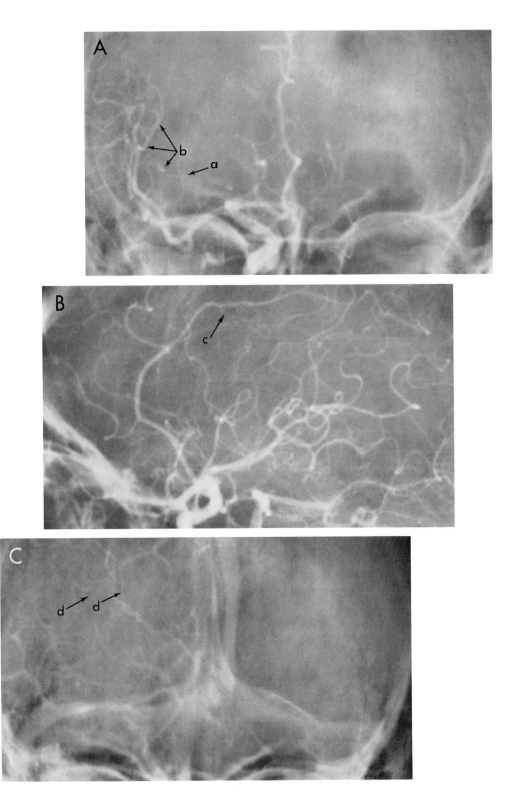

Figure 93 · Oligodendroglioma / 283

Figure 93 (cont.).—Intraventricular oligodendroglioma.

D, venogram, lateral view, succeeding **B:** There is marked flattening of the internal cerebral vein (**e**). The subependymal tributaries are elongated (**d**). There is a local mass effect with lifting and stretching of the subependymal branch coursing in a vertical direction above the foramen of Monro (**f**).

E, pneumoencephalogram, reverse Towne projection, brow-up position: Inasmuch as there was no clinical contraindication to pneumoencephalography, radiographs were made after the displacement of 40 cc of cerebrospinal fluid by gas on lumbar puncture. Air entered the ventricular system readily, and in the position illustrated it outlined the right lateral and third ventricles. The third ventricle is widened but remains in the midline. No gas entered the left lateral ventricle. A large lobulated tumor (**x**) is sharply outlined by the gas in the right lateral ventricle, which is present above, beneath and on the right side of the tumor, the mass apparently being based medially.

F, pneumogram, lateral view, matching **E:** The large irregular tumor (**x**) is situated above the foramen of Monro. It extends into the frontal horn and ventricular body, and cords of tumor also reach the ventricular roof (**f**). The roof of the third ventricle is shown to be conspicuously flattened by the tumor and hydrocephalus, recalling the markedly flattened internal cerebral vein illustrated in **D.** A large amount of gas has also entered the subarachnoid space and reveals atrophic gyri in the frontal regions.

At operation a large cauliflowerlike tumor was found, apparently arising from the septum pellucidum and extending through the septum into the left lateral ventricle. The lesion infiltrated the caudate nucleus, and these portions could not be removed. A large defect remained in the septum pellucidum, and a unilateral ventriculo-atrial shunt was inserted. The patient received postoperative radiation therapy and was greatly improved when last seen nine months after operation.

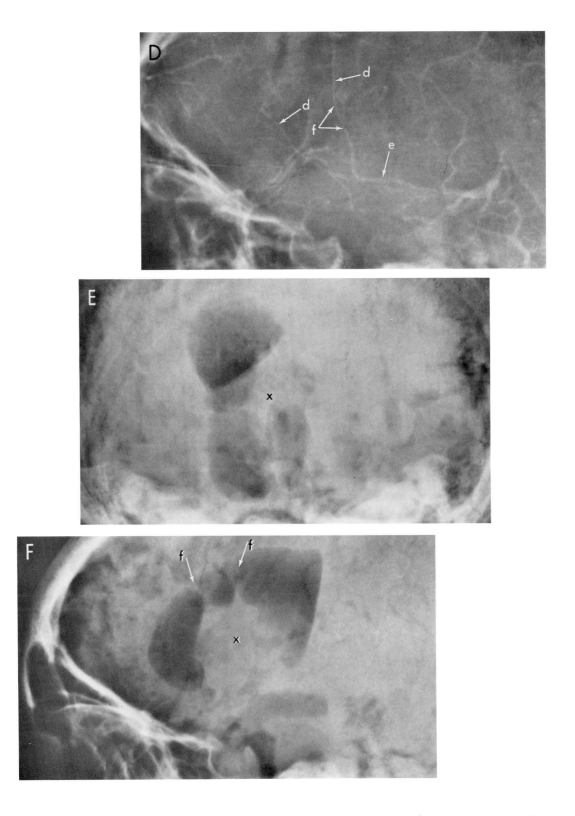

Figure 93 · Oligodendroglioma / 285

Figure 94.—Intraventricular ganglioglioma.

A 6-year-old boy known to have tuberous sclerosis, mental retardation and a seizure disorder was admitted because of vision loss. Typical lesions of tuberous sclerosis were seen on the face and on ophthalmoscopic examination. Papilledema was also observed.

A, ventriculogram, reverse Towne projection, brow-up position: The right frontal horn and ventricular body are greatly dilated. A large mass extends into the ventricular lumen from the medial wall of the ventricle. There is a shift of the medial ventricular wall to the right, especially its upper end, constituting an angular shift. Gas enters the third ventricle from the right side, but there is a block of the left side of the foramen of Monro. Apparently the tumor is larger on the left than on the right, or the left lateral ventricle is much larger, to account for the striking angular shift. Nodular deposits of calcium are present within the mass and along the margins of the tumor. There is also a calcified nodule along the lateral wall of the ventricle opposite the tumor (**arrow**).

B, ventriculogram, lateral view, matching **A:** The even, marked ventricular dilatation involving the body and anterior horn is again demonstrated. In this view the tumor appears to lie chiefly along the ventricular floor, extending upward into the lumen of the frontal horn and ventricular body. Numerous grossly nodular calcifications are superimposed on the shadow of the tumor. The anterior wall of the third ventricle is deformed by the downward extension of the neoplasm. The marked widening of the coronal suture seen here was also visible in frontal view.

Because of the well-known association of tuberous sclerosis and intraventricular tumors composed of glial and mature ganglion cells, a diagnosis of ganglioglioma was made, and this was confirmed by biopsy. A ventriculo-atrial shunting procedure was then carried out, following which there was recession of the papilledema and suture diastasis.

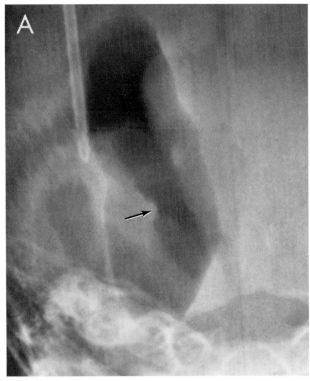

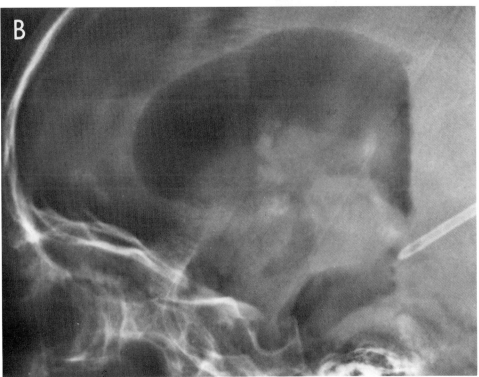

Figure 94 · Ganglioglioma / 287

Figure 95.—Colloid cyst of the third ventricle.

A 53-year-old man had a 15-year history of seizures that usually began in the right arm. He did not complain of headache until one week before hospitalization when severe occipital headache began. On examination he was confused and disoriented and had a very short attention span. Generalized hyperreflexia was demonstrated. No papilledema was found.

A, left carotid angiogram, lateral view, venous phase: The subependymal veins delineate marked hydrocephalus (**a**). In the region of the foramen of Monro and just behind the venous angle there is localized elevation of the internal cerebral vein (**b**). The vein appears to be thin and stretched as it descends (**c**) to a normal level in the roof of the third ventricle and enters the vein of Galen. The sella turcica exhibits demineralization of the cortex of the dorsum and sellar floor.

B, ventriculogram, lateral autotomogram, hanging-head position: After the replacement of 40 cc of ventricular fluid by gas, the major portion has collected in the dilated anterior horns and rostral parts of the ventricular bodies with the head dependent. A smooth mass is present in the foramen of Monro bulging into the lateral ventricles, where its surface is well defined by gas in contact with the lesion. In this position a channel is present between the lateral and third ventricles anterior to the cyst, allowing filling of the third ventricle, which is not dilated.

A right frontal craniotomy was performed and the right lateral ventricle entered through a transcortical incision. A large bluish gray mass was seen in the region of the foramen of Monro bulging into the right lateral ventricle. Approximate diameter was 2 cm. The cyst was removed without difficulty, leaving a wide opening between the lateral and the third ventricles. The mental disturbance, headache and seizures progressively diminished, and 3 years after removal of the cyst he was normal.

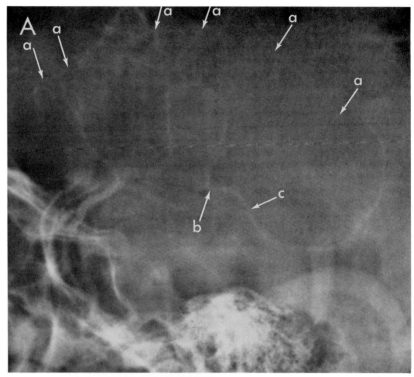

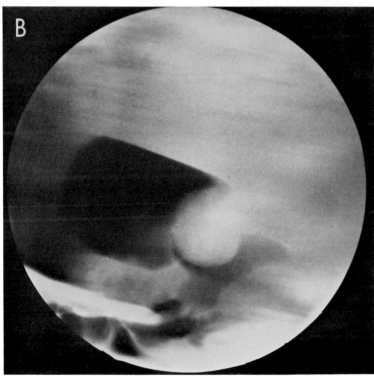

Figure 95 · Colloid Cyst / 289

Figure 96.—Pinealoma.

A 17-year-old boy complained of intermittent headache for several months prior to the onset of persistent and severe headache, vomiting and obtundation that led to hospitalization. He was lethargic, had a stiff neck and papilledema, and there was some fluctuation in pupillary size. Right superior quadrantanopia was elicited. Generalized hyperreflexia was present, with ankle clonus.

Routine skull radiographs revealed a heavily calcified pineal which measured 12 mm in diameter (well shown in **I** and **J**). The center of the pineal gland was 7 mm to the right of the midline, and in lateral views it was displaced far downward and forward. Some atrophy of the cortex of the anterior wall of the dorsum sellae was present, but there was not the pronounced erosion of the top of the dorsum commonly seen with enlargement of the anterior part of the third ventricle.

A, left carotid angiogram, frontal projection, arterial phase: A large medial tentorial artery (**a**) outlines the free edge of the tentorium and extends to the tentorial apex. The anterior cerebral artery is in the midline. Lateral displacement of the lenticulostriate vessels (**b**) suggests ventricular enlargement.

B, left carotid angiogram, lateral view, arterial phase: The medial tentorial artery is shown arising from the cavernous portion of the internal carotid artery. The position of the left tentorial leaf outlined by the artery (**arrows**) indicates its low placement. The anterior cerebral artery describes a wide arc, indicating hydrocephalus. No localized mass effect can be made out among the branches of the middle cerebral artery.

(*Continued.*)

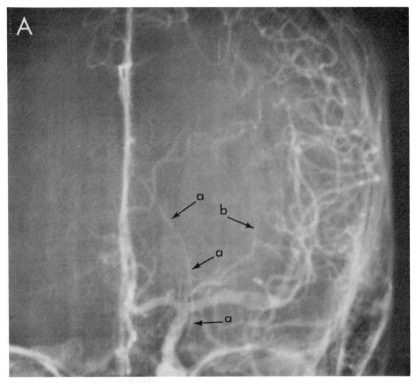

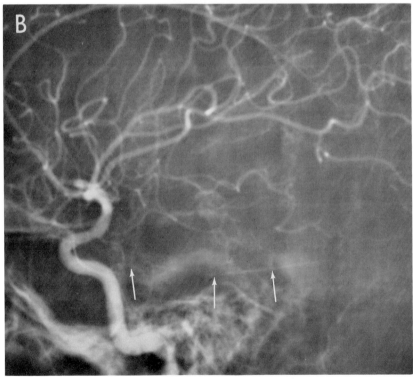

Figure 96 · Pinealoma / 291

Figure 96 (cont.).—Pinealoma.

C, left carotid angiogram, frontal view, venous phase: An enlarged medial atrial vein (**c**) is sharply displaced to the right. The basal vein of Rosenthal (**d**) is straightened and displaced medially in its distal portion. The thalamostriate vein (**e**) is elongated and at a low angle, indicating marked lateral ventricular enlargement on the left.

D, left carotid angiogram, lateral view, venous phase: Marked forward and downward displacement of the posterior part of the internal cerebral vein (**f**) is present. There is also a local mass effect on the medial atrial vein (**c**), which follows an angular course as it extends over the tumor.

(*Continued.*)

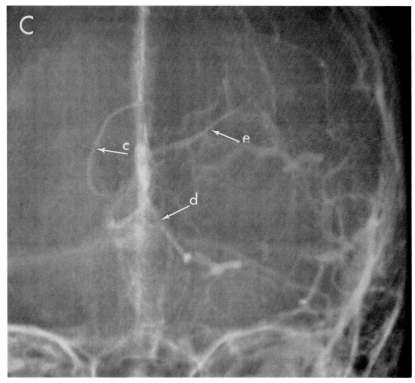

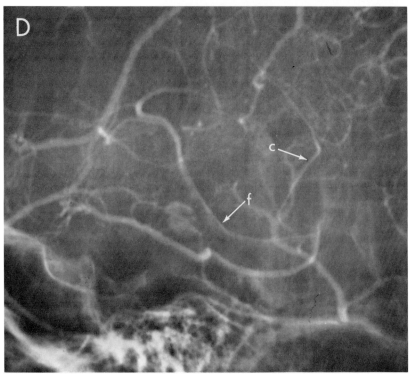

Figure 96 · Pinealoma / 293

Figure 96 (cont.).—Pinealoma.

E, left brachial angiogram, Towne projection, arterial phase: The superior vermian branches (**g**) of the superior cerebellar arteries are widely separated because of infratentorial extension of the tumor posteriorly through the incisural apex. There is also widening of the space between the posterior cerebral arteries (**h**) produced by the supratentorial mass. A mass effect and lateral displacement of the calcarine (**i**) and parieto-occipital branches (**j**) are also evident.

F, left brachial angiogram, lateral projection, arterial phase: The perforating thalamic arteries (**k**) are stretched and displaced forward. The medial and lateral choroidal arteries (**l**) are also displaced forward. The proximal portions of the posterior cerebral arteries are stretched, and numerous branches exhibit local deformities. The superior cerebellar artery, as it begins its ascent toward the culmen of the upper vermis, is locally deformed and displaced downward (**g**). The top of the basilar artery is low, and the vessel is closer than usual to the clivus.

G, left brachial angiogram, Towne projection, venous phase: The perimesencephalic veins (**m**) are separated, and an ill-defined tumor stain is present in the midline.

H, left brachial angiogram, lateral view, venous phase: The medial and lateral choroidal veins (**n**) are markedly deformed, being displaced forward and downward. The precentral vein (**o**) is straightened and displaced downward and backward. The lateral mesencephalic vein (**p**) is displaced forward to a marked degree and the anterior pontomesencephalic vein (**q**) is forward, these changes resulting from tumor extension in front of the upper vermis and behind the midbrain.

(Continued.)

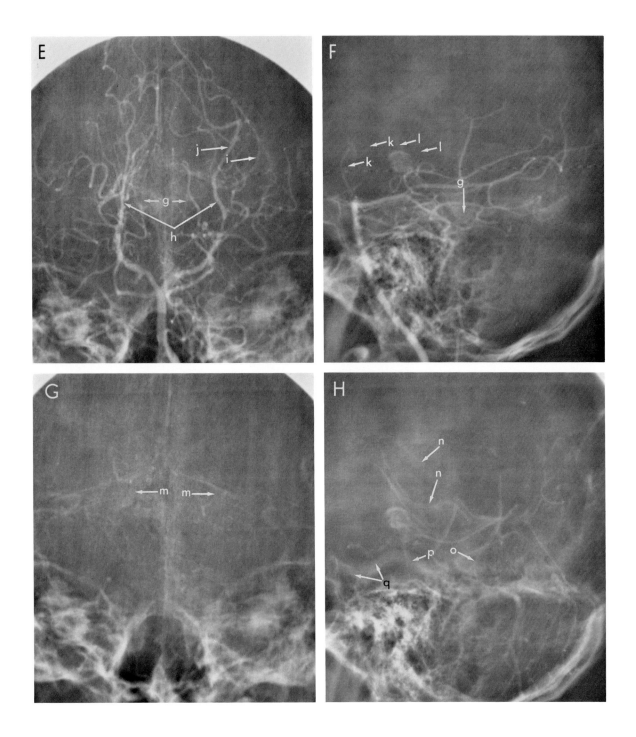

Figure 96 · Pinealoma / 295

Figure 96 (cont.).—Pinealoma.

I, pneumoencephalogram, upright position, reverse Towne projection: Ventricular filling was relatively poor. Some gas that reached the lateral ventricles shows the extent of hydrocephalus. There was also an uneven distribution of gas in the subarachnoid space outlining the Sylvian fissure on the left, a few medial and lateral sulci, but partially outlining the tumor along its inferior and right lateral margins (**r**).

J, lateral autotomogram, filling position: Air that reached the quadrigeminal cistern partially outlines the tumor, as does the retropulvinar collection. The calcified portion of the pineal is shown to be in the lower anterior part of the mass.

Through a transcortical incision the left lateral ventricle was opened. A large soft tumor bulged into the atrium but was covered by ependyma. By cautery, a large grayish necrotic tumor was entered. In the depths of the lesion a large amount of old dark blood filled a 40 cc cavity, indicating hemorrhage within the mass. After further removal of tumor by suction and cautery, it was possible to see pia-lined brain at the margins of the cavity, indicating that the tumor was essentially *extracerebral*. On pathologic examination the cellular structure was that of pineal glia.

After radiotherapy consisting of 5,000 rads the patient did very well for a year. Then multifocal neurologic deficits developed, including back pain and pain and paresthesias of the left lower extremity. A radioactive nuclide brain scan suggested recurrence of the tumor, smaller than before, at the original site. A myelogram revealed a block at L-1/L-2 with multiple filling defects in the Pantopaque outline, indicating spinal metastases. He again responded well to radiation to the head and spine but died 1½ years later.

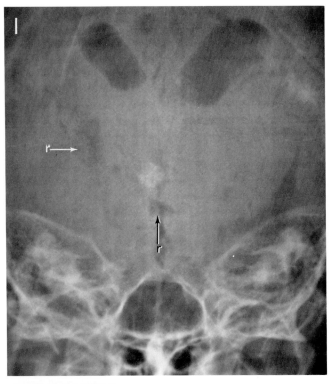

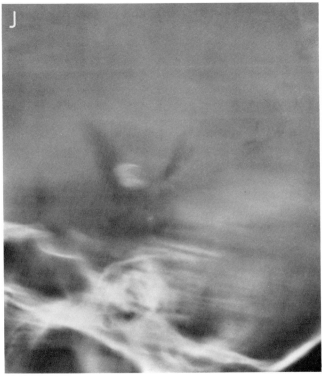

Figure 96 · Pinealoma / 297

Figure 97.—Pinealoma.

A 34-year-old man had a history of frontal headache of increasing severity for a year. For 10 months he noted awkwardness progressing to poor coordination. Examination revealed papilledema, mild intention tremor and ataxia.

A, routine skull radiograph, lateral view: A cluster of calcium deposits of varying size is seen in the region of the pineal gland over an area that measured 1.0×1.5 cm. Advanced changes of increased intracranial pressure are present at the sella turcica, with complete absence of the dorsum sellae of the type seen with an enlarged third ventricle (see Fig. 13). Marked thinning of all cortical borders of the sella turcica is also shown.

B, autotomogram at ventriculography, lateral view, inverted position: A catheter was placed in the right lateral ventricle and 25 cc of ventricular fluid replaced by air. The patient was then taken through a partial backward somersault from brow-up position to upside down. A large amount of gas entered the greatly distended third ventricle. (Some gas is in the temporal horns and atrial areas partially superimposed on the third ventricle.) There was an obstruction at the outlet of the third ventricle, only a very small amount of air reaching the aqueduct and fourth ventricle. In the region of the pineal a fairly smooth mass is outlined projecting into the third ventricle just forward of the more rostral calcific shadows (**a**). A second lobule (**b**) without calcium is also shown ahead of the primary pineal mass; it extends as far forward as the massa intermedia. There is ballooning of the anterior part of the third ventricle into the sella turcica (**c**). A pressure diverticulum of the lamina terminalis is present (**d**).

C, reverse Towne projection, matching **B**: The greatly widened third ventricle is seen in frontal view. The anterior lobulation of the tumor extends along the floor and right wall of the ventricle (**x**) so that gas half-envelops the mass, accounting for its sharp delineation in the lateral view (**B**).

D, autotomogram, lateral view, filling position, made after additional injection of gas via the lumbar route: The fourth ventricle is foreshortened by pressure from above, and the slope of the anterior medullary velum is exaggerated. The aqueduct is displaced forward and downward and is kinked. The iter is locally indented beneath the center of the main pineal mass (**e**). No air entered the third ventricle from below.

The patient underwent a Torkildsen shunt and then received radiation therapy.

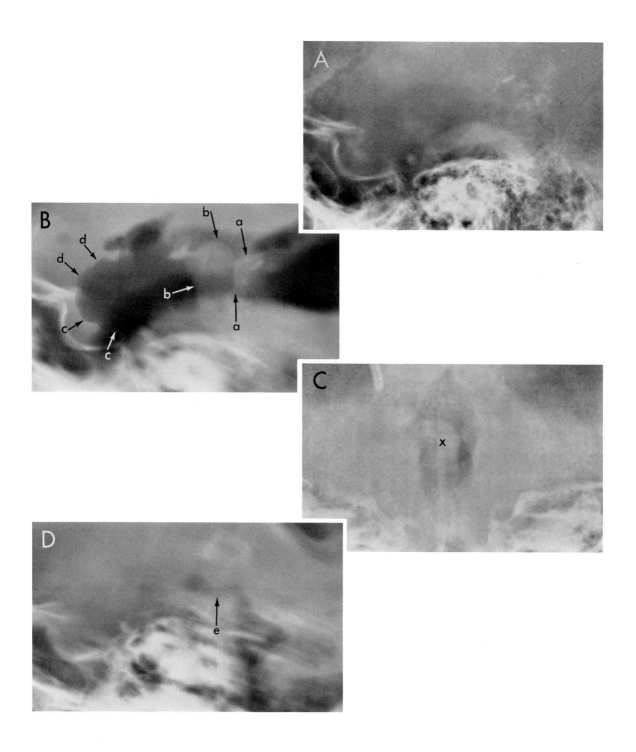

Figure 97 · Pinealoma / 299

PART 11

Intra-axial Posterior Fossa Tumors

Characteristics

The approach to posterior fossa neoplasms has changed in recent years in that the contrast procedure of choice is now angiography rather than pneumography as the primary study. The reason for this is twofold. First, a greater understanding of the normal and deranged anatomy has developed and, second, there have been technical advances in selective opacification of the vertebral arteries and the use of smaller focal spots for magnification serial radiography. From the surgical point of view the advanced knowledge of the relationship of a tumor to adjacent vascular structures is an obvious advantage. In addition, angiography will tell whether or not hydrocephalus and herniation are present, thereby indicating the danger or safety of subsequent pneumography and which route of air injection should be used.

A brain stem glioma usually produces a symmetrical enlargement of the brain stem. When the tumor is eccentric in its growth it has often spread laterally via the cerebellar peduncles. In eccentric cases, section of the brain stem at autopsy often shows that the border of the tumor stops sharply at the median raphe. The growth may become exophytic; although uncommon, this may be diagnosed angiographically because of the paradoxical backward displacement of the basilar artery, while the pontomesencephalic vein is brought forward with the tumor toward the clivus.

Approximately 75% of brain stem tumors occur in childhood and adolescence. The lesion may grow between neural structures without destruction, so that the signs are often the result of pressure phenomena with a patchy presentation of nuclear and tract deficits. Clinically, papilledema is a late development, although angiographically the finding of at least a mild degree of hydrocephalus is an expected occurrence.

The cerebellar astrocytoma has an age incidence similar to that of the brain stem glioma. It has a slightly higher occurrence rate in the hemispheres and has a definite tendency to be cystic. A surprisingly high percentage of the cerebellar astrocytomas have leptomeningeal involvement, but this apparently has little prognostic significance, as distant metastasis and multiplicity are not common.

In children, tumors within the fourth ventricle are of three types: medulloblastoma, ependymoma, and subependymal astrocytoma. A clinical and radiologic distinction may be made because of the rapid growth rate of medulloblastoma, producing acute increased intracranial pressure. Although subacute pressure changes may sometimes occur with medulloblastoma, this is more often found with the ependymoma. A medulloblastoma usually grows from the posterior fourth ventricular roof. Subependymal astrocytomas appear to have the slowest biologic growth rate, and some pathologists believe they may actually represent a form of hamartoma since the tumors are often of mixed cellular type, containing astrocytes and oligodendroglial cells. They usually arise along the fourth ventricular floor and grow posteriorly. Choroid plexus papillomas of the fourth ventricle (and occasionally arising from the choroid tissue of the lateral recesses and cerebellopontine angles) are tumors of adult life.

A hemangioblastoma usually arises adjacent to the midline, although any part of the cerebellum or vermis may be its site of origin. The tonsils and brain stem are infrequent areas in which a hemangioblastoma develops. The lower posterior portion of the medulla oblongata is an exception. There is a familial association with angiomatosis retinae, renal and pancreatic cysts, renal and adrenal neoplasms, polycythemia and pheochromocytoma.

Some downward displacement of the cerebellar tonsils is associated with a fairly high percentage of tumors of the cerebellum and a smaller percentage of tumors of the brain stem and extra-axial structures. Tonsillar herniation is discussed by Epstein in *The Vertebral Column* (An Atlas of Tumor Radiology, 1974).

Figure 98-1.—Brain stem glioma.

A 30-year-old man had had double vision for a month, and for two weeks, weakness of the left hand followed by weakness of the left leg. For several days he had a dull constant headache, primarily bifrontal, and for two days had a number of 5-min episodes of vertigo while walking. Funduscopic examination revealed no spontaneous venous pulsations. He had fine sustained nystagmus bilaterally on horizontal gaze. Eye movements showed incomplete abduction of the right. He had a decreased response to pinprick over the left side of the face and decreased sensation to light touch. Lower facial movement on the left was impaired. He had a decreased shoulder shrug on the left. Left hemiparesis was present. Reflexes were generally hyperactive bilaterally, with bilateral Hoffman and left Babinski responses. After diagnosis, steroid therapy was started, and a course of cobalt to 5000 rads to the entire brain stem.

A, right vertebral angiogram via femoral catheter, subtracted lateral view, arterial phase: There is reflux into the left vertebral artery. Both posterior inferior cerebellar arteries are thus filled and showing the choroidal points (**a**) to be displaced posteriorly. Very fine choroidal vessels outline the position of the choroidal loop. The basilar artery is displaced forward.

B, right vertebral angiogram, frontal view, with subtraction, arterial phase: There is separation of the superior cerebellar (**b**) and posterior cerebral (**c**) arteries as they course around the midbrain. There appears to be attenuation of the superior cerebellar arteries in their perimesencephalic course, particularly on the right.

C, right vertebral angiogram, lateral view with subtraction, venous phase: The pontomesencephalic vein (**d**) is displaced forward and the distance between it and the precentral vein (**e**) is increased. However, there appears to be preservation of the relationship between the lateral mesencephalic (**f**) and precentral veins. This means that there is no gross involvement of the tectum and tegmentum of the midbrain although there is expansion more anteriorly.

(Continued.)

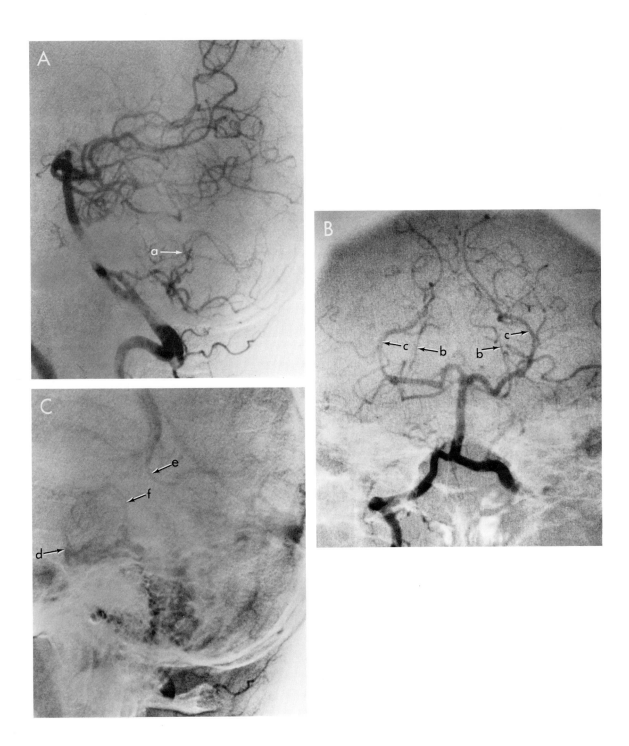

Figure 98-1 · Brain Stem Glioma / 305

Figure 98-1 (cont.).—Brain stem glioma.

D, right vertebral angiogram, frontal view with subtraction, venous phase: The left and right brachial veins (**g**) are separated. The veins of the lateral recess (**h**) bilaterally are also separated. The latter structures cannot be outlined on the lateral view because of superimposition of incompletely subtracted petrous bones.

E, pneumoencephalogram, lateral view: The prepontine and medullary cisterns are markedly compressed. Air in the interpeduncular cistern (**i**) reveals forward displacement and narrowing of this area. The fourth ventricle is displaced backward throughout its course.

F, pneumoencephalogram, frontal view: The fourth ventricle appears symmetrically widened. Air passing over the superior cerebellar peduncle in the inferior portion (**j**) of the perimesencephalic cisterns is bowed outward by the increased mass of the brain stem. Mild hydrocephalus enlarges the lateral ventricles.

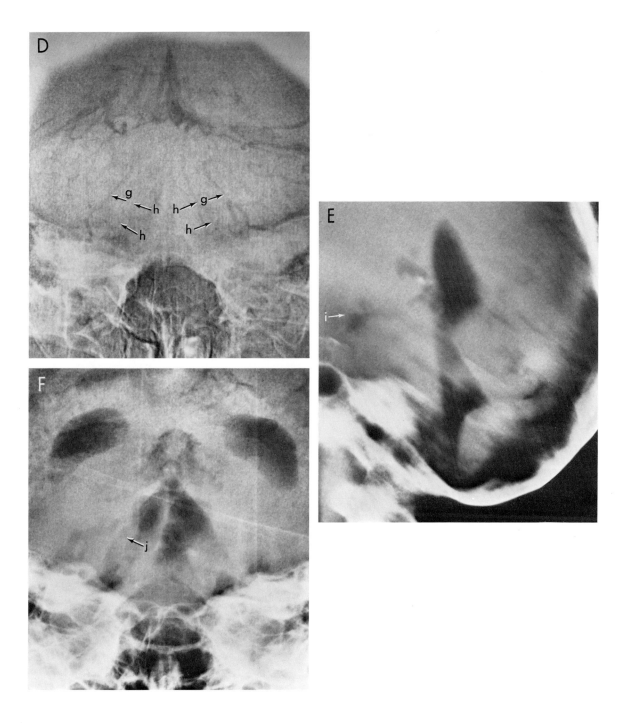

Figure 98-1 · Brain Stem Glioma / 307

Figure 98-2.—Tumor of the brain stem extending into the right cerebellar peduncle.

This 48-year-old woman had a progressive history of dizziness, incoordination, dysarthria, weakness in both arms, inability to walk unaided, dysphagia and inappropriate laughter for four to five months. There were bilateral ptosis, marked limitation of eye movement in all directions, slightly diminished corneal reflex on the left, bilateral facial paresis, decreased gag reflex bilaterally and tongue deviation to the left. Trial of ACTH for a suspected subacute demyelinating process resulted in no improvement. Following radiographic diagnosis of a brain stem lesion, high doses of steroids and radiotherapy seemed effective, but suddenly respiratory distress developed and she died two months after hospitalization.

A, bilateral brachial arteriogram with right carotid compression, frontal view (following pneumoencephalography): There is right-to-left displacement of the posterior inferior cerebellar artery on the left (**a**). The right posterior inferior cerebellar artery is not present; instead a large anterior inferior cerebellar artery is seen which supplies the inferior aspect of the right cerebellar hemisphere. The right superior cerebellar artery (**b**) is slightly elevated.

B, bilateral brachial arteriogram with right carotid compression, lateral view: The ascending limb of the choroid loop (**c**) is displaced posteriorly. The basilar artery is forward in position. There is slight upward stretching of the superior vermis branches (**d**) of the superior cerebellar arteries.

C, bilateral brachial arteriogram, frontal view, venous phase: The vein of the left lateral recess (**e**) is displaced to the left. The distal portions (**f**) of the inferior vermian veins are slightly separated and displaced to the left and the suprapyramidal loop (**g**) on the right is seen end-on, indicating a right-sided mass effect.

(Continued.)

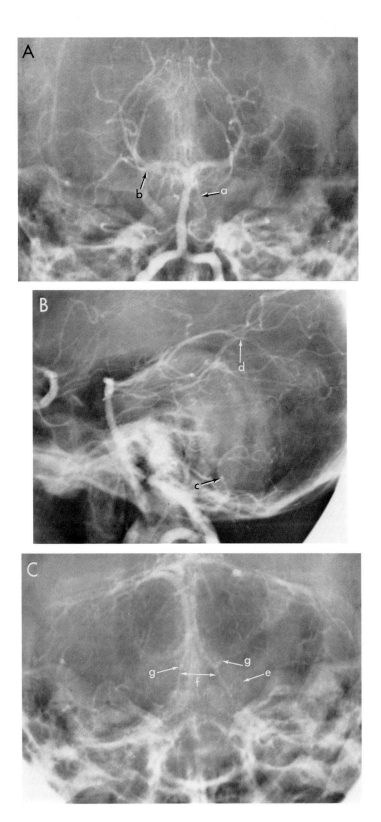

Figure 98-2 · Brain Stem Tumor / 309

Figure 98-2 (cont.).—Tumor of the brain stem extending into the right cerebellar peduncle.

D, bilateral brachial arteriogram, lateral view, venous phase: The pontomesencephalic vein (**h**) and tributaries are forward in position. The precentral vein (**i**) is displaced markedly backward. The inferior vermian vein (**g**) is also displaced posteriorly. The vein of the lateral recess (**e**) is well seen as it is displaced posteriorly free from the overlying air cells in the mastoid region.

E, pneumoencephalogram, filling position, frontal view: The fourth ventricle and aqueduct are displaced to the left, with most marked displacement at the level of the lateral recesses (**j**). The vallecula (**k**) is closer to the midline, indicating a lesser mass effect at the low stem level. The rostral portion of the fourth ventricle and aqueduct are splayed, indicating an intraaxial stem lesion in the pontine and midbrain level.

F, autotomogram during pneumoencephalography, lateral view: The fourth ventricle and aqueduct are displaced posteriorly with greatest displacement at the pontomesencephalic junction (**j**). The proximal portion of the fourth ventricle is not well delineated, being displaced outside of the midline plane.

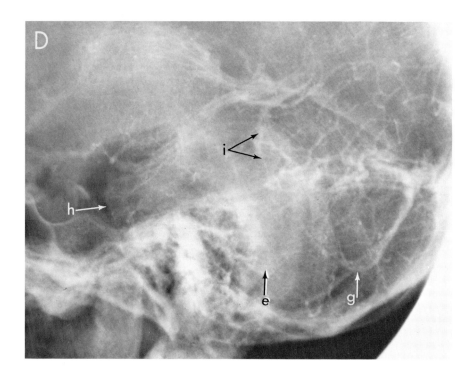

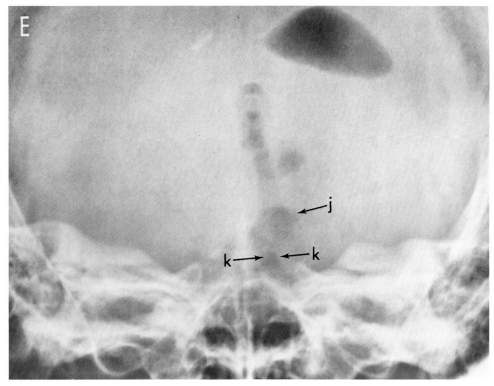

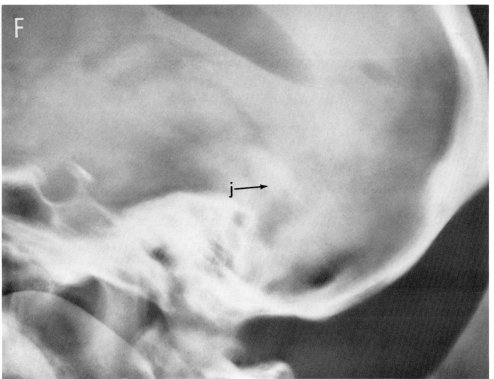

Figure 98-2 · Brain Stem Tumor / 311

Figure 99.—Midbrain metastases.

A 64-year-old man had a three-month history of increasingly severe throbbing bifrontotemporal headaches and some ill-defined dimness of vision. A few days before hospitalization he was obviously slowed, confused and only partially oriented. Neurologic examination revealed only a suggestion of a left homonymous field defect on gross testing. In particular, extraocular movements and other cranial nerves revealed no abnormalities.

A, autotomogram during pneumoencephalogram, filling position, lateral view: The proximal portion (**a**) of the Sylvian aqueduct is partially effaced because of the mass adjacent to it, displacing it away from the midline plane of the tomogram. The bend at the midaqueductal level appears to be increased. This is due to the lateral displacement rather than to a mass effect posterior to the aqueduct.

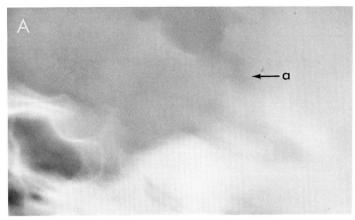

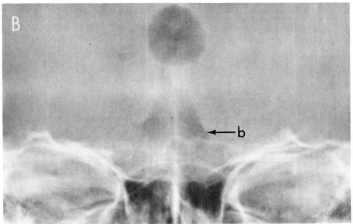

B, same procedure, frontal view: There is a very local displacement of the aqueduct from right to left by the midbrain tumor. Slight downward tilting of the left lateral recess (**b**) is also a reflection of the left-sided midbrain mass.

C, anteroposterior, and **D,** lateral views, right brachial arteriogram, arterial phase: These reveal no definite abnormality aside from mild hydrocephalus. The superior cerebellar vessels ascending and descending in the region of the centrum (**c**) and culmen (**d**) of the vermis seem somewhat depressed, but in view of the generalized vascular tortuosity this finding of itself is not diagnostic.

(Continued.)

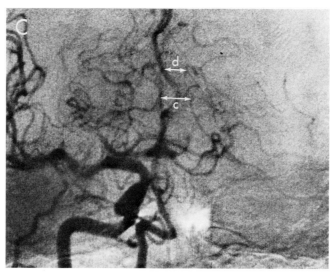

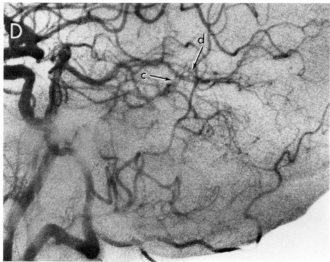

Figure 99 · Midbrain Metastases / 313

Figure 99 (cont.).—Midbrain metastases.

E, right brachial arteriogram, frontal view, venous phase: The precentral vein (**e**) is displaced to the right. The lateral mesencephalic vein on the left side (**f**) is slightly displaced laterally, although the brachial vein (**g**) appears to be in normal position.

F, right brachial arteriogram, subtracted lateral view, venous phase: The distance between the lateral mesencephalic (**f**) and precentral vein (**e**) is increased. Slight but definite local mass effect with forward displacement of the lateral mesencephalic vein is seen. The precentral vein is mildly straightened and displaced posteriorly.

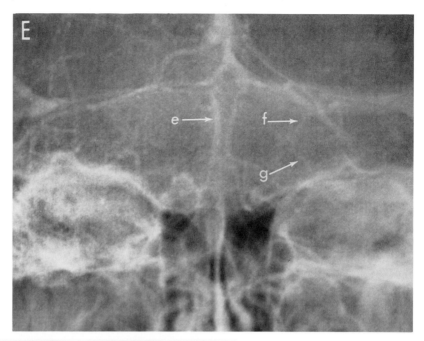

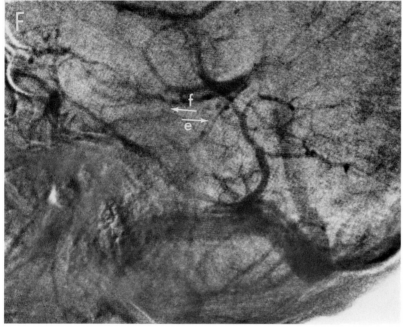

Figure 99 · Midbrain Metastases / 315

Figure 100.—Ependymoma of the fourth ventricle invading the brain stem.

A 49-year-old man had a 14-month history, beginning with vertigo, progressive gait disturbances and, before admission, vertical diplopia, slurred speech and difficulty in swallowing. There were no signs of intra-cranial pressure. Striking findings were ataxia of gait and of the upper extremities, more pronounced on the left than the right. Diplopia was present in all fields of gaze and the gag reflex was greatly decreased. A sub-occipital craniectomy and upper cervical laminectomy revealed an extremely large tumor arising from the floor of the fourth ventricle but subependymal in location and thought to represent a subependymal astrocytoma. The medulla appeared to be grossly enlarged by the tumor; this unusual large invasive aspect of the tumor caused the angiographic changes to resemble those of a brain stem astrocytoma. The tumor was soft, relatively avascular and adherent to the lateral margins of the obex and to the lateral region of the fourth ventricle rostral to the obex. The tumor extended forward to the midportion of the fourth ventricle superiorly to the vermis and lay up against the choroid plexus. Branches from the posterior inferior cerebellar artery were seen at surgery to course down over the tumor, which extended to C-1/C-2.

A, bilateral brachial arteriogram, frontal subtracted view, Caldwell projection: There is marked separation of the portion of the posterior inferior cerebellar arteries (**a**) coursing around the stem, particularly dorsally. The vermian branches (**b**) finally achieve a midline position. Cerebellar hemispheric branches are normal. However, small vessels are seen from the inferior aspect of the posterior inferior cerebellar artery extending into the cervical region and represent tumor vessels (**t**).

B, bilateral brachial arteriogram, subtracted lateral view: There is pronounced elongation of the portion of the posterior inferior cerebellar arteries (**a**) coursing around the brain stem. The choroidal loops (**c**) of the arteries are accordioned together. The vermian (**b**) and hemispheric branches are unremarkable. It is difficult to identify the tumor branches (**t**) into the upper cervical region because of the muscular and meningeal branches overlying the area.

(Continued.)

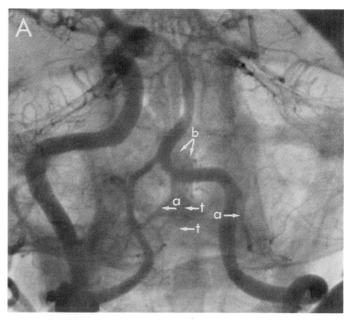

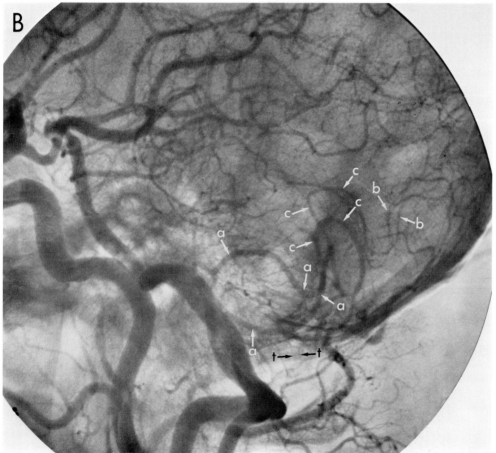

Figure 100 · Ependymoma of the 4th Ventricle / 317

Figure 100 (cont.).—Ependymoma of the fourth ventricle invading the brain stem.

C, bilateral brachial arteriogram, frontal view, venous phase: There is slight spreading apart of the inferior portion of the inferior vermian veins (**d**). The two thin midline veins (**e**) are probably on the tumor surface. No other stretched or displaced venous structures are seen.

D, bilateral brachial arteriogram, lateral view, venous phase: Marked backward displacement of the inferior vermian veins (**d**) is demonstrated. The precentral (**f**), lateral mesencephalic (**g**) and pontomesencephalic (**h**) veins appear to be normal. The cerebellar hemisphere veins are also unremarkable.

E, Pantopaque myelogram, lateral view: The tumor (**x**) is capped at the level of C-1 by the Pantopaque. The sharp rounded appearance is reminiscent of an intradural extramedullary lesion, but this is not unusual with exophytic tumors.

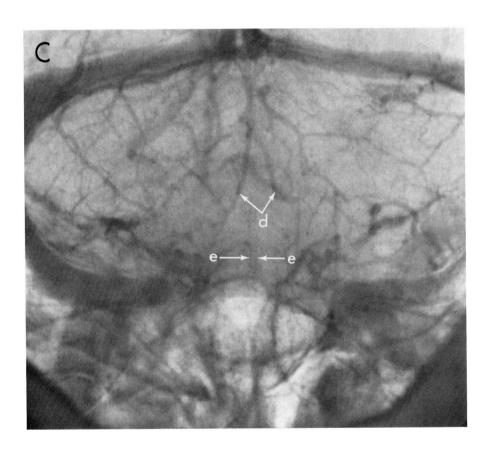

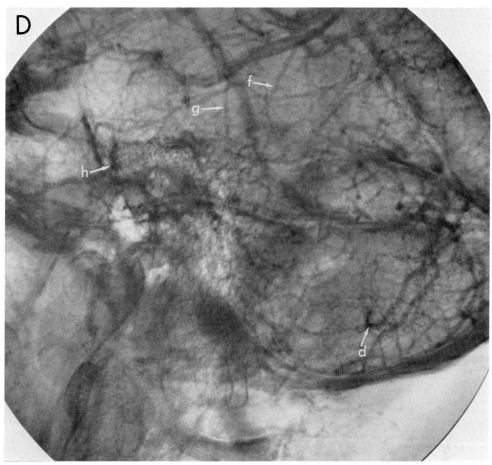

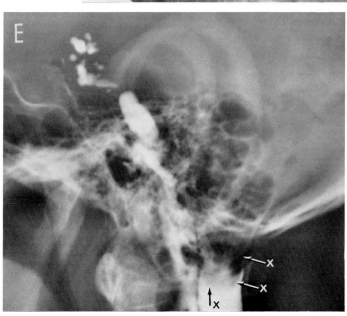

Figure 100 · Ependymoma of the 4th Ventricle / 319

Figure 101.—Cystic astrocytoma of the right cerebellum.

This 8-year-old girl was hospitalized because of increasing incoordination and evidence of raised intracranial pressure on physical examination. Ventriculography revealed a large right cerebellar hemisphere mass. On suboccipital craniotomy a large cystic tumor was removed except for a small portion which appeared to extend toward the brain stem on the right side. She received radiotherapy postoperatively. Four years later she again had signs of increasing intracranial pressure. Restudy and reoperation revealed recurrence of the cystic astrocytoma.

A, skull radiograph, frontal view, Caldwell projection: The right occipital bone (**arrows**) is markedly thin and displaced outward. The ballooning of the right side of the posterior fossa extends laterally to the mastoid process and medially to the midline, which is actually displaced to the left.

B, skull radiograph, lateral view: The thinned and expanded right occipital bone (**arrows**) is evident. In addition there are marked thinning and a slight forward concavity of the basiocciput (**a**). The calcification (**b**) in the upper midportion of the posterior fossa is within the tumor wall. Generalized signs of increased intracranial pressure are also evident.

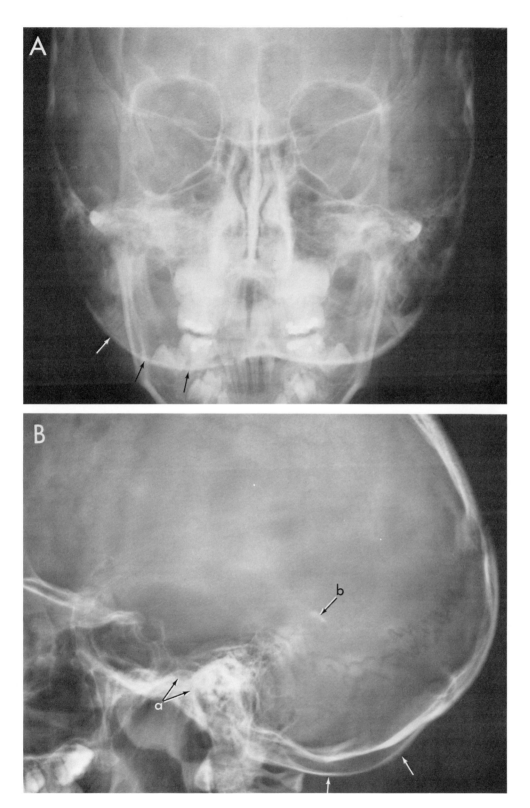

Figure 101 · Cystic Astrocytoma / 321

Figure 102.—Cystic metastatic carcinoma of the left cerebellar hemisphere.

A 58-year-old man had posterior cervical and suboccipital pain for six weeks, and for four weeks, dizziness, nausea and vomiting. Several days before admission he became stuporous and the day before was unable to move his right arm and hand. Examination disclosed Cheyne-Stokes respirations, weakness of the left V, VII, VIII, IX, X and XI cranial nerves, right hemiparesis and papilledema. Following ventricular drainage for approximately 24 hours, a ventriculogram was obtained and arteriography performed. At operation a 13-cc cystic lesion containing xanthochromic fluid was found. Radiotherapy was given to the posterior fossa as well as to the apex of the left lung, where the primary carcinoma was discovered.

A, left brachial arteriogram, frontal view, arterial phase: There is marked displacement to the right of the posterior inferior cerebellar artery (**a**). In addition there are stretching and elevation of the anterior inferior cerebellar artery (**b**) just above the petrous pyramid.

B, left brachial arteriogram, lateral view, arterial phase: Branches to the tonsil (**c**) of the posterior inferior cerebellar artery are seen to be below the foramen magnum practically reaching the arch of C-1. The inferior vermian artery is normal in position and height. The anterior inferior cerebellar artery (**b**) coursing around the biventral lobule is markedly arced.

(Continued.)

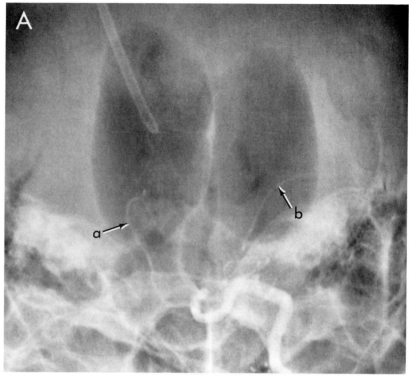

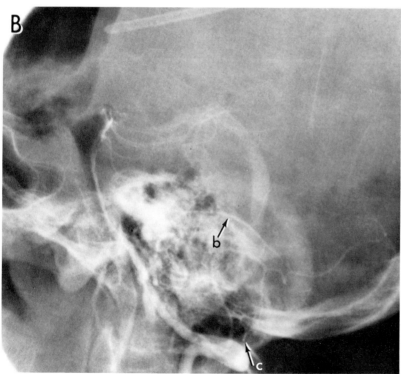

Figure 102 · Cystic Metastatic Carcinoma / 323

Figure 102 (cont.).—Cystic metastatic carcinoma of the left cerebellar hemisphere.

C, bilateral brachial arteriogram, frontal view, arterial phase: In addition to the findings in **A** and **B,** marked arcing upward of the marginal branch (**d**) of the superior cerebellar artery is evident. There is a relative sparseness of filling of superior cerebellar artery branches on the left side. The basilar artery is displaced slightly to the right.

D, bilateral brachial arteriogram, arterial phase, lateral view. A small tumor stain (**x**) is seen within the choroidal loop of the posterior inferior cerebellar artery. (This small vascular nodule associated with the larger mass effect can also be found in cystic astrocytomas and hemangioblastomas.) The basilar artery is displaced forward. There is slight upward herniation of the superior cerebellum, as outlined by the slightly elevated branches coursing over the superior vermis (**e**).

E, bilateral brachial arteriogram, frontal view, venous phase: There is a relative paucity of venous filling on the left. The small tumor nodule (**x**) close to the midline on the left side is probably within the tonsil. The precentral vein (**f**) is displaced to the right. The brachial tributary (**g**) to the left petrosal vein is straightened. The inferior portion of the inferior vermian vein (**h**) is displaced to the right.

(Continued.)

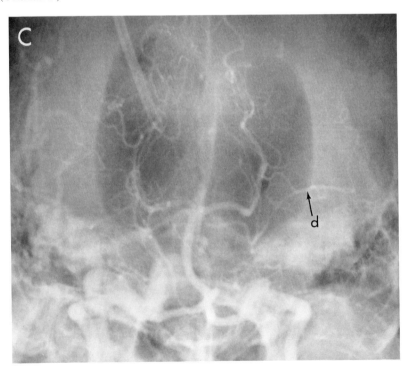

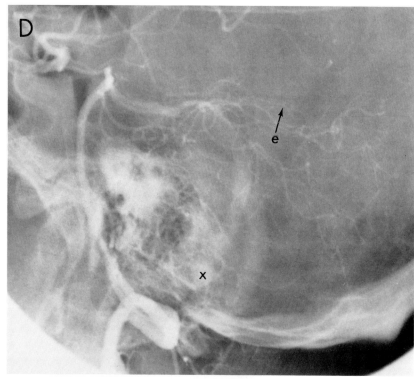

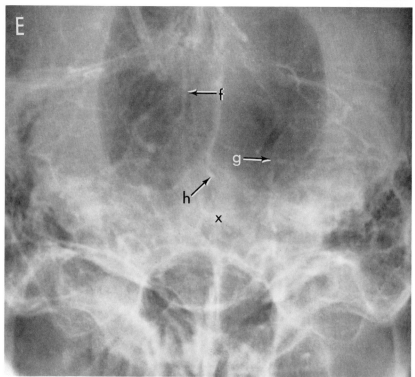

Figure 102 · Cystic Metastatic Carcinoma / 325

Figure 102 (cont.).—Cystic metastatic carcinoma of the left cerebellar hemisphere.

F, bilateral brachial arteriogram, lateral view, venous phase: The pontomesencephalic vein (**h**) is displaced forward and the precentral vein (**f**) upward and forward. A collection of venous structures (**i**) just above the transverse sinus can be seen to be stretched. There is a small residuum of contrast material in the vascular tumor nodule (**x**).

G, ventriculogram, frontal view: The aqueduct (**j**) and fourth ventricle (**k**) are markedly displaced to the right. The third ventricle and lateral ventricles are dilated because of the obstruction. Most of the mass effect is in the inferior half of the cerebellar hemisphere.

H, autotomogram on ventriculography, lateral view: The aqueduct (**j**) and rostral fourth ventricle are kinked and displaced forward. The more proximal portions of the fourth ventricle are not seen because they are out of the plane of view.

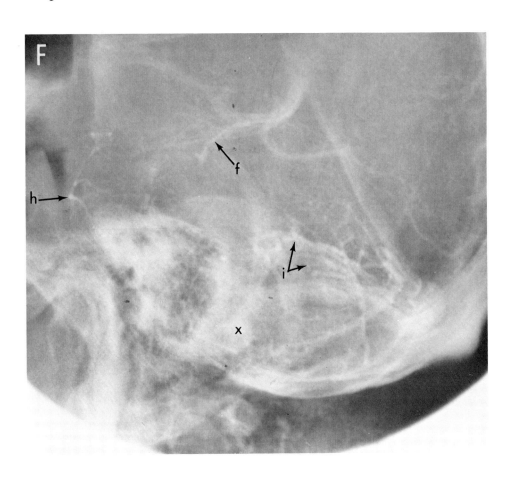

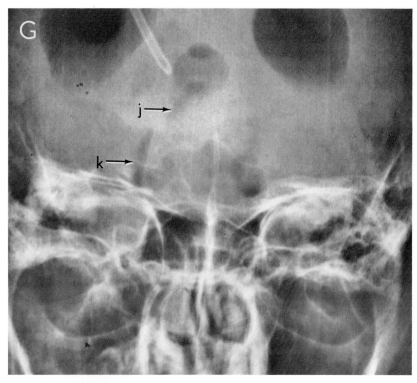

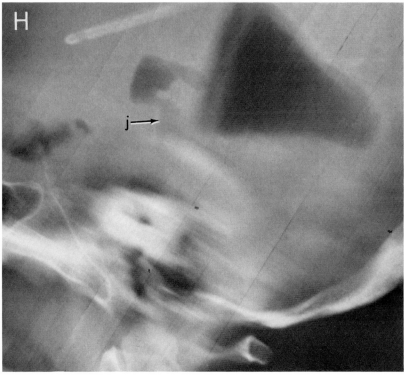

Figure 102 · Cystic Metastatic Carcinoma / 327

Figure 103.—Right cerebellar hemisphere metastasis.

This 59-year-old woman had had a carcinoma resected from the colon four years previously. For four weeks she had increasingly severe head-aches, unsteady gait, vomiting and, recently, irritability and confusion. Examination revealed considerable gait difficulty and unsteadiness on turns, mild nuchal rigidity, early papilledema, mild nystagmus on right lateral gaze and dysmetrial finger-to-nose and finger-to-finger responses on the right. There was no other focal deficit. A hilar mass was noted in the chest radiograph. At operation a 3 × 4 cm mass which was pseudoencapsulated was removed from the inferolateral margin of the right cerebellar hemisphere.

A, left vertebral arteriogram, subtracted frontal view: The left posterior inferior cerebellar artery (**a**) is displaced to the left. No obvious deformity is seen in the superior cerebellar branches. This is because the tumor is low in position and the vessels supplying the inferior portion of the cerebellar hemisphere on the right are not filled.

B, left vertebral arteriogram, subtracted lateral view: The basilar artery and the choroidal loop (**b**) of the posterior inferior cerebellar artery are displaced forward. No definite tonsil branches are seen arising from the choroid loop. No upward herniation of the superior cerebellar branches is evident.

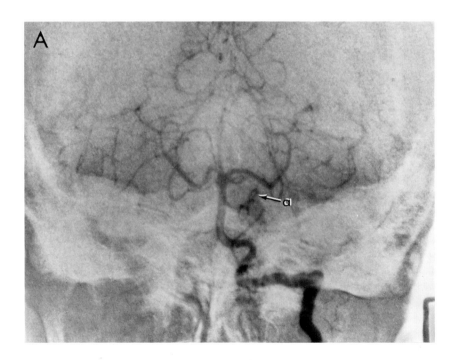

C, left vertebral arteriogram, frontal view, venous phase: The precentral vein (**c**) is well seen and is displaced to the left. There is suggestion of stretching of several incompletely filled right cerebellar hemisphere veins (**d**).

(*Continued.*)

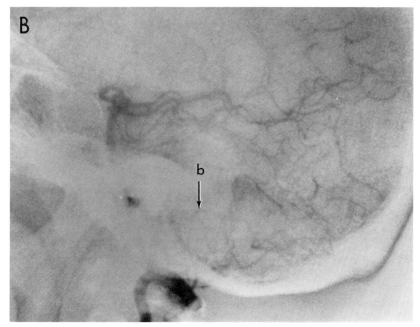

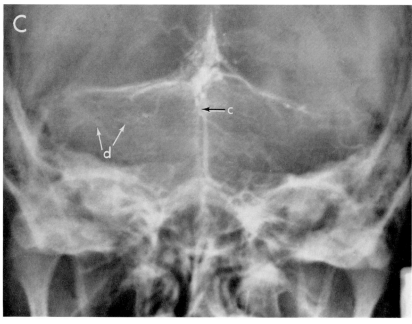

Figure 103 · Cerebellar Metastasis / 329

Figure 103 (cont.).—Right cerebellar hemisphere metastasis.

D, left vertebral arteriogram, lateral view, venous phase: The precentral vein (**c**) is displaced forward, as is the pontomesencephalic vein (**e**). Some stretching is seen of horizontally coursing veins (**d**) in the vicinity of the transverse sinus. There is good demonstration of several venous structures on the surface of the cerebellar tonsils (**f**), which are herniated to the level of C-1. This was confirmed at operation as well as by ventriculography.

E, ventriculogram, frontal view following backward somersault to brow-down position: The aqueduct (**g**) and fourth ventricle (**h**) are displaced to the left, with the greatest shift at the proximal fourth ventricular level.

F, autotomogram, lateral view: The fourth ventricle (**h**) is displaced forward and marked compression of the brain stem is evident. The cerebellar tonsils (**f**) are again seen to be herniated to C-1.

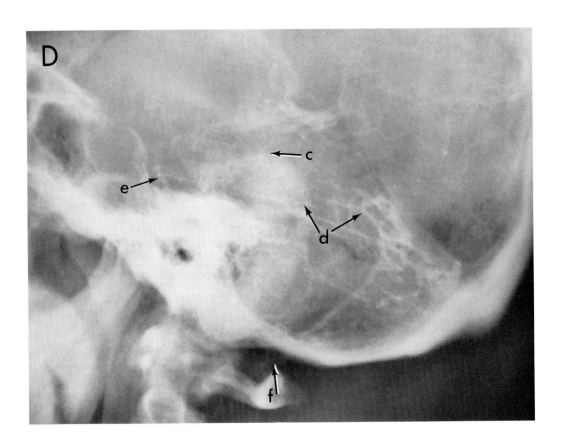

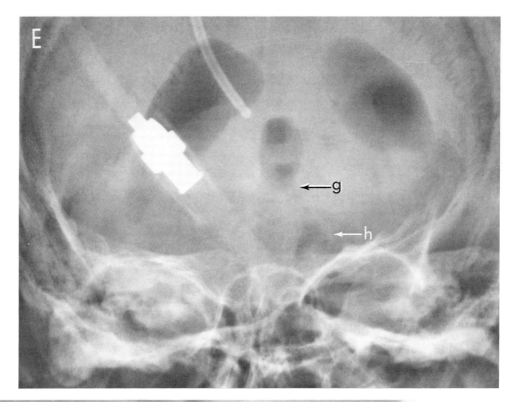

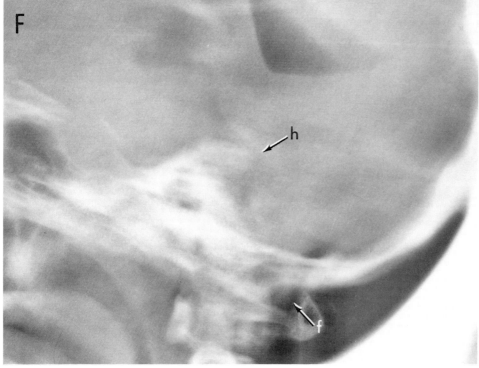

Figure 103 · Cerebellar Metastasis / 331

Figure 104.—Metastatic melanoma of the right cerebellar hemisphere.

This 68-year-old man had a one-month history of increased fatigue and difficulty with gait. Some deterioration of handwriting as well as occipital headaches and morning nausea were noted a week prior to admission. Examination showed the optic discs to be hyperemic with slight venous engorgement. Gait was slightly wide-based and unsteady, but no Romberg sign or nystagmus was found. There was a trace of dysmetria on finger-to-nose examination, but succession movements were preserved. A chest radiograph showed two noncalcified nodules in the right lung field. At operation, about 1.5 cm within the right cerebellar hemisphere, a large bluish-red friable highly vascular tumor was encountered. Gross total removal was effected and a tantalum-type mesh was placed on the tumor bed. Search for the site of the melanoma was unrewarding.

A, right brachial arteriogram with right carotid compression, subtracted frontal view: A faint tumor stain (**x**) overlies the superior aspect of the right petrous pyramid. The right superior cerebellar artery (**a**) is displaced slightly medially and two of its branches are markedly stretched in the immediate vicinity of the tumor. Several vessels lateral and inferior to the tumor stain are also markedly stretched.

B, right brachial arteriogram, lateral view: A tonsillar branch (**b**) arising from the ascending limb of the choroidal loop (**c**) is seen below the foramen magnum. The choroidal loop itself is depressed. A faint tumor stain (**x**) is seen in the area immediately below the transverse sinus being fed by superior cerebellar artery branches. The marginal branch (**d**) of the superior cerebellar artery is conspicuously stretched adjacent to the tumor. Slight upward herniation of the superior vermis (**e**) is evident.

(Continued.)

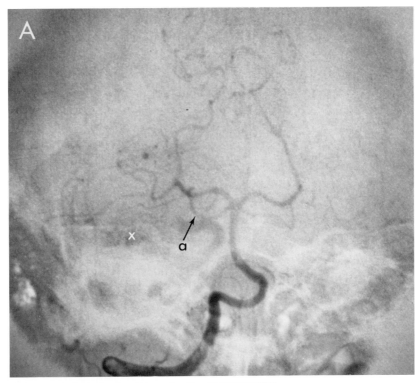

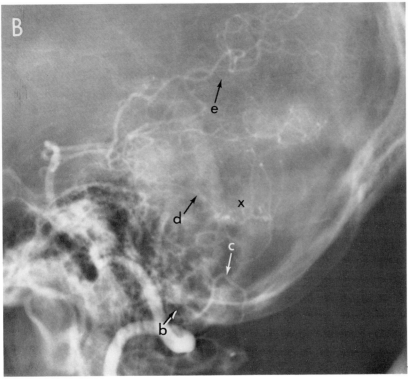

Figure 104 · Metastatic Melanoma / 333

Figure 104 (cont.).—Metastatic melanoma of the right cerebellar hemisphere.

C, right brachial arteriogram, frontal view, venous phase: Several large venous structures drain the vascular portion of the tumor into the transverse sinus. The precentral vein (**f**) is at the midline. Poor filling of the left side of the posterior fossa is technical, as only one vertebral artery was opacified.

D, right brachial arteriogram, lateral view, venous phase: Several stretched veins enter the transverse sinus on the upper pole of the tumor. The precentral (**f**), lateral mesencephalic (**g**) and pontomesencephalic (**h**) veins are in normal position.

E, pneumoencephalogram, frontal view: The fourth ventricle (**i**) is displaced to the left, with lessening degrees of displacement of the aqueduct which reaches the midline as it enters the third ventricle.

(*Continued.*)

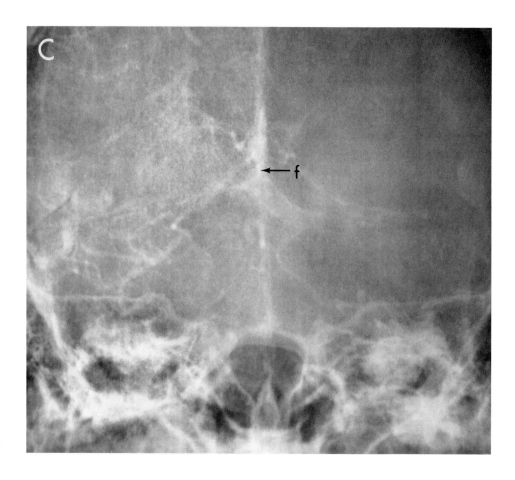

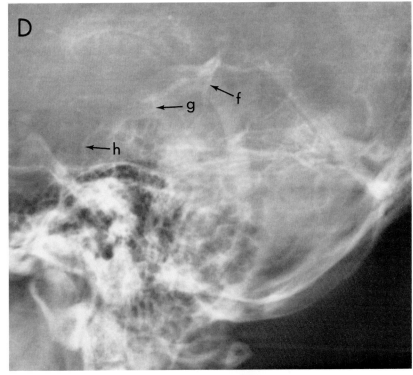

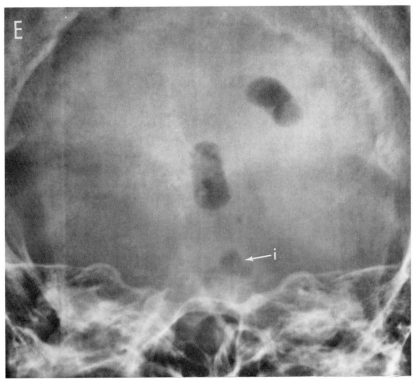

Figure 104 · Metastatic Melanoma / 335

Figure 104 (cont.).—Metastatic melanoma of the right cerebellar hemisphere.

F, autotomogram during pneumoencephalography, lateral view: The fourth ventricle (**i**) is within normal limits here, being displaced directly laterally by the rather low-lying cerebellar mass.

G, pneumoencephalogram, lateral view: Air in the cervical region outlines the herniated tonsils (**b**) and confirms the arteriographic finding.

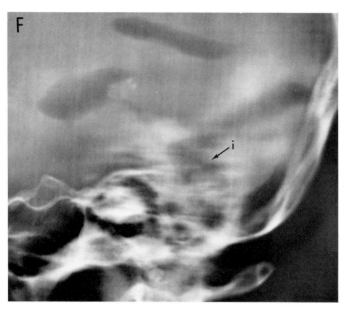

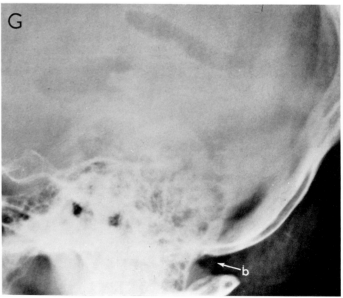

H, frontal, and **I,** lateral views of postoperative skull radiographs: Showing the tantalum mesh in the right cerebellar hemisphere from which the tumor was excavated.

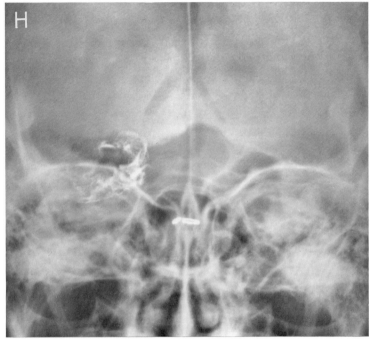

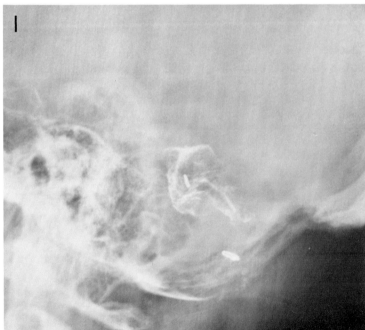

Figure 104 · Metastatic Melanoma / 337

Figure 105.—Left cerebellar hemisphere metastasis.

A 71-year-old man had received radiotherapy seven months previously for an inoperable oat cell carcinoma of the upper lobe of the left lung with mediastinal metastases. He did well until one month before this study, when he experienced vomiting, vertigo and marked ataxia. Examination revealed generalized wasting and proximal weakness, particularly in the lower extremities without fasciculations or myotonia. This was considered to be secondary to carcinomatous neuromyopathy (Lambert-Eaton syndrome). He was markedly ataxic; finger-to-nose and finger-to-finger ataxia was greater on the left than on the right. He was slightly dysphasic, and coarse horizontal nystagmus was present on left lateral gaze. At operation, gross total removal was accomplished of a partially necrotic metastatic nodule about 4 cm in diameter from the midsuperior portion of the left cerebellar hemisphere.

A, bilateral brachial arteriogram, frontal view, arterial phase: The right posterior inferior cerebellar artery (**a**) is displaced to the right. The left posterior inferior cerebellar artery is small, but one of its branches (**b**) can be made out just to the left and then through the basilar artery, which is also displaced to the right. The left anterior inferior cerebellar artery is large and its branches show no definite evidence of direct mass effect. The left superior cerebellar artery in its perimesencephalic portion (**c**) is conspicuously arced, and the superior vermis branch (**d**) is displaced to the right.

B, bilateral brachial arteriogram, subtracted lateral view, arterial phase: The choroidal loop (**e**) of the posterior inferior cerebellar artery is markedly displaced down and forward. The basilar artery is also forward in position. There is no angiographic evidence of tonsillar herniation.

C, bilateral brachial arteriogram, frontal view, venous phase: There is striking lack of venous filling in the superior portion of the left cerebellar hemisphere. A few veins seen in the area appear stretched. The brachial tributary (**f**) to the left petrosal vein is taut.

(Continued.)

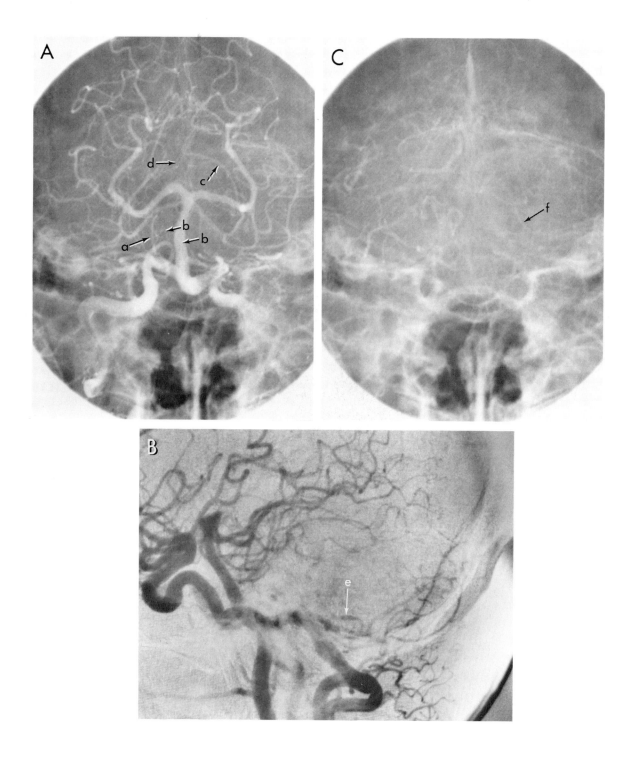

Figure 105 · Cerebellar Metastasis / 339

Figure 105 (cont.).—Left cerebellar hemisphere metastasis.

D, bilateral brachial arteriogram, lateral view, venous phase: The precentral (**g**) and lateral mesencephalic (**h**) veins are displaced forward. The pontomesencephalic vein (**i**) in its course around the pons is displaced forward but appears to be in normal position within the interpeduncular fossa. This may be due to enlargement of the third ventricle with imposition of its inferior portion behind the sella turcica within the interpeduncular fossa in a fashion similar to that commonly seen in aqueduct stenosis. Stretching of a hemispheric vein (**j**) above the transverse sinus is the only evidence of direct mass effect seen.

E, ventriculogram following a nonventricular filling pneumoencephalogram, frontal view: The aqueduct (**k**) and fourth ventricle (**l**) are displaced to the right. The proximal portion of the fourth ventricle is not filled. The vallecula (**m**) is compressed and also displaced to the right. There is marked compression of the left cerebellopontine angle (**n**).

F, same procedure as **E,** lateral view: The aqueduct (**k**) and rostral fourth ventricle (**l**) are displaced forward. Air in the prepontine cistern (**o**) is compressed by the forward displacement of the pons.

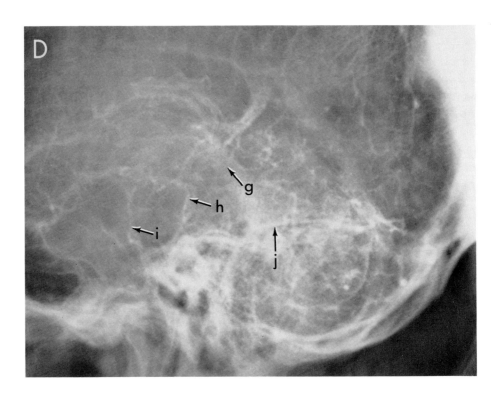

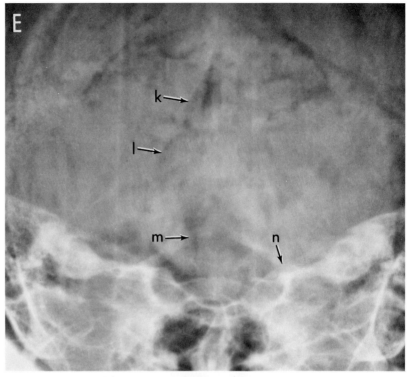

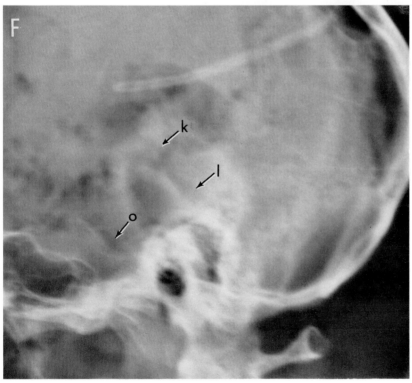

Figure 105 · Cerebellar Metastasis / 341

Figure 106.—Cerebellar hemangioblastoma.

This 64-year-old man had bilateral occipital headaches and gait disturbance for two months. Family history was significant in that three relatives had a gait disturbance and died before age 50 without definite diagnosis. Examination revealed bilateral dysmetria and an ataxic gait. Hematocrit read 53. A suboccipital decompressive craniotomy was done. Postoperatively the patient developed a urinary tract infection, gram-negative sepsis and pulmonary emboli, and died. At autopsy the hemangioblastoma was found, as well as multiple simple cysts of the kidney and telangiectasia of the intestine. Angiomatosis retinae was not found, although this case probably represents a modified form of Hippel-Lindau syndrome.

A, simultaneous bilateral brachial arteriogram with right carotid compression, frontal view: The right superior cerebellar artery is enlarged, and numerous tortuous vessels arise as the artery reaches the back of the midbrain.

B, simultaneous bilateral brachial arteriogram, lateral view: The large vascular channels fed by the superior cerebellar artery are seen in the region of the superior vermis, which is expanded. Definite upward herniation of the cerebellum is outlined by stretched and upwardly displaced superior vermis arteries (**a**). Posterior inferior cerebellar artery is abnormal in that its choroidal point (**b**) is displaced downward along with the inferior vermian branch (**c**). Tonsillar herniation is outlined by tonsillar branches (**d**) seen 2 mm beneath the foramen magnum.

(Continued.)

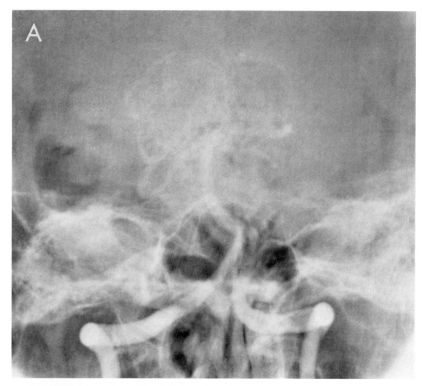

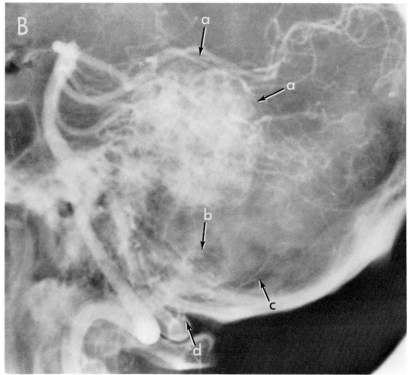

Figure 106 · Cerebellar Hemangioblastoma / 343

Figure 106 (cont.).—Cerebellar hemangioblastoma.

C, bilateral brachial arteriogram, frontal view, venous phase: The venous drainage of this hemangioblastoma involving the vermis and right cerebellar hemisphere is via numerous midline vessels overlying the vermis and right side of the hemisphere as well as into the petrosal venous system, which is seen well on the left side, where there is a prominent brachial vein (**e**).

D, bilateral brachial arteriogram, lateral view, venous phase: The extensive vascular nature of the tumor is well depicted. Its venous drainage is via hemispheric veins and a forward-displaced precentral vein (**f**) into the Galenic system. Enlarged tributaries (**g**) to the petrosal system are also seen anteriorly.

E, pneumoencephalogram, lateral view: A compressed pontine cistern is well outlined. Tonsillar herniation (**d**) approximately 2 mm beneath the foramen magnum confirms the arteriographic finding. There is no ventricular filling.

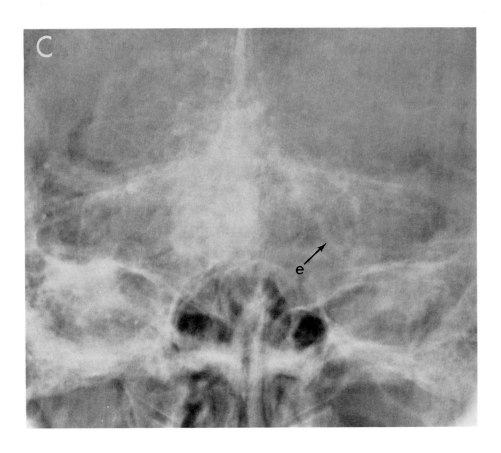

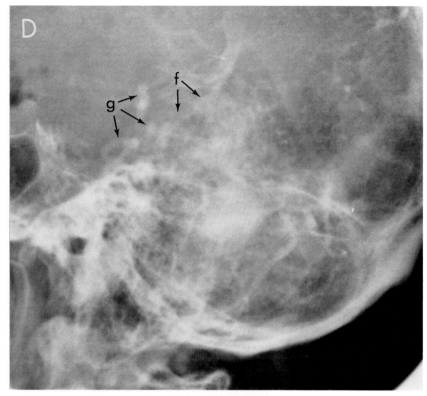

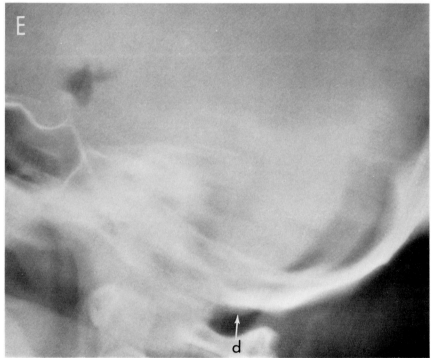

Figure 106 · Cerebellar Hemangioblastoma / 345

Figure 107.—Medulloblastoma.

This 8-year-old boy had a 3½-month history of headache, vomiting and weight loss. Examination revealed marked papilledema, right sixth nerve palsy and fluctuating cerebellar signs, more prominent on the left. Suboccipital craniotomy disclosed a large tumor in the fourth ventricle with tumor seeding over the surface of the cerebellum, cervical spinal cord and medulla. Involvement of the inferior vermis with extension into the right cerebellar hemisphere was noted. Postoperatively the patient received radiotherapy to the entire neural axis.

A, left vertebral arteriogram, frontal view: There is good reflux into the right vertebral artery. The two posterior inferior cerebellar arteries are only very slightly displaced to the left at the point where very small choroidal vessels (**a**) are seen exiting from the arteries. The inferior vermian arteries (**b**) are midline. The anterior inferior cerebellar arteries (**c**) are taut as the ventral portion of the cerebellar hemispheres (biventral lobules) are displaced forward en bloc bilaterally.

B, left vertebral arteriogram, lateral view, arterial phase: The basilar artery is displaced forward against the clivus. The perimedullary portion (**d**) of the two posterior inferior cerebellar arteries is markedly accordioned forward. Abnormally enlarged choroidal vessels (**a**) extend from the proximal portion of the choroidal loop to the tumor in the fourth ventricle. Supratonsillar segments (**e**) of the choroidal loop are elongated, and abnormal vessels (**f**) arise just as the posterior inferior cerebellar artery begins its course around the inferior vermis. The inferior vermian arteries (**g**) seem somewhat taut. The tonsillar branches (**h**) extend to the inferior lip of the foramen magnum; this position of the tonsils was confirmed at surgery. The superior cerebellar arteries are displaced upward secondary to transtentorial herniation. The medial and lateral posterior choroidal vessels are compressed together and the splenial vessels displaced posteriorly. These latter changes are secondary to hydrocephalus.

(Continued.)

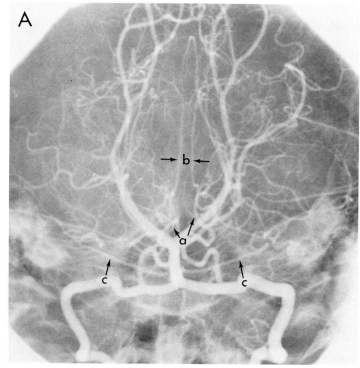

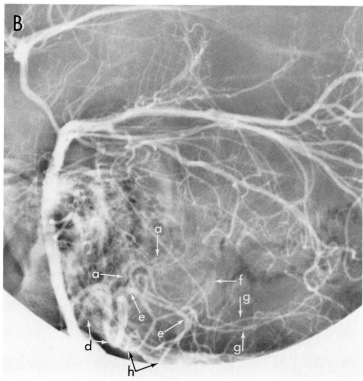

Figure 107 · Medulloblastoma / 347

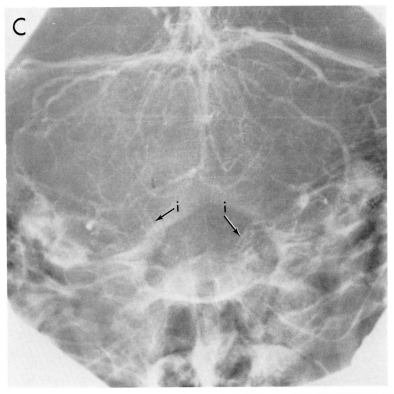

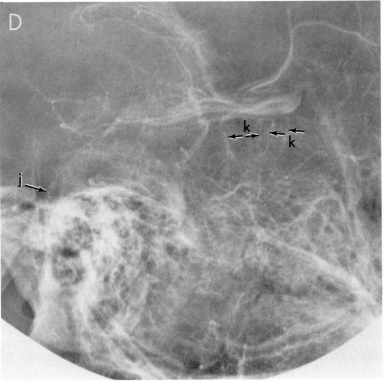

Figure 107 (cont.).—Medulloblastoma.

C, left vertebral arteriogram, frontal view, venous phase: Perimedullary veins (**i**) are enlarged bilaterally due to increased blood flow through the bed of this rather vascular medulloblastoma.

D, left vertebral arteriogram, lateral view, venous phase: Pontomesencephalic vein (**j**) shows the belly of the pons displaced markedly forward against the clivus. The veins extending over the posterior surface of the cerebellar hemisphere (**k**) toward the superior vermis outline the upward herniation of this structure. The separation of the choroidal and splenial veins secondary to the hydrocephalus is also apparent.

E, ventriculogram, frontal view following a backward somersault: The fourth is obstructed by a tumor within it. The tumor is greater on the right side as it obliterates more of the fourth ventricle outline. The rest of the ventricular system is also dilated.

F, ventriculogram, lateral view following backward somersault to brow-down position: The upper pole of the tumor in the fourth ventricle is well capped. Forward displacement of the brain stem is evident. Air posteriorly at the cervicomedullary junction reveals the position of the tonsils extending to the foramen magnum.

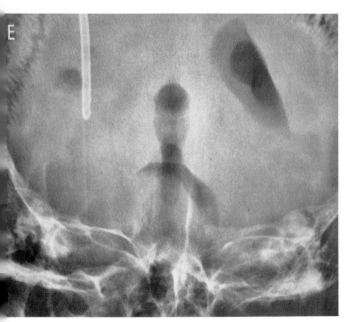
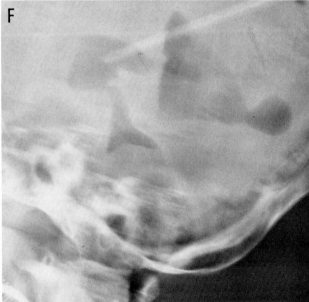

Figure 107 · Medulloblastoma / 349

Figure 108-1.—Ependymoma probably arising from the floor of the fourth ventricle.

A 29-year-old woman had mild left occipital headache for two years. Nausea and vomiting occurred four months before this study and she experienced slight nocturnal diplopia. Neurologic examination was remarkable for its relative normality. There was a question of old healed bilateral papilledema. She had minimal difficulty with tandem walking with her eyes closed. No other cranial nerve, reflex, motor or sensory abnormalities were found. At operation a large fleshy tumor was found in the midline immediately below the cerebellum. It extended dorsally over the medulla and upper spinal cord. The cerebellum, including the cerebellar tonsils, was pushed upward symmetrically. The tumor appeared to arise from the floor of the fourth ventricle.

A, ventriculogram, frontal view, brow-down position: The extraventricular air remains from an attempt at pneumoencephalography which failed to fill the ventricular system. The third and lateral ventricles are dilated. The aqueduct is in the midline. The fourth ventricle is mildly dilated with its right side slightly tilted upward. A tumor (**x**) is outlined at the very inferior aspect of the fourth ventricle centrally, and another nodule (**y**) is seen to the right.

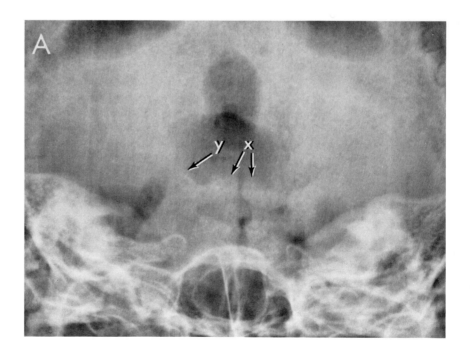

B, ventriculogram, lateral view: The fourth ventricle is elevated and mildly dilated. An obstructing mass (**x**) obliterates the obex of the fourth ventricle.

C, autotomogram in the filling position of a pneumoencephalogram, lateral view: A mass (**x**) extending below C-1 has rather sharply angular borders which are more consistent with a sheet of tumor extending downward than with herniated tonsils.

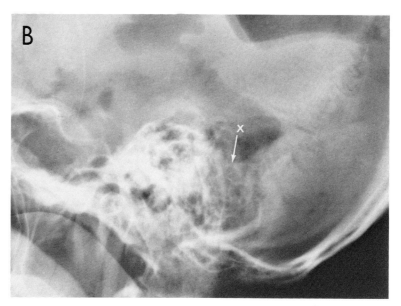

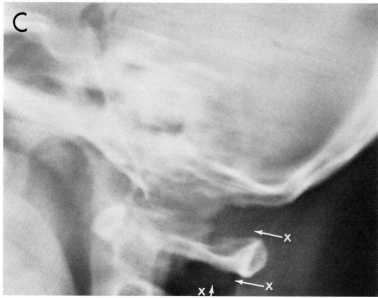

Figure 108-1 · Ependymoma / 351

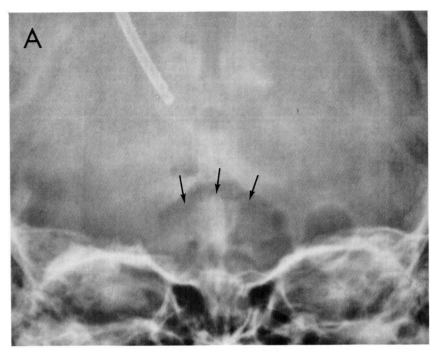

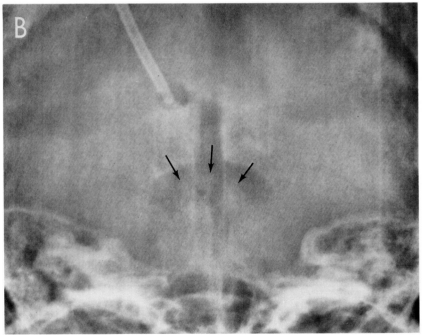

Figure 108-2.—Choroid plexus papilloma of the fourth ventricle.

A 34-year-old woman had gradual progressive vision loss over four years. Examination revealed only a trace of nystagmus on right lateral gaze, obvious chronic papilledema and the presence of multiple drusen bodies on the nerve heads and retinal surfaces. A suboccipital craniotomy was performed, the inferior vermis split and the tonsils separated. A tumor filling the lower portion of the fourth ventricle was found which was not adherent to the ependyma. The tumor was removed piecemeal with coagulation of feeding vessels seen within capillary tufts of the tumor.

A, Granger, and **B,** Towne views of ventriculogram, following backward somersault: A mass (**arrows**) within the fourth ventricle is expanding the side-to-side dimension of this structure, particularly at the plane of the lateral recesses. The third ventricle is also slightly dilated secondary to the partially obstructive nature of the tumor.

C, ventriculogram, lateral view, following backward somersault: A lobulated tumor (**arrows**) in the floor of the lateral ventricle is causing enlargement of the rostral portion of the fourth ventricle and aqueduct. Small lobulations (**l**) of the tumor can be seen within the vallecular space. Chronic increased intracranial pressure changes are present within the sella turcica.

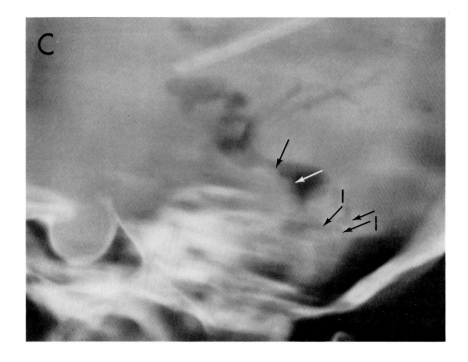

Figure 108-2 · Choroid Plexus Papilloma / 353

PART 12

The Posterior Fossa:
Extra-axial Tumors

Types and Diagnostic Procedures

MOST EXTRA-AXIAL TUMORS of the posterior fossa occur in the ventral compartment of the fossa; that is, they are related to the anterior aspect of the brain stem and cerebellar hemispheres. The occasional dorsal tumors are usually either meningiomas related to the transverse sinus or exceptional congenital tumors associated with midline posterior defects.

The midline tumors in the ventral compartment arise from the clivus, its meningeal coverings or congenital rests. Chordomas are tumors of notochordal tissue that are usually found at either end of the vertebral column. Although they are occasionally seen in a parasellar location, they are most often observed in the midline arising from the basisphenoid or basiocciput. Origin as low as the foramen magnum and odontoid process is not uncommon. They are prone to extend into the nasopharynx. These lesions rarely metastasize but because of their regional invasiveness are extremely difficult to control.

The tumor most often found in the ventral compartment is the neurinoma or Schwannoma. It is a tumor of adulthood and occurs one and a half to two times as often in women as in men. It has a striking tendency to arise from sensory nerve coverings, particularly of the eighth nerve. However, in von Recklinghausen's disease, multiplicity and origin from motor nerves is common. They may be intra- or extradural in location but almost always arise after the nerve has pierced the pia mater. The commonest neurinoma is acoustic.

In the diagnosis of cerebellopontine angle tumors the selection of procedures from among the several contrast methods commonly available—arteriography, venography, pneumoencephalography and Pantopaque cisternography—is often confusing. A useful approach to the patient with a cerebellopontine angle syndrome follows: If the bone erosion is confined to the intracanalicular portion of the canal, Pantopaque cisternography is performed to cap the lesion. However, if bone erosion involves the suprameatal portion of the porus, or if there is no bone erosion, one assumes that the tumor may be of significant size. In this case the initial procedure should be selective vertebral angiography. This is done for two reasons: first, to confirm the mass effect, and second, to delineate the venous and arterial landmarks, which will be of utmost help to the surgeon at operation. Pneumoencephalography may be done especially in conjunction with tomography if the results of angiography are equivocal or if it is thought that the entire extent of the lesion has not been outlined. The presence of an incisural block and hydrocephalus will of course also be demonstrated, although the latter may also be assessed by obtaining a right carotid arteriogram at the time of the vertebral angiography. If the tumor is a meningioma, selective internal and external carotid angiography is required to demonstrate the entire possible dural blood supply.

Jugular venography is done to assess the involvement inferiorly in order to assist in surgical planning, since lesions within the jugular foramen and more caudally may require an anatomic approach different from that to lesions confined to the cerebellopontine angle.

Glomus jugulare tumors are the most common cause of a jugular foramen syndrome. They arise from glomus bodies found along the tympanic branch of the glossopharyngeal nerve (nerve of Jacobson) and the auricular branch of the vagus nerve (nerve of Arnold). A distinction is usually made between a glomus tympanicum of the middle ear and a glomus jugulare, although a glomus jugulare may invade the middle ear and resemble the former on otoscopic examination.

Figure 109.—Glomus jugulare tumor.

A, lateral polytomogram: A large area of destruction is evident in the external auditory canal. Inferiorly the defect has extended into the glenoid fossa.

B, polytomogram during pneumoencephalography: This reveals the extensive destruction of the base of the petrous bone, enlargement and destruction of all but the medial aspect of the jugular fossa and extension laterally to the temporomandibular joint and superiorly into the middle ear and external auditory canal.

C, left common carotid arteriogram, arterial phase: A large tumor stain (**arrows**) occupies the eroded area and is supplied by branches of the external carotid artery.

(Continued.)

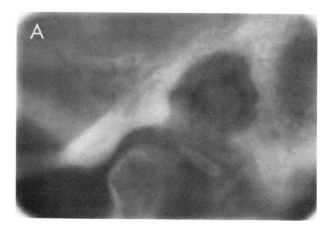

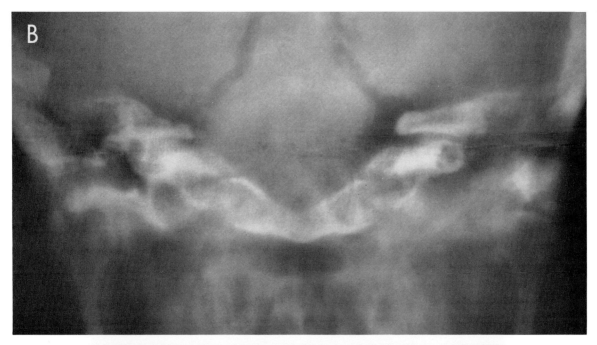

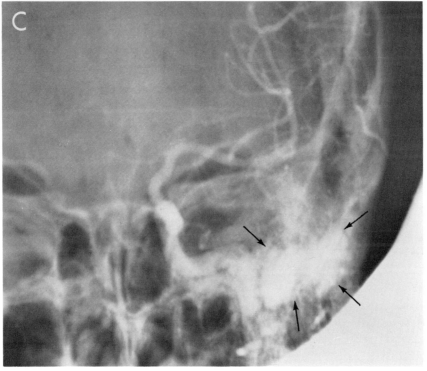

Figure 109 · Glomus Jugulare Tumor / 359

Figure 109 (cont.).—Glomus jugulare tumor.

D, vertebral arteriogram: A large muscular branch (**a**) is seen arising from the vertebral artery, giving off some small branches (**b**) in the postauricular region which go to supply the tumor.

E, left jugular venogram, lateral view: The jugular vein is occluded prior to its reaching the jugular fossa, and an ill-defined filling defect (**c**) is seen within it.

F, left jugular venogram, frontal view: The filling defect (**c**) is seen as a well-circumscribed multilobulated lesion expanding the obstructed end of the jugular vein.

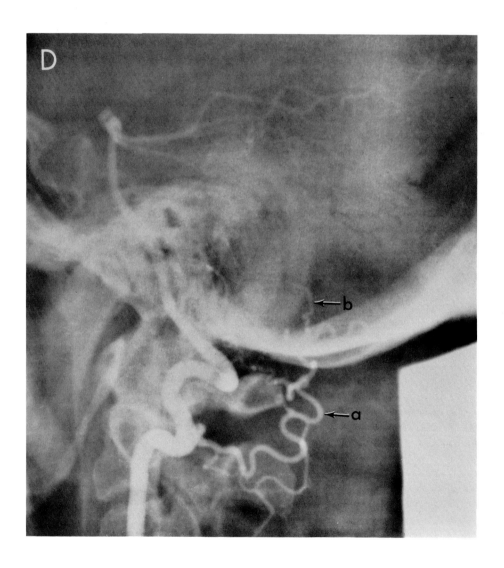

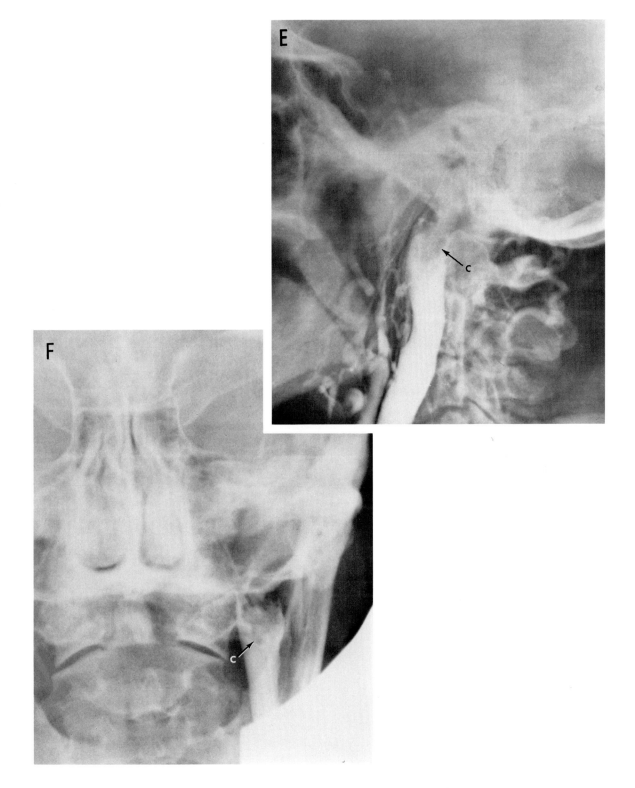

Figure 109 · Glomus Jugulare Tumor / 361

Figure 110.—Glomus jugulare tumor.

A, polytomogram at the level of the internal and external auditory canals, frontal view: A large erosive defect is seen in the jugular fossa on the right side extending medially into the inferior aspect of the petrous bone but not obviously involving the jugular tubercle. The larger portion of the tumor extends into the middle ear and external auditory canal, the margins of which are obliterated.

B, right brachial arteriogram, subtracted frontal view, arterial phase: A large tumor stain (**arrows**) fed by hypertrophied external carotid vessels (**a**) occupies the region of the jugular fossa, middle and external ear. A muscular branch (**b**) of the right vertebral artery is also enlarged and supplies the tumor. The anterior meningeal artery (**c**) is seen over a somewhat larger than normal extent and probably also gives a small contribution to the tumor.

(Continued.)

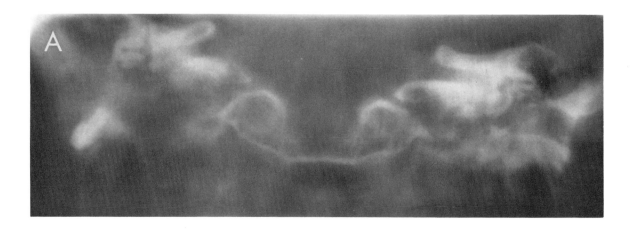

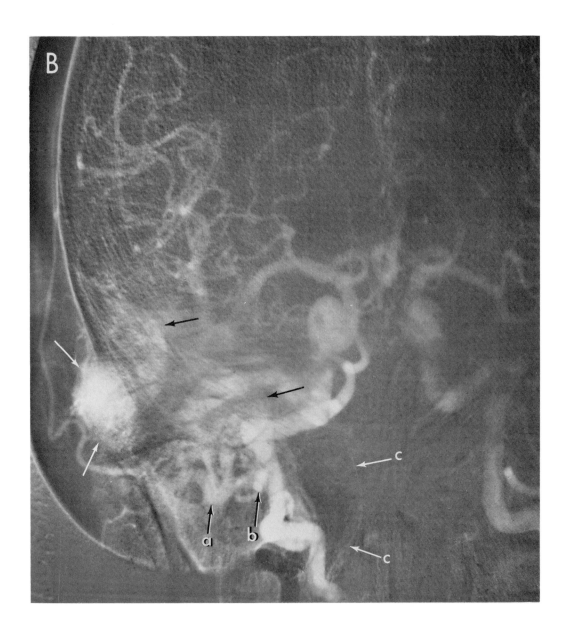

Figure 110 · Glomus Jugulare Tumor / 363

Figure 110 (cont.).—Glomus jugulare tumor.

C, right brachial arteriogram, subtracted lateral view, later arterial phase: More arterial feeders (**a**) are now evident at the base of the lesion. The extensive tumor stain (**arrows**) is well appreciated.

D, right jugular venogram, lateral view: As the jugular vein reaches the jugular fossa there is a cut-off with an area of narrowing which abruptly ceases and shows an ill-defined caplike deformity where tumor (**d**) is obliterating it.

E, right jugular venogram, frontal view: The jugular vein is displaced and compressed medially by the tumor (**d**), which is sharply outlined along its lateral surface in the region of the jugular fossa.

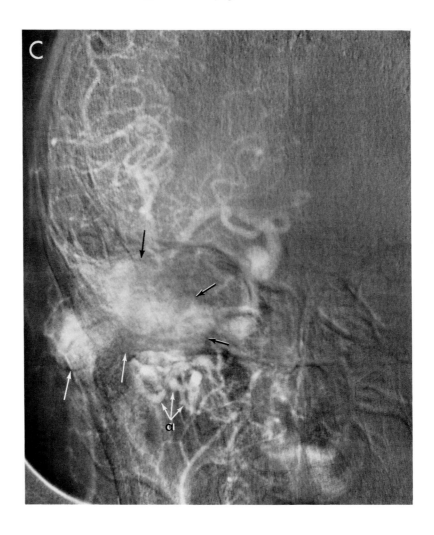

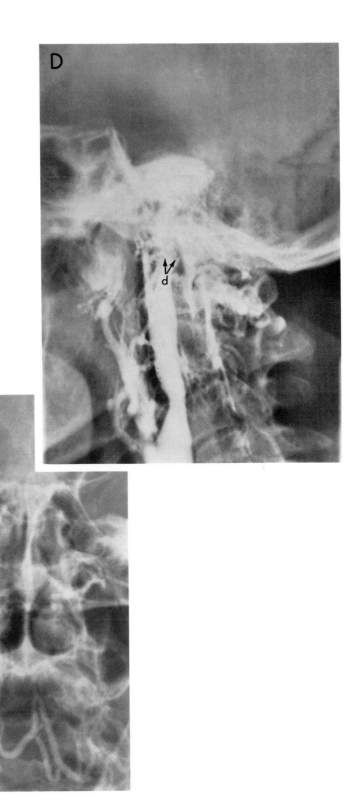

Figure 110 · Glomus Jugulare Tumor / 365

Figure 111.—Glomus tympanicum tumor.

A 55-year-old woman noted tinnitus and pulsation in her left ear for eight months prior to admission. Examination revealed no abnormalities aside from the finding of a pulsatile mass in the floor of the left middle ear.

A, left external carotid arteriogram, subtracted frontal view: A highly

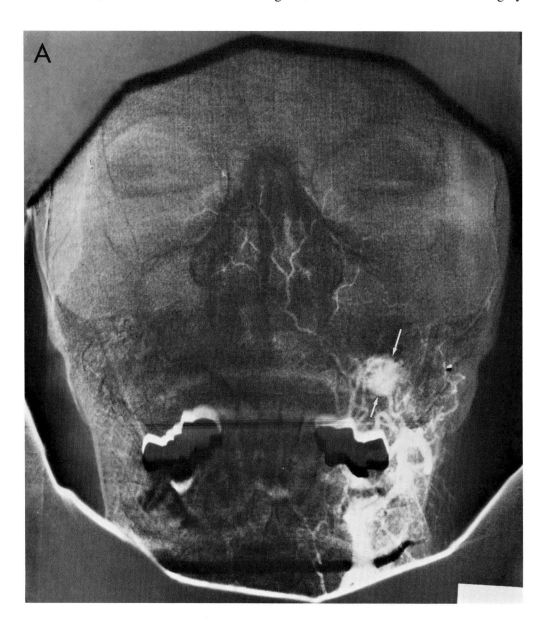

vascular mass (**arrows**) is seen in the temporal bone partly within the middle ear and partly within the jugular fossa.

B, selective left external carotid arteriogram, subtracted lateral view: The vascular mass (**arrows**) is fed by several external carotid branches, the most prominent of which is the ascending pharyngeal artery (**a**). In addition, preauricular (**b**) and postauricular (**c**) branches of the external occipital artery enter the glomus tumor.

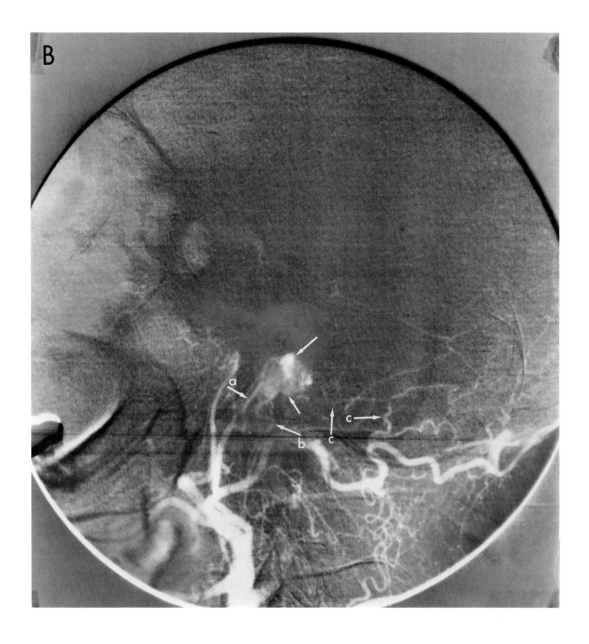

Figure 111 · Glomus Tympanicum Tumor / 367

Figure 112.—Clivus chordoma.

A 30-year-old man was seen because of recent onset of diplopia and slurred speech. Examination revealed diminished gag reflex, atrophy of the right side of the tongue and sixth nerve palsy.

A, right vertebral arteriogram, subtracted frontal view, arterial phase: An enlarged anterior meningeal artery (**solid arrow**) with a small tumor stain (**open arrow**) is evident. The right vertebral artery is displaced to the right as is also the posterior inferior cerebellar artery. A left vertebral arteriogram showed identical changes, that is, splitting of the two vertebral arteries and posterior inferior cerebellar arteries.

B, right vertebral arteriogram, subtracted lateral view, arterial phase: The enlarged anterior meningeal artery (**solid arrow**) and small stain (**open arrow**) are again seen. Marked posterior displacement of the brain stem by the clivus tumor is outlined by the posteriorly displaced vertebral and basilar arteries.

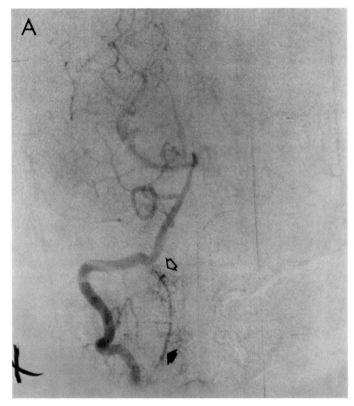

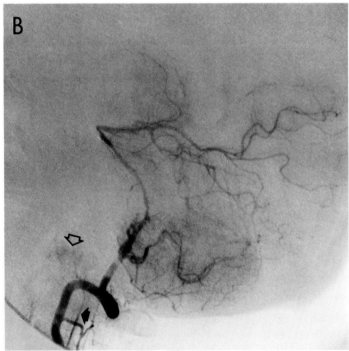

Figure 112 · Clivus Chordoma / 369

Figure 113.—Clivus chordoma.

A 21-year-old man had a left sixth nerve weakness that developed four years prior to admission. More recently he noted a change in his voice and began to have difficulty in swallowing. He also noted weakness in the left arm and shoulder. Examination revealed left sixth nerve palsy, right lateral gaze nystagmus and deficits in the left ninth, tenth and twelfth nerves. At operation gross total removal of the tumor was accomplished. Because of the nature of the tumor the patient also received radiotherapy.

A, lateral laminagram at a left-sided parasellar level: A reasonably well corticated fragment of bone (**a**) is seen behind the sella and above the petrous bone. This is within the chordoma and sequestered off of the clivus.

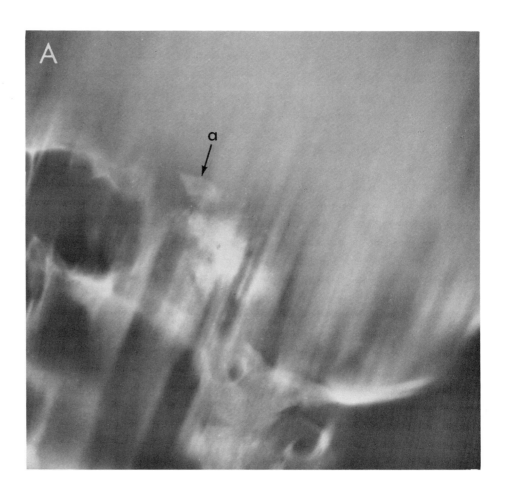

B, bilateral brachial arteriogram with right carotid compression, frontal view: The intracranial portions of the vertebral arteries and the basilar artery are markedly displaced to the right. The posterior inferior cerebellar artery (**b**) also shows right-sided displacement, although to a lesser degree. The left superior cerebellar (**c**) and posterior cerebral arteries (**d**) are elevated.

(Continued.)

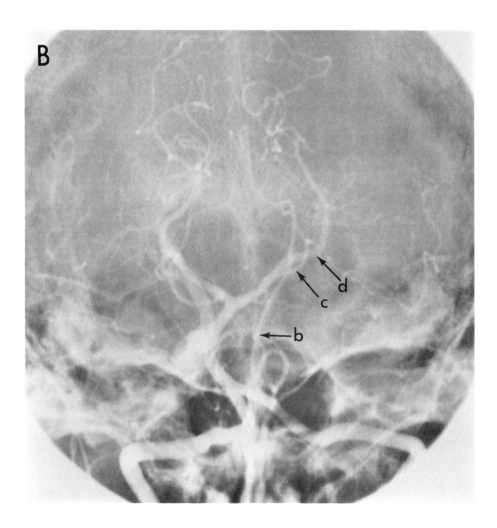

Figure 113 · Clivus Chordoma / 371

Figure 113 (cont.).—Clivus chordoma.

C, bilateral brachial arteriogram, lateral view, arterial phase: The normal anterior convexity of the basilar artery has been lost. No meningeal blood supply to the tumor is seen.

D, bilateral brachial arteriogram, frontal view, venous phase: There is displacement of the left cerebellar hemispheric vein (**e**) in its proximal portion. However, the two inferior vermian veins (**f**) show no evidence of displacement. The cerebellar hemisphere vein is lower and more ventral in location and is therefore closer to the tumor.

(Continued.)

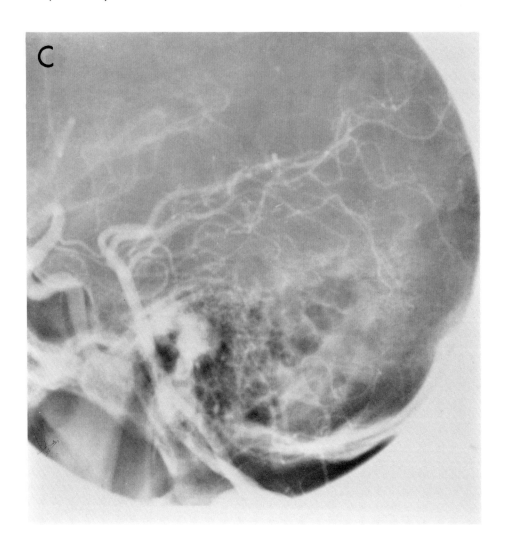

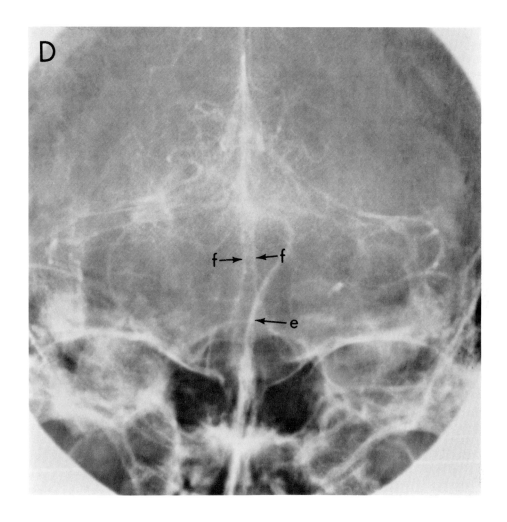

D

Figure 113 · Clivus Chordoma / 373

Figure 113 (cont.).—Clivus chordoma.

E, bilateral brachial arteriogram, lateral view, venous phase: A local deformity of the pontomesencephalic vein (**g**) at the level of the belly of the pons is seen. No other local deformity of venous structures is apparent. Small tonsillar veins (**h**) outline very mild tonsil herniation.

F, frontal laminagram during pneumoencephalography: The upper portion of the tumor (**i**) is capped by air. The left perimesencephalic cistern (**j**) is mildly dilated and is mildly displaced medially.

G, pneumoencephalogram, lateral view: The tonsils are mildly herniated (**h**). A soft tissue mass fills the pontine cistern, and the upper border of the mass (**i**) is capped in the interpeduncular fossa.

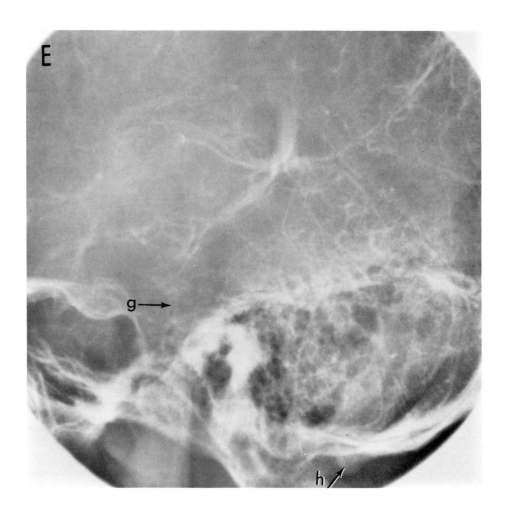

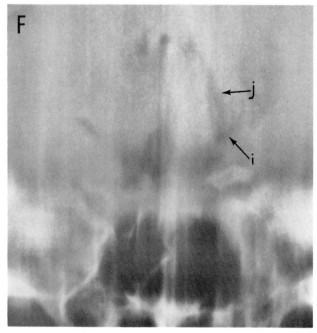

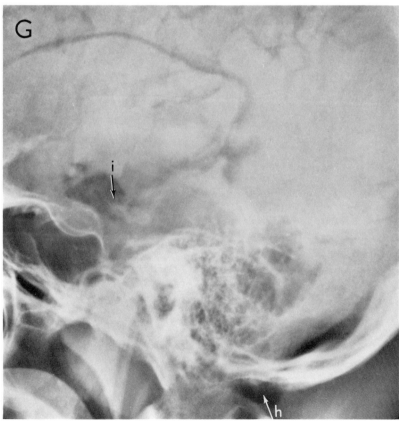

Figure 113 · Clivus Chordoma / 375

Figure 114.—Neuroepithelial cyst.

This patient was first studied at age 2 because of third nerve palsy on the left. A mass was found in the interpeduncular region. A cystic mass excised at surgery was described by the pathologist as a neuroepithelial cyst. Microscopically the specimen consisted of a narrow band of loose-meshed fibrous tissue in which some of the fibers were calcified. A layer of high columnar epithelium lined one surface of the cyst wall; in other areas there was considerable pseudostratification. The patient was rehospitalized 11 years later because of difficulty in controlling seizures of a psychomotor nature which had developed 1 year after surgery. The seizures were quite well controlled in the hospital so surgical intervention was not recommended.

A, pneumoencephalogram, frontal view, brow-up position: A rounded calcified lesion (**arrow**) just to the right of the midline is causing a very minimal deformity of the anterior tip of the third ventricle.

B, pneumoencephalogram, lateral view, filling position: The irregular mass (**arrow**) is outlined in the pontine and interpeduncular cisterns. Air within the cisterns completely separates the upper half of the mass from the clivus. However, a soft tissue component inferiorly is contiguous with the clivus. The midbrain and pons are slightly displaced posteriorly, with consequent straightening of the aqueduct. There is, however, no evidence of obstruction to flow of cerebrospinal fluid as there is no enlargement of the third and lateral ventricles.

C, laminagram at the level of the clivus during pneumoencephalography, frontal view, filling position: The mass (**arrows**) is well outlined by air within the interpeduncular and pontine cisterns laterally and superiorly. The attachment appears inferiorly on the clivus.

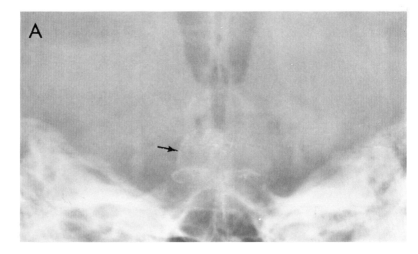

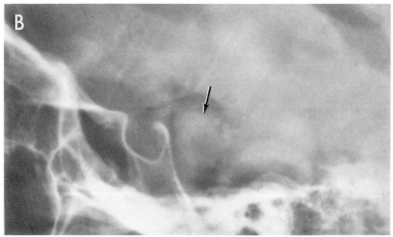

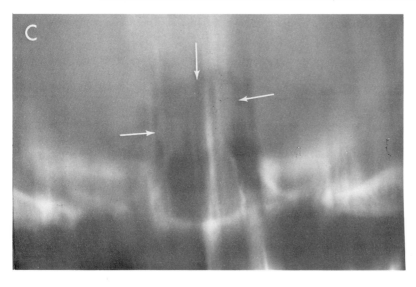

Figure 114 · Neuroepithelial Cyst / 377

Figure 115.—Acoustic neurilemmoma.

A, pneumoencephalogram, erect position: Tonsillar herniation (**a**) is evident, with mild forward displacement of the cervical cord (**b**). The coning effect of the tonsils has trapped this air in spite of the patient's being in an erect position.

B, pneumoencephalogram: There are marked deformity and compression with displacement of the fourth ventricle (**c**) to the left side. There is filling of the left cerebellopontine angle (**d**). The right cerebellopontine angle is completely obliterated.

C, autotomogram, brow-down position: The fourth ventricle (**c**) is displaced posteriorly.

D, autotomogram, brow-up position: There is elevation of the floor of the third ventricle (**e**) and midbrain secondary to the upward transtentorial herniation.

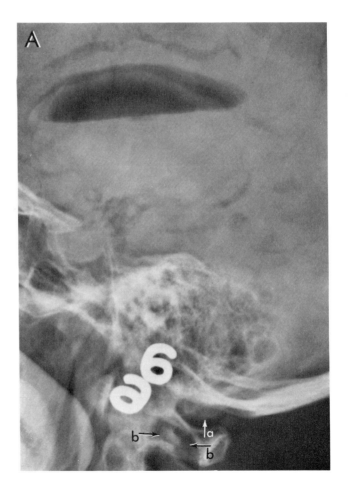

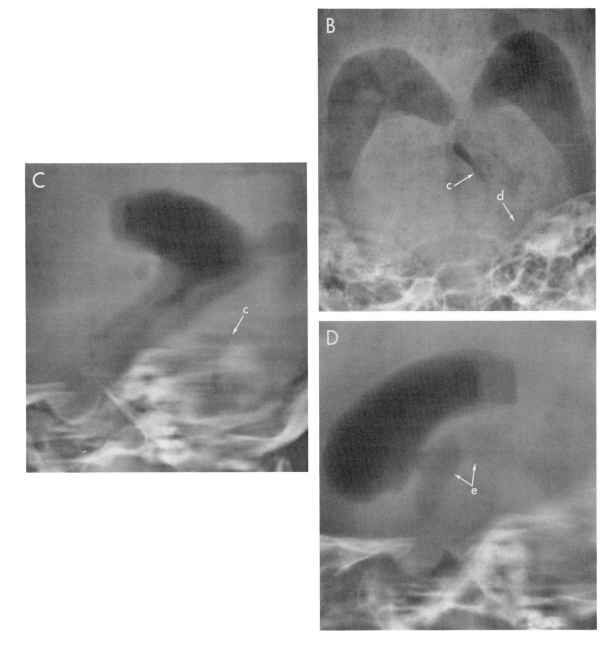

Figure 115 · Acoustic Neurilemmoma / 379

Figure 116.—Acoustic neurilemmoma.

A, polytomograms of the right and left auditory canals: The right canal is normal. The left canal shows expansion of the intracanalicular portion (**a**) and erosion of the posterior wall (**b**) and suprameatal portion (**c**).

B, pneumoencephalogram, frontal view: The fourth ventricle is tilted upward on its left side (**d**). Mild left-to-right displacement is also present.

C, pneumoencephalogram following increased injection of air, frontal view: This reveals widening of the left perimedullary cistern and capping of the medial surface of the acoustic neurilemmoma (**arrows**).

D, autotomogram during pneumoencephalography, filling position, lateral view: The fourth ventricle is in normal position but is enlarged in its antero-posterior diameter. The tonsils are not herniated. Increased intracranial pressure changes are evident in the sella turcica.

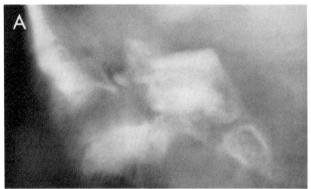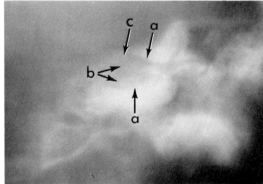

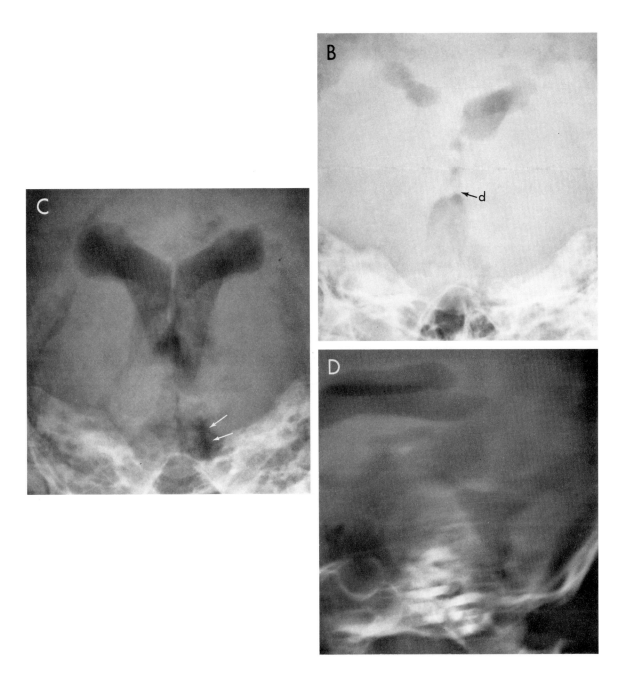

Figure 116 · Acoustic Neurilemmoma / 381

Figure 117.—Acoustic neurilemmoma.

A, polytomograms of the right and left internal auditory canals: The right canal is normal. The left canal shows persistent enlargement from the region of the intracanalicular portion (**a**) to the porus acousticus (**b**). Undercutting of the suprameatal portion (**c**) of the canal is also evident.

B, pneumoencephalogram, filling position, frontal view: There is slight left-to-right displacement of the vallecula (**d**) and fourth ventricle (**e**). The infratentorial perimesencephalic cistern on the left (**f**) stops at the upper pole of the tumor (**arrows**), which is faintly outlined by air within the cerebellopontine angle cistern. It is interesting that the tumor has caused so little deformity of the fourth ventricle in spite of its large size (2.5 cm).

C, pneumoencephalogram, filling position, lateral view: No deformity or enlargement of the fourth ventricle is seen.

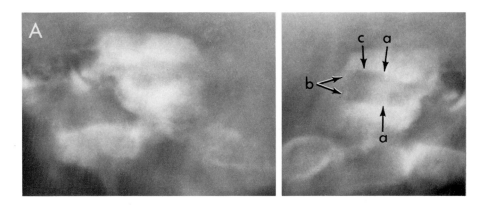

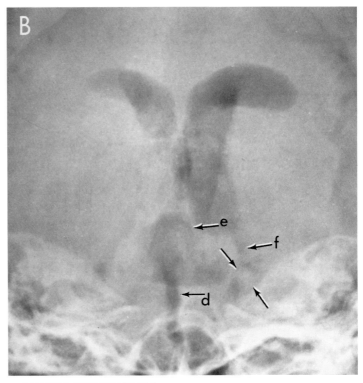

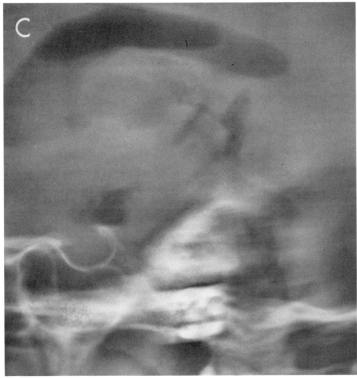

Figure 117 · Acoustic Neurilemmoma / 383

Figure 118.—Left acoustic neurinoma, partially cystic.

A 37-year-old man had a 10-year history of decreased hearing on the left and a 1-year history of ataxia. On examination palsies involving the left fifth, sixth and seventh cranial nerves were found. Bilateral papilledema was evident. Surgery disclosed a large vascular gritty tumor extending out from the internal auditory meatus. Ventrally and medially there was a cystic component containing about 60 cc of xanthochromic fluid. The lower end of the tumor was decompressed; the superior portion extending into the incisura could not be approached. Postoperatively the patient did well but developed signs of increased intracranial pressure secondary to an incisural block; following ventriculoatrial shunt, he showed further improvement.

Bibrachial arteriogram, subtracted Caldwell view, arterial phase. There is displacement of the posterior inferior cerebellar arteries (**a**) to the right. The left anterior inferior cerebellar artery (**b**) is attenuated and displaced inferiorly, and several small branches (**c**) are seen to enter the tumor. Mild medial and upper displacement of the left superior cerebellar artery (**d**) is evident. There is also mild elevation of the left posterior cerebral artery (**e**).

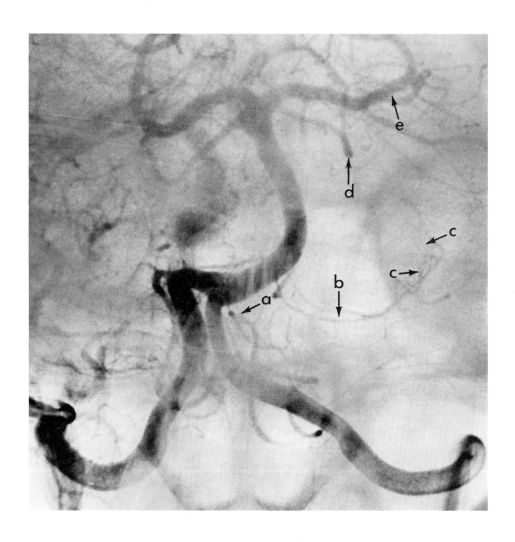

Figure 118 · Left Acoustic Neurinoma / 385

Figure 119.—Left acoustic neurinoma.

A 65-year-old woman with long-standing decreased hearing in the left ear complained of recent onset of numbness of the left side of the face and unsteadiness of gait. Examination revealed nystagmus in all directions, most pronounced on left lateral gaze. No papilledema was present. Numbness was present in all divisions of the fifth cranial nerve, and taste was absent on the anterior portion of the left tongue. Hearing was decreased on the left side, and there was no left caloric response to ice water. At operation a moderately vascular neurinoma was removed from the left cerebellopontine angle.

A, selective right vertebral arteriogram, Towne projection, subtracted

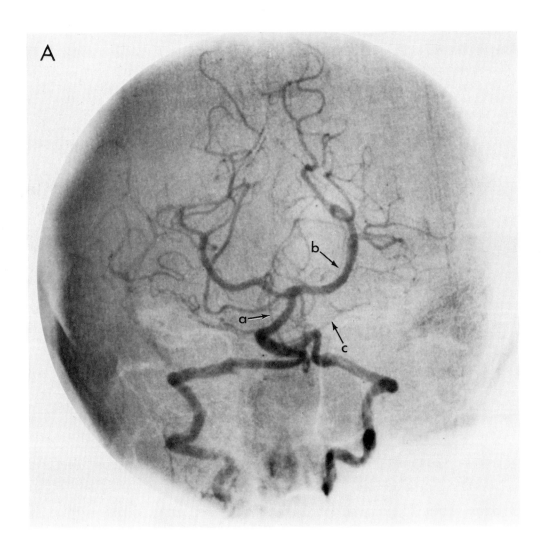

frontal view, arterial phase: The posterior inferior cerebellar artery is displaced to the right (**a**), and the superior cerebellar artery on the left (**b**) is elevated and partially obscured by the posterior cerebral artery. The left anterior inferior cerebellar artery shows an area of straightening (**c**).

B, selective right vertebral arteriogram, Caldwell projection, subtracted frontal view: The changes of the left anterior inferior cerebellar artery (**c**) are better appreciated here, with local mass effect seen as it courses behind the left petrous bone. A small area of tumor stain (**x**) is seen at the peripheral portion of the lower branch; **a,** posterior inferior cerebellar artery; **b,** superior cerebellar artery.

(*Continued.*)

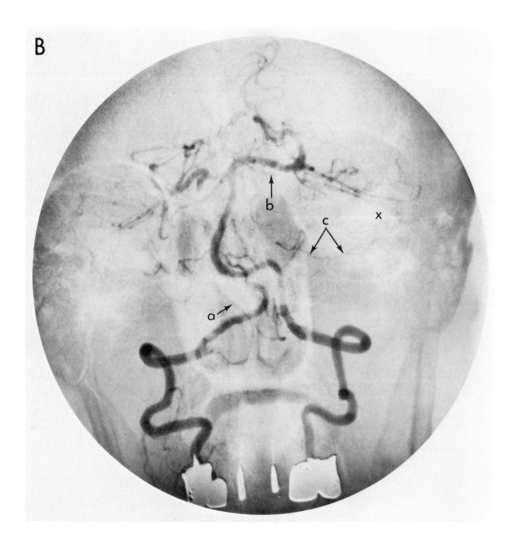

Figure 119 · Left Acoustic Neurinoma / 387

Figure 119 (cont.).—Left acoustic neurinoma.

C, right vertebral arteriogram, subtracted lateral view, arterial phase: There is mild posterior displacement of the choroidal loop (**a**) of the posterior inferior cerebellar artery. The position of the basilar artery appears to be normal. One superior cerebellar artery (**b**) is elevated above the other and represents the displaced left-sided vessel. The stretched vessel seen through the petrous bone represents the anterior inferior cerebellar artery (**c**) on the

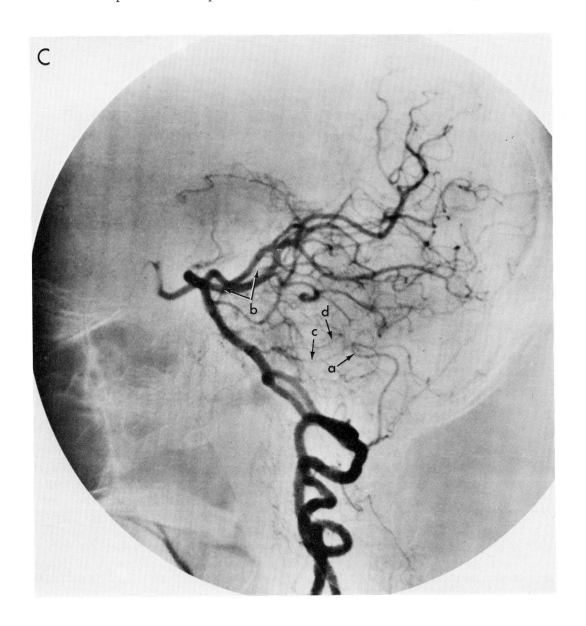

left. Compare it with the more ambling course of the normal right-sided anterior inferior cerebellar artery (**d**).

D, right vertebral arteriogram, Towne projection, frontal view: The left petrosal vein (**e**) is elevated. A small area of tumor staining (**x**) with small venous structures draining the tumor is seen in the region of the cerebello-pontine angle. The left crural vein (**f**) is flattened; compare to the normal right crural vein (**arrow**).

(Continued.)

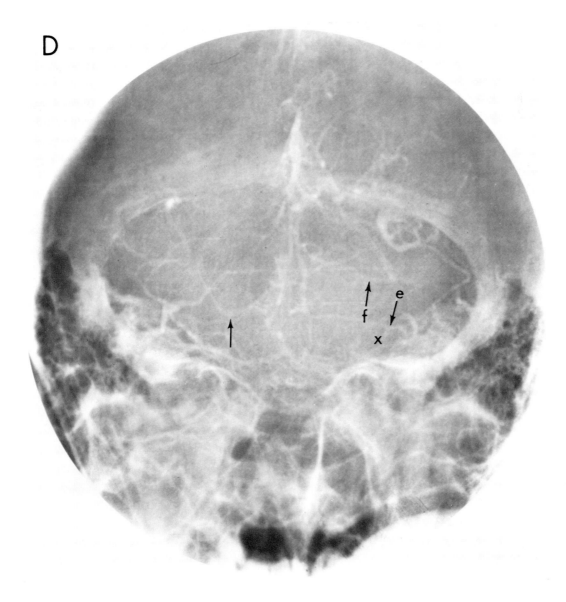

Figure 119 · Left Acoustic Neurinoma / 389

Figure 119 (cont.).—Left acoustic neurinoma.

    E, right vertebral arteriogram, Caldwell projection, subtracted frontal view, venous phase: The elevation of the left petrosal vein (**e**) with a normal superior petrosal sinus indicates the intradural position of the lesion.

    F, right vertebral arteriogram, subtracted lateral view, venous phase: Several arcuately coursing veins (**g**) cap the upper and posterior portions of the angle neurinoma.

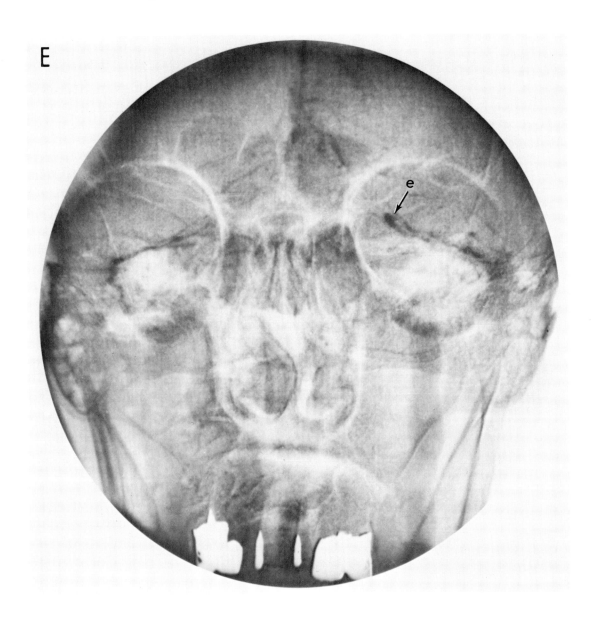

F

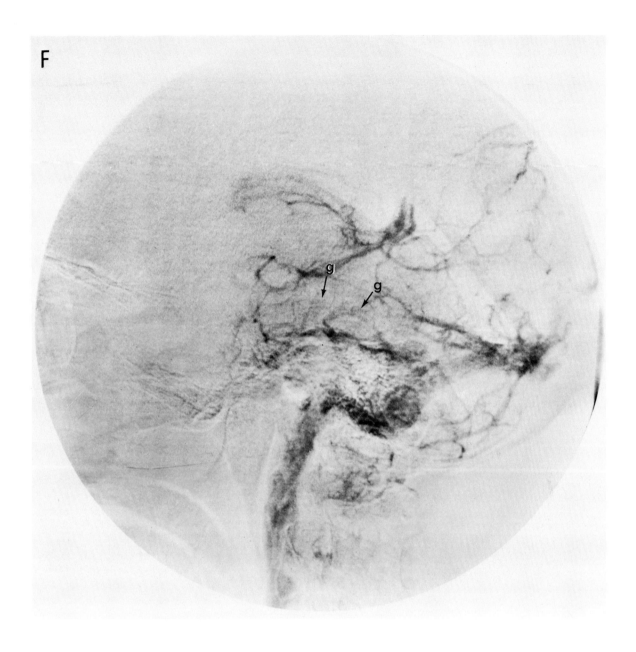

Figure 119 · Left Acoustic Neurinoma / 391

Figure 120.—Left cerebellopontine angle meningioma.

A 39-year-old woman had a 2½-year history of progressive hearing loss in the left ear. In the previous year, she had had episodes of pain in the back of the neck followed by headache. She had also noted infrequent occurrences of blurred vision. Her gait was slightly broad-based, and she was unsteady on tandem walking. Hearing was diminished on the left. Advanced papilledema with hemorrhage was seen on funduscopic examination. At operation the tumor was found to involve the dura, extending laterally over the sigmoid sinus inferiorly into the foramen magnum and medially to the midline.

A, left brachial arteriogram, frontal view, arterial phase: There is marked elevation of the left anterior inferior cerebellar artery (**a**). The opposite one (**b**) is in normal position. There is minimal medial displacement of the left superior cerebellar artery (**c**).

B, left brachial arteriogram, frontal view, venous phase: A faint but definite tumor stain (**arrows**) is seen in the cerebellopontine angle with elevation of the petrosal vein (**d**) and its tributaries. There is slight displacement to the right of the cerebral peduncles as outlined by the crural veins (**e**).

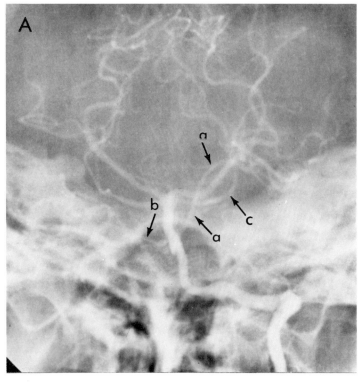

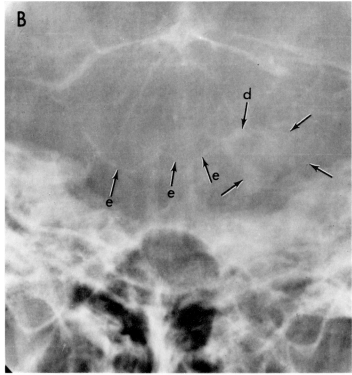

Figure 120 · Cerebellopontine Angle Meningioma / 393

Figure 121.—Cerebellopontine angle cholesteatoma.

A 29-year-old woman had hearing loss on the right and uncontrollable episodes of blinking of the right eyelid. At craniotomy the contents of a cholesteatoma were evacuated and partial removal of the lining was effected.

A, modified Towne view: A smooth area of destruction of the medial aspect of the right petrous tip is seen. A curvilinear calcification (**a**) outlines the upper portion of the cholesteatoma.

B, base view: A smoothly outlined erosive defect (**b**) involves the floor of the middle fossa extending into the body of the sphenoid bone medially as well as the petrous bone laterally.

C, frontal laminagram: At the level of the clivus the smoothly outlined erosion of the basisphenoid (**c**) and basiocciput (**d**) is well appreciated. Calcification (**a**) in the upper pole of the mass is seen as well as the petrous bone erosion laterally.

D, right carotid arteriogram, frontal view: There is marked compression of the internal carotid artery in the cavernous (**e**) and precavernous (**f**) portions and to a lesser extent as it enters the base of the skull and within the carotid canal.

(Continued.)

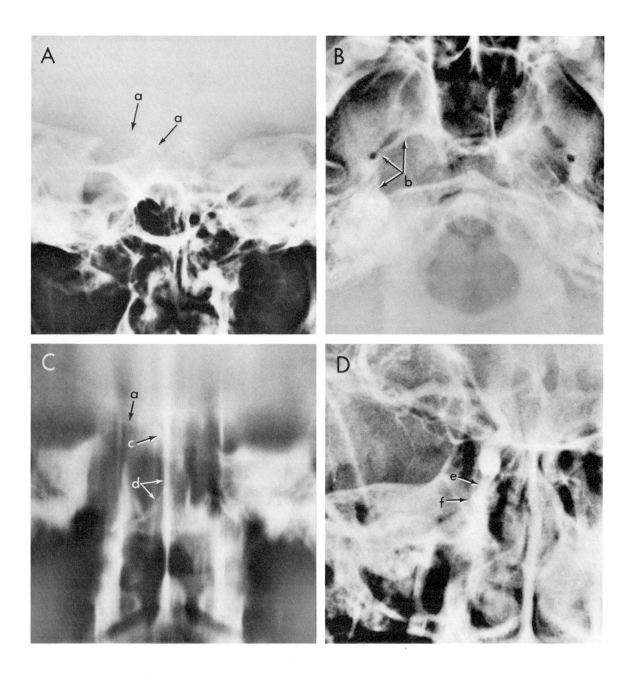

Figure 121 · Cerebellopontine Angle Cholesteatoma / 395

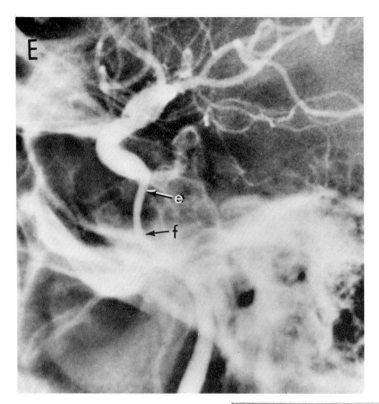

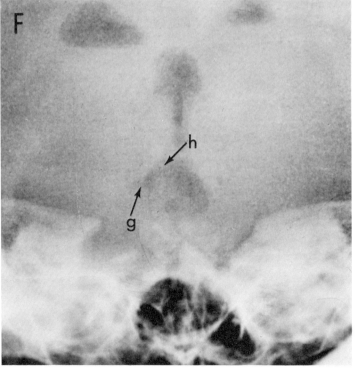

Figure 121 (cont.).—Cerebellopontine angle cholesteatoma.

E, right carotid arteriogram, lateral view: Forward displacement of the cavernous (**e**) and precavernous (**f**) portions is evident. The carotid artery is narrowed in this area as well as the more proximal portions within the carotid canal and skull base.

F, pneumoencephalogram, frontal view: There is slight blunting of the right side of the fourth ventricle with elevation of the lateral recess (**g**) and a minimal upward tilt of the right side of the superior medullary vellum (**h**). No significant displacement of the fourth ventricle is seen. Because of the extradural position of the lesion, one does not expect large displacements of the posterior fossa contents.

G, autotomogram, lateral view, filling phase of pneumoencephalogram: The fourth ventricle is in normal position. Vertebral arteriography, also performed, showed only minimal changes on the basilar artery and its branches.

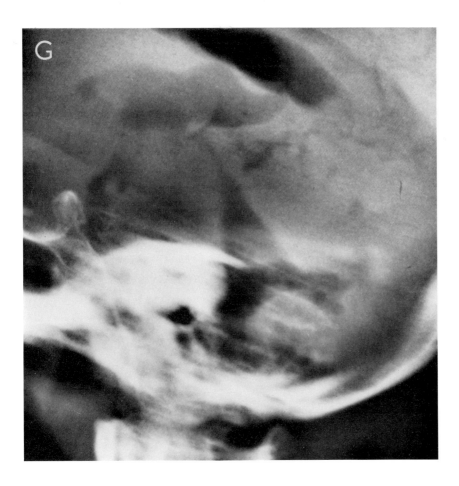

Figure 121 · Cerebellopontine Angle Cholesteatoma / 397

Figure 122.—Tenth nerve neurinoma.

A 32-year-old woman noted speech difficulty during pregnancy five years prior to admission. A year later, study revealed deficits of the left ninth, tenth, eleventh and twelfth cranial nerves. More recently tinnitus, hearing loss and diplopia on left lateral gaze had developed. At craniotomy a completely extradural neurinoma involving the tenth nerve was found and partially removed.

A, skull radiograph, Caldwell projection: There is diminished density of the medial portion of the left petrous bone seen through the maxillary sinus.

B, laminagram through the petrous bones, frontal view: There is a large area of destruction (**a**) in the left jugular fossa involving the floor of the internal auditory canal superiorly and extending medially to destroy the cortical border superiorly of the left jugular tubercle.

C, right and left Stenvers projections: These give a clearer appreciation of the destruction (**a**) of the inferior surface of the left petrous bone.

(*Continued.*)

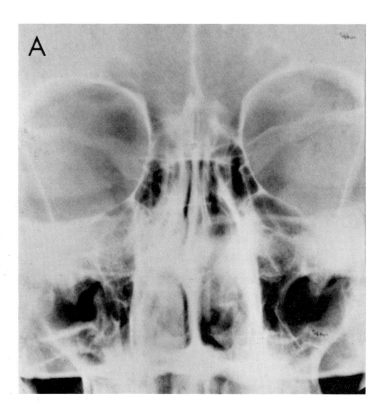

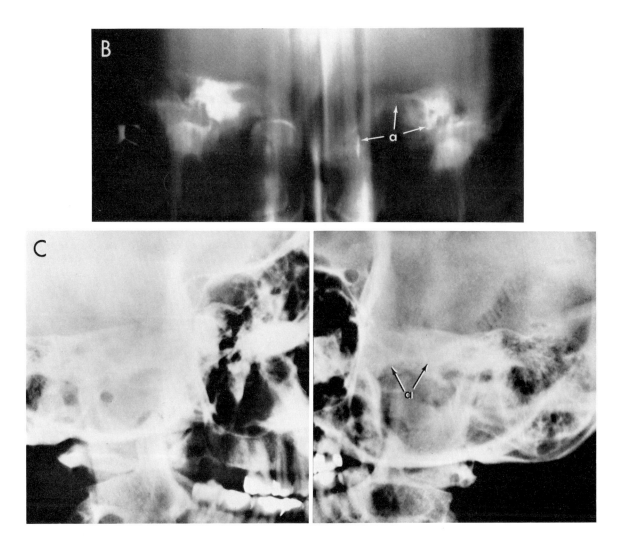

Figure 122 · Tenth Nerve Neurinoma / 399

Figure 122 (cont.).—Tenth nerve neurinoma.

D, lateral view: A soft tissue density is seen in the region of the naso-pharynx but not representing the nasopharynx, as one can see its inferior border (**b**) extend to the bony border of the body of C-2.

E, base view: The anteromedial border (**c**) of the neurinoma is outlined within the left side of the nasopharyngeal air shadow.

F, left common carotid arteriogram, lateral view: There is mild anterior bowing of the distal cervical portion (**d**) of the internal carotid artery.

(Continued.)

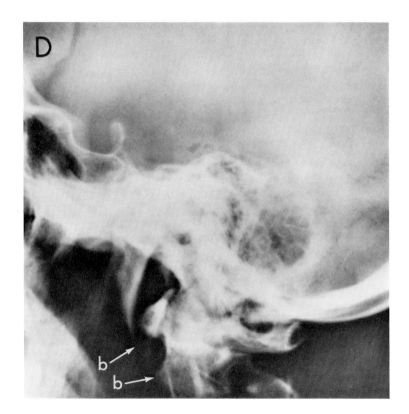

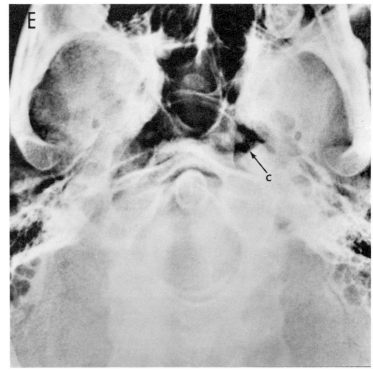

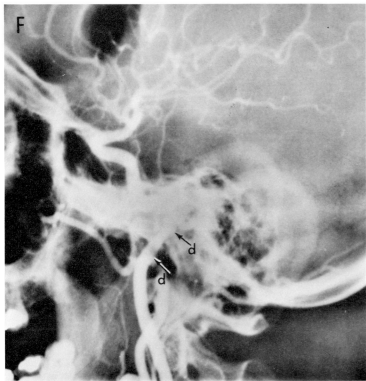

Figure 122 · Tenth Nerve Neurinoma / 401

Figure 122 (cont.).—Tenth nerve neurinoma.

G, left external carotid arteriogram, lateral view: Marked forward bowing of the ascending pharyngeal artery (**e**) is seen with several small branches arising from it supplying small areas of neovascularity (**arrows**) in the neurinoma.

H, left vertebral arteriogram, subtracted frontal view, arterial phase: The anterior meningeal artery becomes tortuous as it extends toward the region of the neurinoma (**arrows**). Small tortuous vessels (**f**) arising from the posterior inferior cerebellar artery also extend to the lesion. The posterior inferior cerebellar arteries (**g**) are slightly displaced to the right of the midline.

I, pneumoencephalogram, frontal view: No ventricular or cisternal abnormality is seen aside from changes compatible with mild hydrocephalus. The lack of displacement of the fourth ventricle is not uncommon with extradural tumors and particularly in this case, in which the tumor is situated more anteriorly.

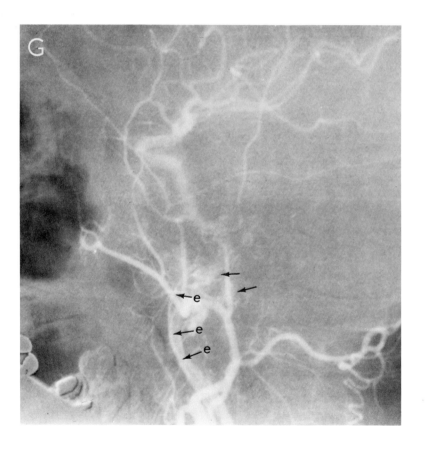

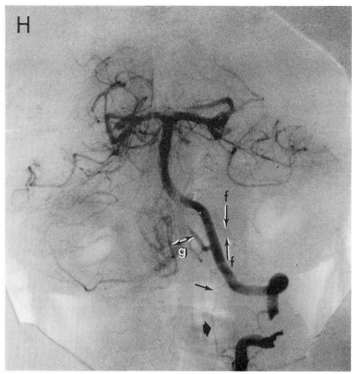

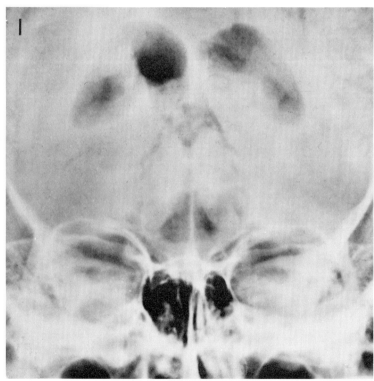

Figure 122 · Tenth Nerve Neurinoma / 403

Figure 123.—Fifth nerve neurinoma.

A 73-year-old man had had failing vision in the right eye for about one year. Visual acuity was diminished to counting fingers. There was a mild Horner's syndrome on the right, with slight sixth nerve weakness on the right, definite hypalgesia and diminished corneal reflex and diminished motor action involving the fifth nerve on the right.

A, Towne projection: The pineal gland is displaced slightly to the left. The medial aspect of the right petrous pyramid is destroyed. An ill-defined soft tissue density (**arrows**) is seen in the region of the sella turcica extending from the right to just beyond the left side of the midline.

B, optic canal views: The left side is normal; a discrete optic strut (**a**) divides the optic canal and superior orbital fissure. The right side shows marked enlargement of the superior orbital fissure (**b**), with loss of the entire lateral boundary of the optic canal.

(Continued.)

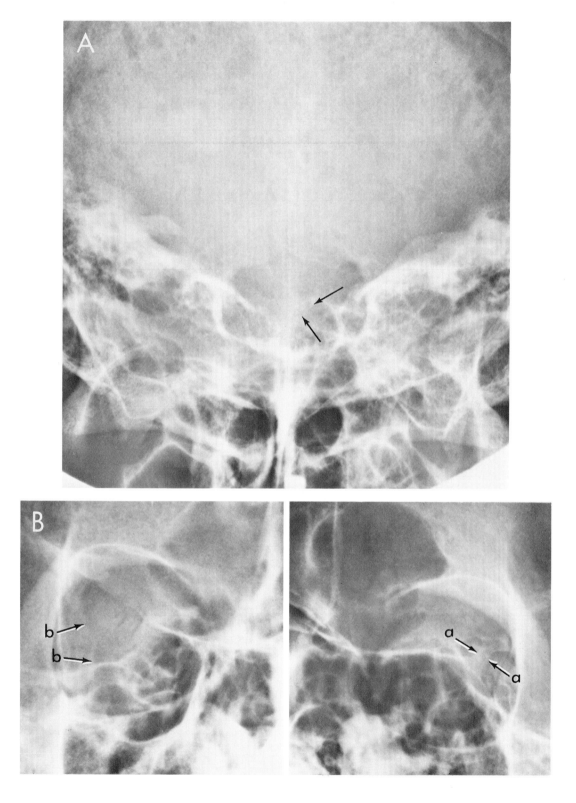

Figure 123 · Fifth Nerve Neurinoma / 405

Figure 123 (cont.).—Fifth nerve neurinoma.

C, laminagram at the level of the body of the sphenoid, frontal view: A soft tissue mass´ (**arrow**) is seen in the right and middle thirds of the body of the sphenoid obliterating the floor of the sella turcica.

D, laminagram just to the right of the midline, lateral view: The floor of the pituitary fossa is markedly deepened. A soft tissue mass presents anteriorly with a thin cortical remnant (**arrows**) just behind the greater wing of the sphenoid.

E, right brachial arteriogram, frontal view, early arterial phase: The right superior cerebellar (**c**) and posterior cerebral (**d**) arteries are elevated. Beginning filling of the right carotid circulation delineates the marked medial displacement of the cavernous (**e**) and supraclinoid (**f**) portions of the internal carotid artery as well as elevation of the middle cerebral artery (**g**).

F, right brachial arteriogram, frontal view, midarterial phase: Displacement upward and medially of the anterior and midportions of the middle cerebral artery and its branches is evident. The displacement of the anterior cerebral artery (**h**) is disproportionately small in comparison with the local mass effects.

(Continued.)

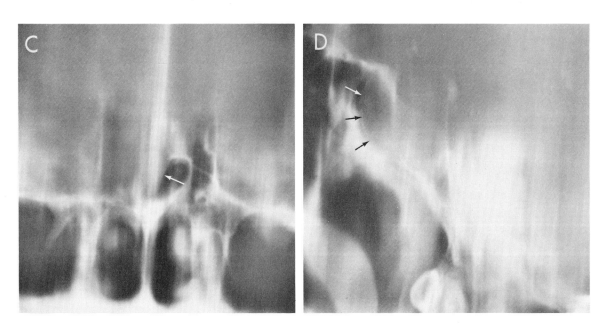

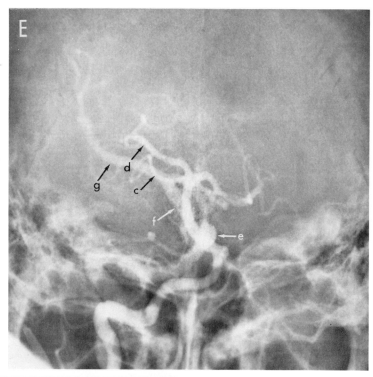

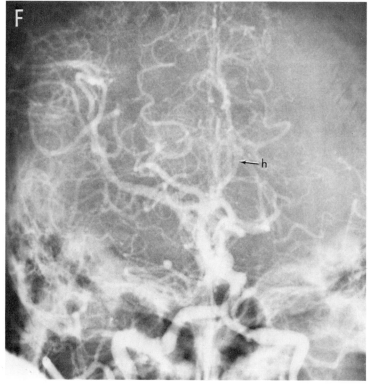

Figure 123 · Fifth Nerve Neurinoma / 407

Figure 123 (cont.).—Fifth nerve neurinoma.

G, right brachial arteriogram, Caldwell projection: The middle cerebral vessels going toward the temporal tip are definitely elevated (**i**) by the extra-axial mass.

H, right brachial arteriogram, lateral view, arterial phase: Elevation of the right superior cerebellar (**c**) and posterior cerebral (**d**) arteries is again evident; these vessels are seen to be displaced posteriorly as well. The middle cerebral artery group is strikingly elevated.

(Continued.)

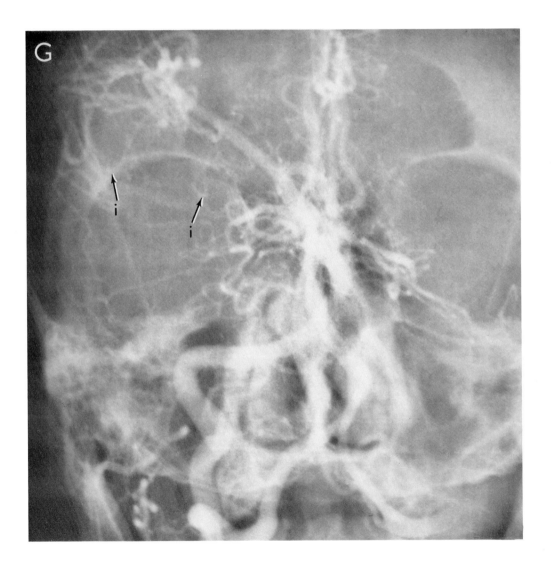

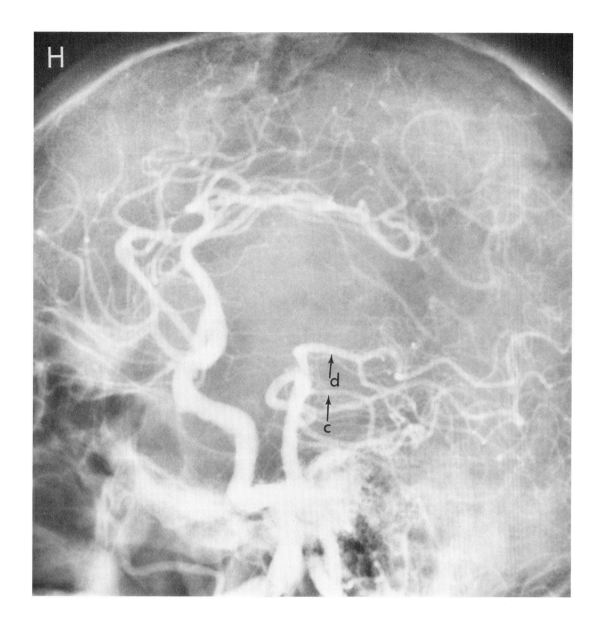

Figure 123 · Fifth Nerve Neurinoma / 409

Figure 123 (cont.).—Fifth nerve neurinoma.

l, right brachial arteriogram, frontal view, venous phase: There is mild displacement of the internal cerebral vein (**j**). The veins draining into the petrosal vein (**k**) on the right are higher in position than those on the left secondary to the extension of the fifth nerve neurinoma into the petrous apex. The tumor has probably occluded the venous outflow in the right petrosal

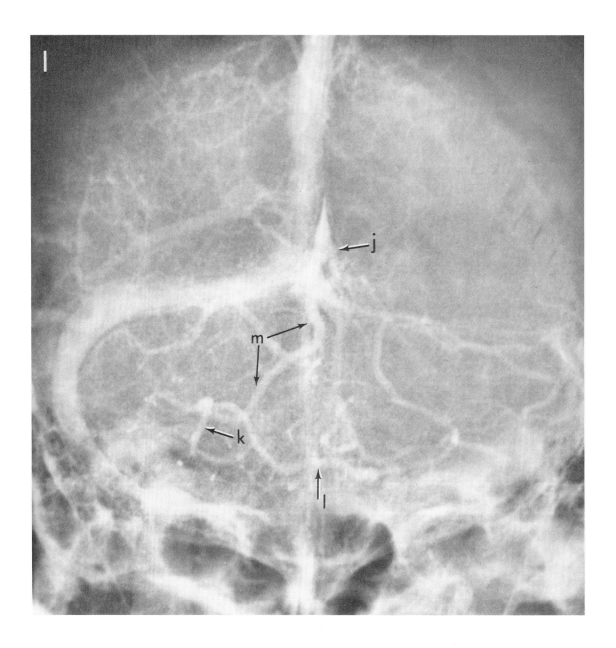

sinus as there is a large transverse pontine vein (**l**) coursing across the midline toward the opposite petrosal vein. **m**, great cerebellar vein.

J, right brachial arteriogram, lateral view, venous phase: The basal vein of Rosenthal (**n**) is conspicuously elevated, particularly in its proximal portion. The great cerebellar vein (**m**) is a right-sided vein; the large venous structure in the prepontine region represents the anastomotic channel (**l**) from the right petrosal vein to the left petrosal vein.

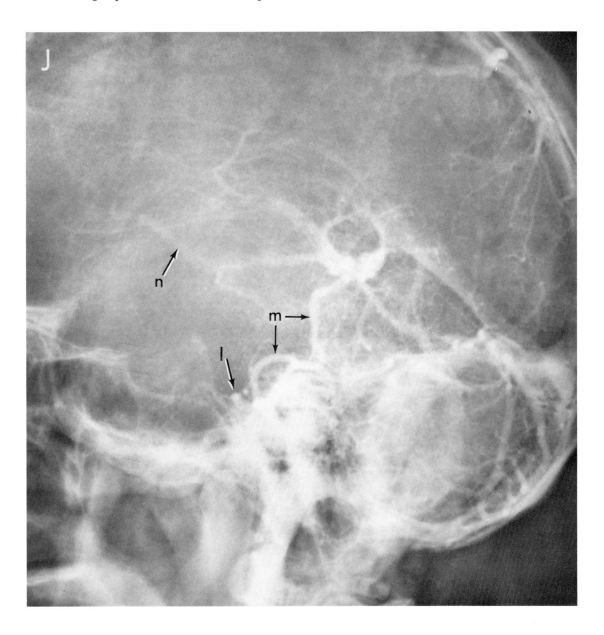

Figure 123 · Fifth Nerve Neurinoma / 411

Figure 124.—Fifth nerve neurinoma.

A 43-year-old woman had a one-year history of progressive numbness on the right side of the face and right-sided facial pain. Examination revealed altered taste sense on the right side of the tongue, slight weakness and atrophy of the orbicularis oris on the right and numbness in the second division of the right fifth nerve. Masseter muscle weakness was also evident on the right. There were no eighth nerve symptoms or signs. At operation a small tumor surrounding the fifth nerve was removed.

A, Pantopaque cisternogram, anteroposterior view: A prominent defect (**a**) is seen in the upper outer aspect of the Pantopaque column on the right side, just beneath the outline of the superior cerebellar arteries in the expected anatomic location of the fifth nerve. A smaller normal defect (**b**) is present on the left side.

B, cisternogram, oblique view, right side down: This shows the oval filling defect (**a**) of the right fifth nerve enlarged by the neurinoma.

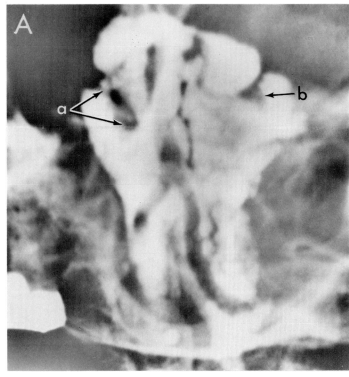

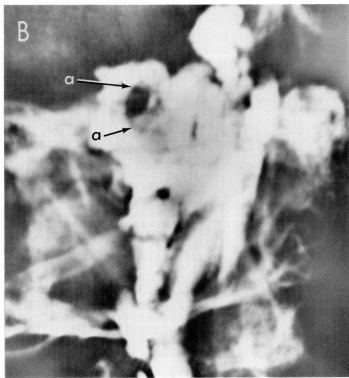

Figure 124 · Fifth Nerve Neurinoma / 413

PART 13

Meningiomas

General Characteristics

HISTORICALLY, meningiomas are among the best-known tumors, probably because they occasionally present as palpable protuberances on the cranial vault. With the advent of radiographic examination they could be diagnosed because of characteristic changes of the cranial vault such as hyperostosis, "blistering," erosive changes and increased vascular markings. In addition, calcification within the tumor ranging from fine psammomatous type to dense accumulation is seen. The incidence of meningiomas is wide, ranging from childhood to the later decades of life. The peak incidence is in the forties, and there is a slightly greater incidence in females than in males (4:3). The location of meningiomas is definitely associated with the distribution of the arachnoid granulations and so they are found most commonly in the parasagittal region. Supratentorially they are also common along the convexity, sphenoid ridge, subfrontal regions from the olfactory groove,

TABLE 6.—DURAL BLOOD SUPPLY (ARTERIAL)

Anterior fossa and frontal bone
  Ophthalmic artery branches
    Anterior ethmoidal
    Posterior ethmoidal
    Anterior falx
    Anterior meningeal
    Lacrimal
    Recurrent meningeal
  Superficial temporal artery, frontal branch
  Middle meningeal, anterior division
  Accessory meningeal

Middle fossa, temporal and parietal bones
  Recurrent meningeal
  Accessory meningeal
  Middle meningeal, anterior and posterior divisions
  Ascending pharyngeal
  Superficial temporal artery, temporal branch
  External occipital artery, auricular branch
  Internal carotid artery, precavernous (tentorial) and cavernous branches

Posterior fossa and occipital bones
  Vertebral artery, anterior and posterior meningeal arteries
  Internal carotid artery, cavernous and precavernous (tentorial) branches
  Ascending pharyngeal
  External occipital
  Middle meningeal, posterior division

cribriform plate and tuberculum regions, and less common from the tentorium, falx and temporal fossa and within the ventricles. Subtentorially the most usual site of involvement is the posterior aspect of the petrous bone and subjacent to the transverse and straight sinuses. This is followed by involvement of the foramen magnum and clivus. Because of the dural attachment of these lesions it is extremely important to understand the dural blood supply; for this reason an anatomic listing of that supply is presented in Table 6.

Meningosarcomas and angioblastic meningiomas are more aggressive tumors and are not necessarily characterized by the typical meningioma stain seen angiographically which appears late, is homogeneous and remains late and is often surrounded by a capping of veins around the tumor. Partial or complete occlusion of the sinus by a meningioma is also noteworthy and critical to surgical planning. The establishment of well-developed collaterals will permit resection of a portion of a sinus provided the collaterals are left intact. The meningosarcoma, when vascular, will often show numerous areas of neovascularity from its widespread dural attachment. Sarcoma appears to have a predilection for the middle fossa in children.

Figure 125.—Frontal meningioma.

A 49-year-old woman had a three-month history of personality change and a three-week history of rapid visual deterioration. Examination revealed bilateral papilledema with only light perception in the right eye and macular vision in the left eye. Mildly inappropriate behavior was noted during the examination. At operation a large left-sided parasagittal meningioma was removed. The tumor had a dural attachment extending over an area approximately 4 cm in diameter. It extended from the coronal suture to the frontal pole and down along the falx cerebri. The tumor did not involve the sagittal sinus, and the dural attachment was removed along the sinus without difficulty.

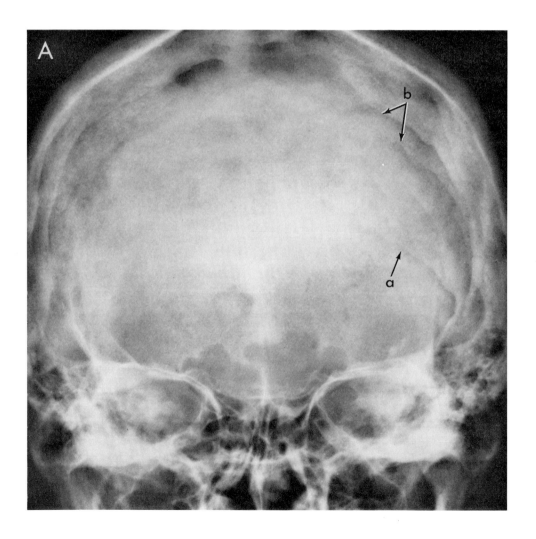

A, skull radiograph, frontal view: A hyperostotic area is present in the left parasagittal area in the frontal bone extending to the midline. One enlarged meningeal groove (**a**) is seen going to the central portion of the hyperostosis and two (**b**) to the upper pole of the hyperostosis. An enlarged vascular channel is evident just to the right of the midline above the frontal sinus.

B, skull radiograph, lateral view: The hyperostotic area is evident frontally. Enlarged grooves are visible going to the area as a single channel in the region of the pterion which then divides into two large and one small channel that progressively enlarge as they extend toward the dural attachment of the tumor.

(Continued.)

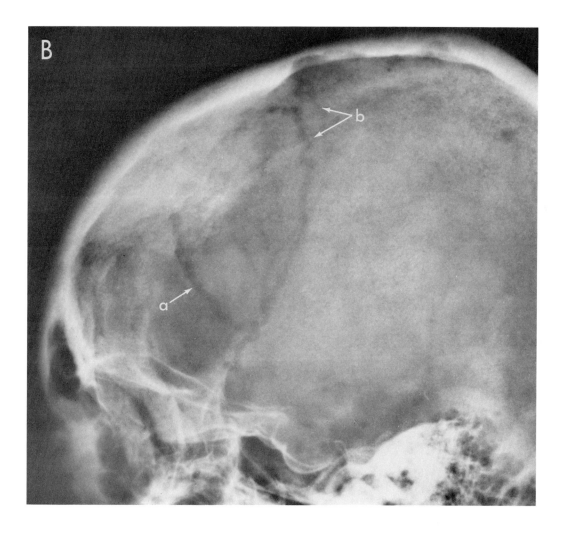

Figure 125 · Frontal Meningioma / 419

Figure 125 (cont.).—Frontal meningioma.

C, left carotid arteriogram, frontal view, arterial phase: The distal internal carotid artery is straightened and there is a pronounced shift of the anterior cerebral artery. Lateral displacement of the middle cerebral vessels, particularly the proximal insular loops, is apparent. An enlarged middle meningeal artery with two large branches (**c**) is visible along the inner table. The more anterior branch (**a**) is seen coursing to the parasagittal area to supply the tumor.

D, left carotid arteriogram, lateral view, arterial phase: The carotid siphon is closed and the Sylvian triangle depressed. There is marked stretching of the anterior cerebral arteries along their interhemispheric course (**d**). Enlargement of the accessory meningeal and middle meningeal vessels is well demonstrated as they course toward the meningioma.

(*Continued.*)

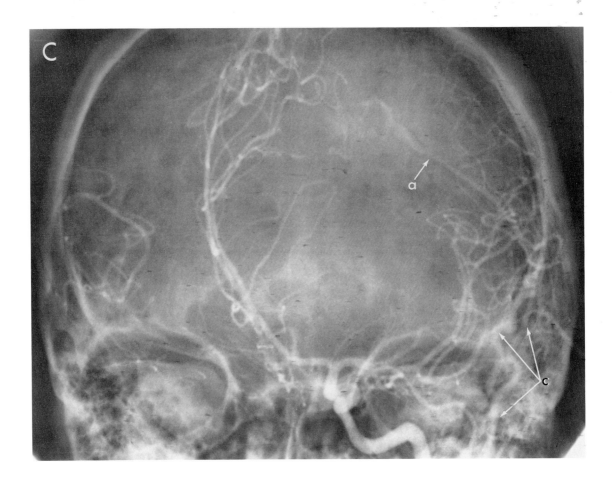

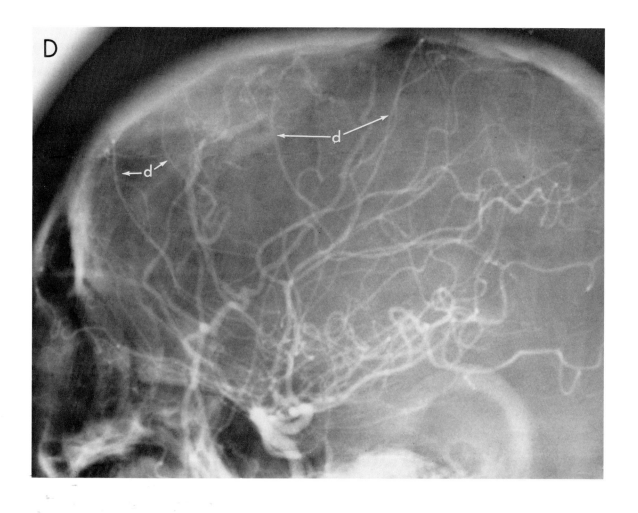

D

Figure 125 · Frontal Meningioma / 421

Figure 125 (cont.).—Frontal meningioma.

E, left carotid arteriogram, lateral view, late arterial phase: Characteristic tumor stain of meningioma is seen as the vessels extend from the dural pedicle and fan out into the vascular tumor bed.

F, left carotid arteriogram, frontal view, late arterial phase: The stellate distribution of the tumor vessels from the central pedicle is again well demonstrated. The tumor is seen to cross the midline.

G, left carotid arteriogram, lateral view, venous phase: There is marked downward displacement of the uncal (**e**) and poorly filled middle cerebral (**f**) veins secondary to trans-sphenoidal herniation. The internal cerebral vein is humped and its subependymal tributaries are markedly flattened. No collateral venous circulation is seen in the frontal region, and the entire frontal portion of the superior sagittal sinus is fragmentarily delineated.

(Continued.)

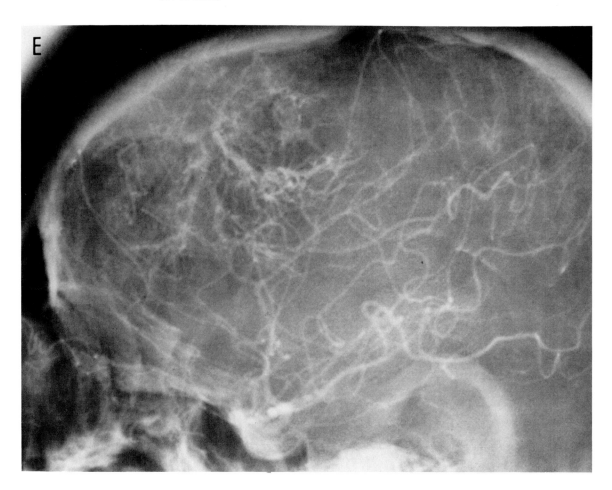

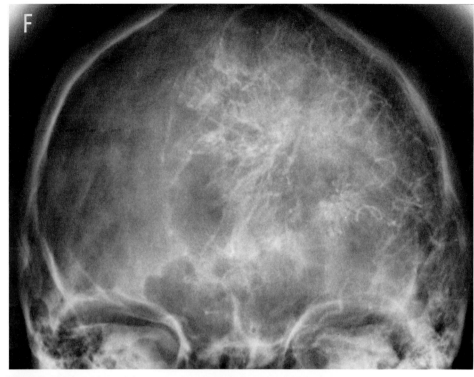

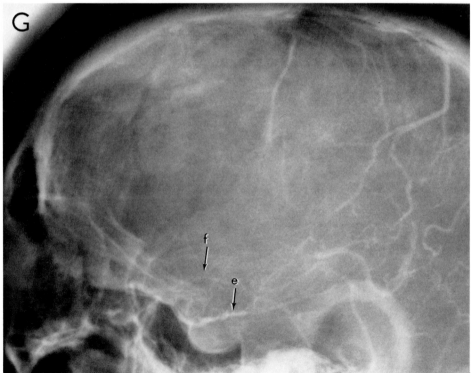

Figure 125 · Frontal Meningioma / 423

Figure 125 (cont.).—Frontal meningioma.

H, right carotid arteriogram, frontal view, arterial phase: A very large midline vessel representing the anterior falx artery (**g**) supplies the tumor.

I, right carotid arteriogram, lateral view, arterial phase: This shows separation and very slight stretching of the anterior cerebral arteries along their interhemispheric course (**h**). This corresponds to the approximate equator of the tumor, which has burrowed through the falx to produce this change. Marked posterior displacement of the vertical portion of the anterior cerebral artery (**i**) is also evident. The anterior falx artery (**g**) is well demonstrated as it arises from the ophthalmic artery and courses along the region of the superior sagittal sinus to supply the tumor. The accessory and middle meningeal arteries do not show evidence of enlargement.

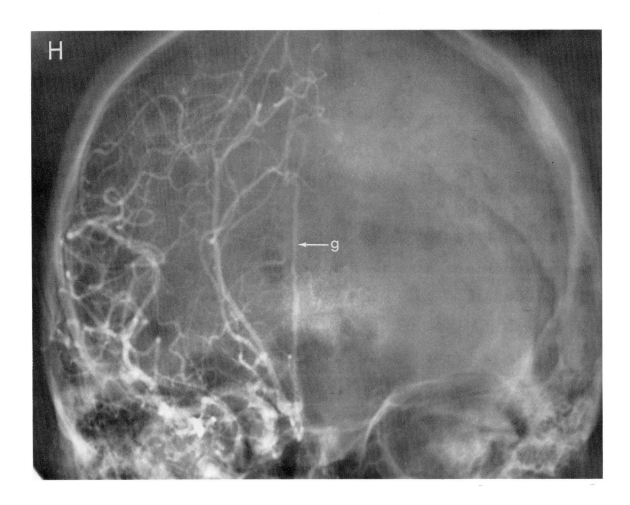

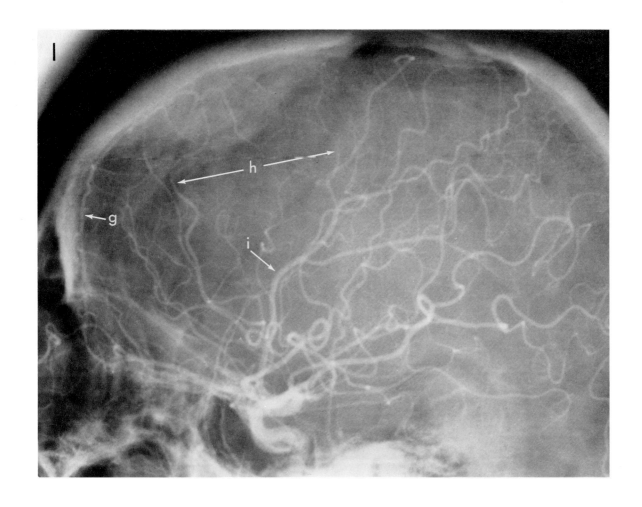

Figure 125 · Frontal Meningioma / 425

Figure 126.—Bifrontal meningioma arising from the left anterior falx.

A 51-year-old woman had decreasing vision in the left eye for six months. Examination revealed bilateral papilledema. Her affect was bland. There was a slightly increased space to the gait and some difficulty was encountered with tandem walking. Titubation of the arms and head was evident. Some extensor weakness was noted in the left arm and leg, as well as a drift of the left arm with a pronator sign. Dysmetria was present in both extremities on cerebellar testing. Total removal of the meningioma was effected. The surgeon stated that the tumor had originated from the falx cerebri.

A, left carotid arteriogram, frontal view, arterial phase: The anterior cerebral artery is displaced from left to right. The pericallosal branches (**a**) on the upper and lower extremities of the mass are displaced to the left side as they are being carried away from the falx by the meningioma which has arisen from there. A faintly filled enlarged anterior falx artery is seen. The blood supply from the pericallosal branches to the tumor is also evident.

B, right brachial arteriogram with cross-compression, frontal view, arterial phase: Extension through the falx to the right side is evident from displacement of a pericallosal branch (**b**) of the right anterior cerebral artery away from the falx. A prominent anterior falx artery (**c**) is also evident on the right side.

(*Continued.*)

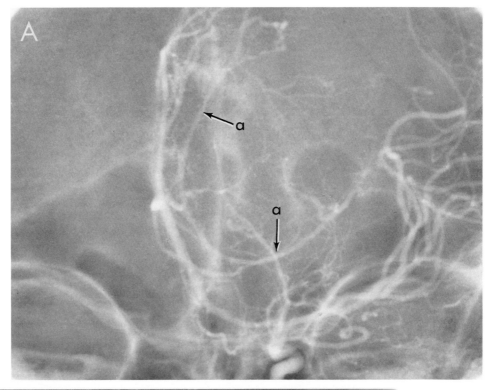

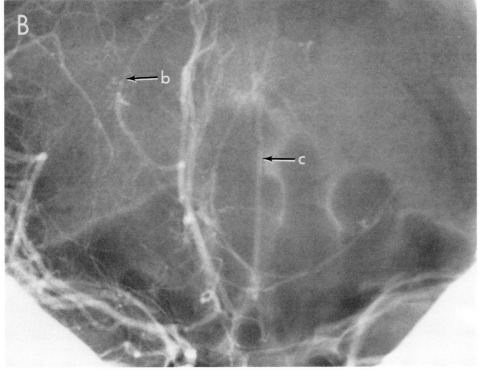

Figure 126 · Bifrontal Meningioma / 427

Figure 126 (cont.).—Bifrontal meningioma arising from the left anterior falx.

C, left carotid arteriogram, lateral view, arterial phase: The carotid siphon is closed. Branches of the pericallosal artery (**a**) that are stretched around the tumor are also displaced posteriorly. Neovascularity into the meningioma arises both from the anterior falx artery (**c**) and from branches of the anterior cerebral arteries. The anterior aspect of the Sylvian triangle is displaced down and backward.

D, right brachial arteriogram, lateral view, arterial phase: Displacements similar to those seen in the left carotid angiogram (**C**) are demonstrated. A prominent anterior falx artery (**c**) is also evident from the right side supplying the meningioma.

E, right brachial arteriogram, lateral view, venous phase: Numerous veins (**d**) enclose the meningioma. The middle cerebral vein (**e**) is displaced down and backward because of the attending transphenoidal herniation. The internal cerebral vein (**f**) is humped backward.

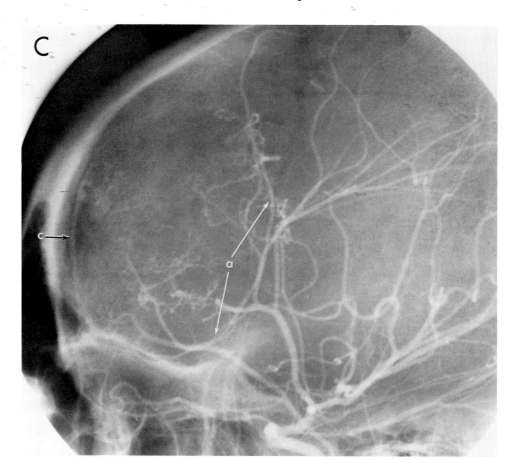

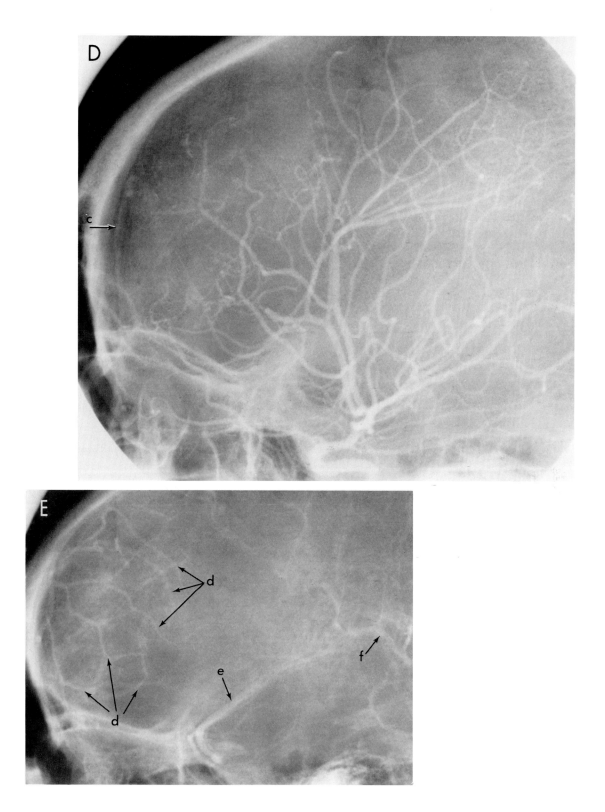

Figure 126 · Bifrontal Meningioma / 429

Figure 127.—Subfrontal meningioma.

A 55-year-old woman had one seizure, characterized by automatic movements, about two months before admission. Results of the neurologic examination were essentially normal. Electroencephalography revealed a left frontotemporal focus, and the brain scan recorded an uptake in the left frontal lobe. At surgery, gross total removal of the tumor was achieved. The patient has done well since. Plain radiographs are shown in Figure 41, page 74.

A, left common carotid arteriogram, frontal view, arterial phase: A cluster of several tortuous vessels (**a**) is seen to enter the meningioma. The parent vessels of this cluster are the anterior ethmoidal (**b**) and anterior meningeal (**c**) vessels which can be seen through the medial air cell of the left frontal sinus. A proximal shift of the anterior cerebral artery is evident.

B, left common carotid arteriogram, lateral view, arterial phase: The ophthalmic artery is enlarged and ethmoidal branches (**b**), both posteriorly and anteriorly, are seen to enter the tumor. Feeders from the anterior meningeal artery (**c**) are also evident. The anterior cerebral artery is not displaced posteriorly because the bulk of the tumor is lateral to it. However, the frontal polar branch (**d**) of the anterior cerebral artery is slightly stretched and elevated as it reaches the distal portion of the interhemispheric fissure. The orbital frontal branch (**e**) of the middle cerebral artery abruptly turns posteriorly on itself as it reaches the tumor in a typical extra-axial fashion. The proximal portion of the Sylvian triangle is depressed.

C, left common carotid arteriogram, frontal view, venous phase: A large homogeneous tumor stain (**f**) extends from the midline to near the lateral margin of the left orbital roof. A stretched and enlarged frontal cortical vein (**g**) caps the meningioma. The internal cerebral vein is midline.

D, left common carotid arteriogram, lateral view, venous phase: The homogeneous stain (**f**) of the meningioma is apparent. Several frontal cortical veins (**g**) are stretched around the periphery of the tumor.

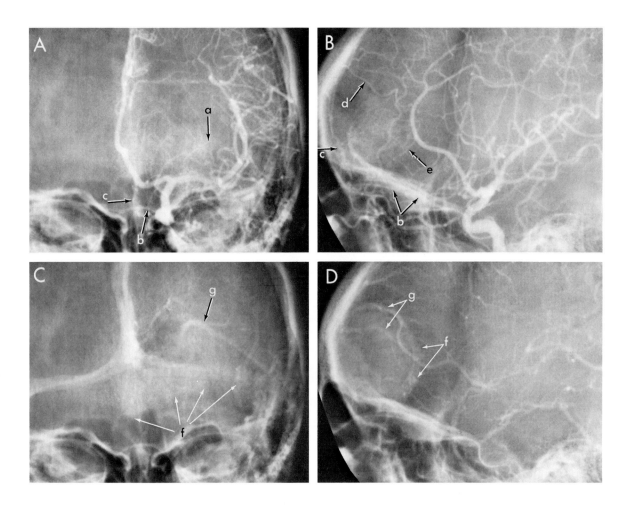

Figure 127 · Subfrontal Meningioma / 431

Figure 128.—Planum sphenoidale meningioma.

A 48-year-old woman noted vision loss, predominantly in the left eye, for six years, and for the past several years had had progressive diminution of visual acuity on the right. On examination only light perception was found on the left. On the right there was a temporal defect, with 20/30 vision. She underwent bifrontal craniotomy with gross total removal of a large meningioma of the planum sphenoidale. Postoperative improvement in visual acuity and fields was dramatic.

A, skull radiograph, frontal view: The region of the planum sphenoidale (**a**) is visible through the frontal sinus and shows some irregular thickening, particularly on the left side.

B, skull radiograph, lateral view: Numerous irregular areas of thickening with underlying blistering are evident over the entire length of the planum sphenoidale (**a**). Posteriorly the blistering is seen as numerous small lytic areas within the hyperostotic bone. Anteriorly, larger lucencies are mixed with the smaller blisters.

C, right common carotid arteriogram, lateral view, arterial phase: The ophthalmic artery gives rise to ethmoidal branches (**b**) supplying the tumor. The horizontal portion (**c**) of the anterior cerebral artery is lifted vertically and displaced posteriorly. The initial vertical portion (**d**) of the anterior cerebral artery is likewise displaced and the orbitofrontal branches (**e**) are lifted upward in typical fashion by this extra-axial lesion.

D, right common carotid arteriogram, lateral view, venous phase: A faint homogeneous tumor stain (**f**) is seen in the suprasellar region. There are marked attenuation and upward displacement of the septal vein (**g**). Although the mass effect is quite near the region of the foramen of Monro, there is no evidence of obstructive hydrocephalus as the subependymal veins outline a ventricle of normal size.

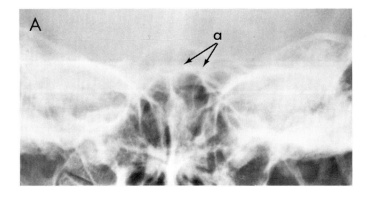

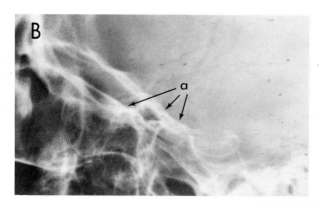

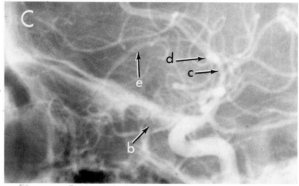

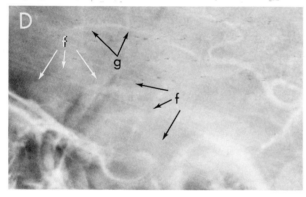

E, right common carotid arteriogram, frontal view: The supraclinoid portion of the internal carotid artery is displaced laterally. The horizontal portion of the anterior cerebral artery is markedly displaced upward. The an-

terior communicating artery and both anterior cerebral arteries are filled. The mass effect from the tumor separates these structures and permits their easy identification.

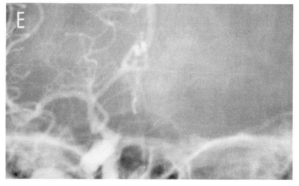

Figure 128 · Planum Sphenoidale Meningioma / 433

Figure 129.—Diaphragma sellae meningioma.

A 44-year-old woman was seen because of progressive failing vision. Examination revealed a marked visual field deficit, with only a medial quadrant remaining on the right side; visual acuity was 20/70. A bifrontal craniotomy was performed with gross total removal of the meningioma, which arose from the diaphragma sellae, elevating and compressing the optic chiasm, as well as both optic nerves. The right optic nerve, in addition, was creased by the anterior cerebral artery. The tumor extended anteriorly on the tuberculum.

A, pneumoencephalogram, frontal view, brow-up position: A horizontal cut-off (**a**) of the anterior portion of the third ventricle is demonstrated. In addition there is mild left-to-right displacement of the third ventricle. The temporal and frontal horns show no displacement.

B, pneumoencephalogram, lateral view, hanging-head position: The anterior portion of the third ventricle is markedly splayed (**a**) by the meningioma impinging on it, with obliteration of both optic and infundibular recesses. Hyperostosis is evident in the region of the planum sphenoidale posteriorly.

C, pneumoencephalogram, frontal view, laminagraphic section at the plane of the planum sphenoidale and origin of the anterior clinoids: Air within the parasellar and suprasellar cisterns outlines all but the right upper aspect of the tumor, which has a smooth border and is slightly lobular. Thickening of the left aspect of the planum sphenoidale is evident.

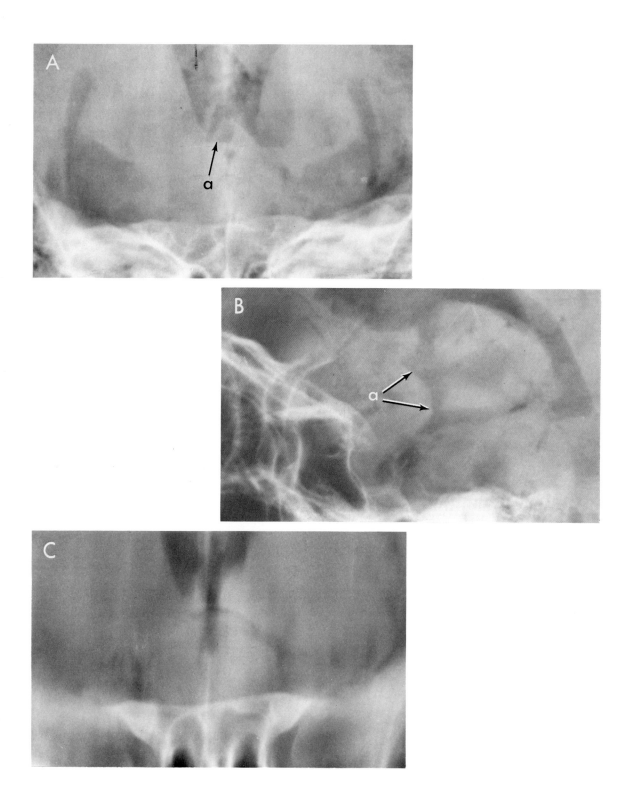

Figure 129 · Diaphragma Sellae Meningioma / 435

Figure 130.—Sphenoid wing meningioma.

A 44-year-old woman had a three-month history of blurred vision. Examination revealed a nasal field deficit on the left side and only an inferior temporal island of vision preserved in the right eye. A left temporal bifrontal craniotomy was performed and a large portion of the tumor removed. Tumor that extended medially beneath the left internal carotid artery, left optic nerve, optic chiasm and right optic nerve was excised, as well as the subfrontal portion and much of the tumor in the middle fossa and sphenoid ridge. The postoperative course was complicated by development of communicating hydrocephalus, controlled by a ventriculoatrial shunt.

A, skull radiograph, base view: A mottled mixed hyperostotic and lucent change involves the floor of the middle fossa and extends anteriorly to involve the greater wing of the sphenoid bone. The lateral wall of the orbit and pterygoid plates are intact. Extension into the left parasellar region is evident from a soft tissue mass (**a**) in the left side of the sphenoid air cell.

B, laminagram, frontal view: Hyperostosis involves the greater wing of the sphenoid and extends medially to involve the bone surrounding the foramen rotundum. Superiorly the lesser wing of the sphenoid bone is affected, with extension into the left side of the planum sphenoidale. The parasellar involvement of the sphenoid body is not seen because the laminagraphic section is too far anterior.

C, left carotid arteriogram, frontal view, arterial phase: The middle cerebral artery is markedly elevated and the distal internal carotid artery displaced medially. A small shift of the anterior cerebral artery is present. Numerous vessels (**b**) arise from the ophthalmic artery supplying the tumor on the sphenoid wing. A cavernous branch (**c**) of the internal carotid artery to the tumor medially is seen.

(Continued.)

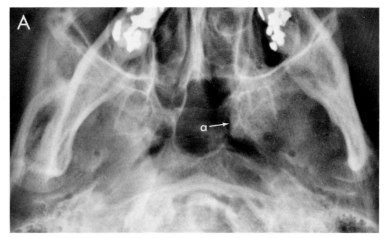

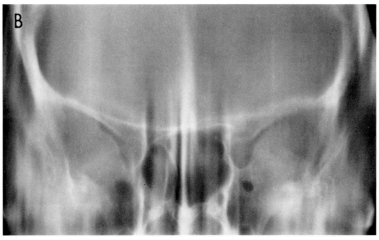

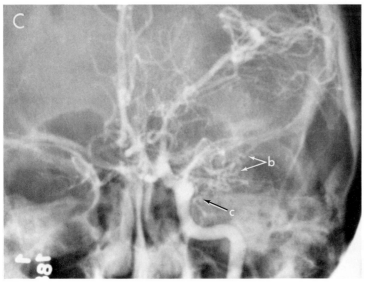

Figure 130 · Sphenoid Wing Meningioma / 437

Figure 130 (cont.).—Sphenoid wing meningioma.

D, left carotid arteriogram, lateral view, arterial phase: The middle cerebral artery is conspicuously elevated. Marked stretching of vessels with a faint tumor stain is seen extending from the posterior temporal region to the pterion. Several medium-filled vessels (**b**) arising from the ophthalmic artery can be seen through the hyperostotic sphenoid bone superiorly and the cavernous branch (**c**) inferiorly.

E, left carotid arteriogram, frontal view, venous phase: Numerous dilated venous channels (**d**) extend nearly to the midline and on the superior aspect of the tumor. The internal cerebral vein is shifted from left to right.

F, left carotid arteriogram, lateral view, venous phase: Tumor stain and venous channels (**d**) that cap the tumor are seen extending from the floor of the middle fossa superiorly and anteriorly to the sphenoid bone to involve the floor of the anterior fossa. This characteristic involvement of adjacent cranial fossae is typical of meningioma and other extra-axial lesions and is distinctly uncommon with intra-axial tumors.

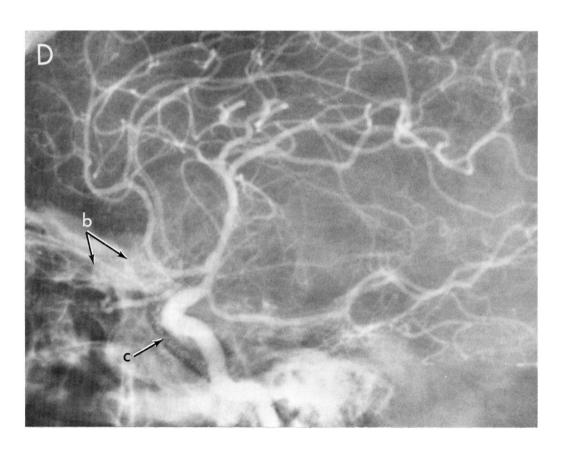

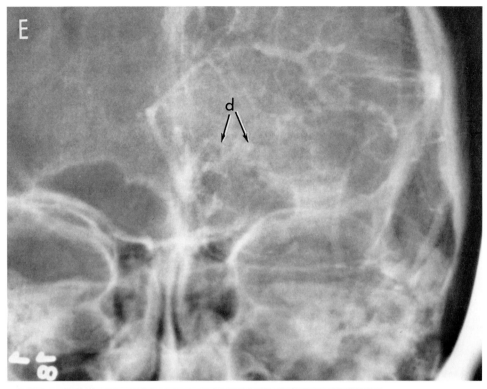

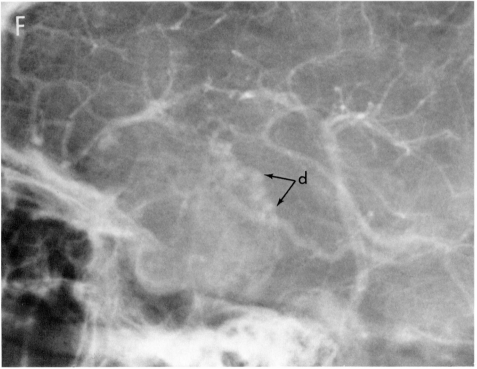

Figure 130 · Sphenoid Wing Meningioma / 439

Figure 131.—Pterion meningioma.

A 70-year-old woman had a four-year history of a swelling in the left temporal region which became occasionally painful. Gradual enlargement of the mass was noted. No neurologic deficit could be found. At operation an en plaque meningioma involving the dura and bone was removed.

A, skull radiograph, base view: A large channel (**a**) extends from the foramen spinosum on the right. Although the foramen itself is not enlarged, the channel for the middle meningeal vessels is abnormally wide and tortuous. There is a slight change in density of the greater wing of the sphenoid as it extends toward the temporal bone. This change is characterized by thickening (**b**) and a local area of hyperostosis (**c**).

B, frontal, and **C,** lateral views, selective carotid arteriogram: The arterial supply to the tumor is via the middle meningeal (**d**) and accessory meningeal (**e**) vessels. Small branches of the superficial temporal artery also extend toward the tumor. The internal carotid arteriogram showed extremely minimal changes adjacent to the brain surface of this basically en plaque extradural meningioma.

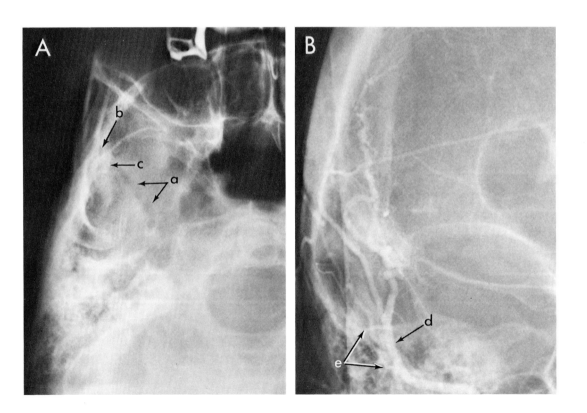

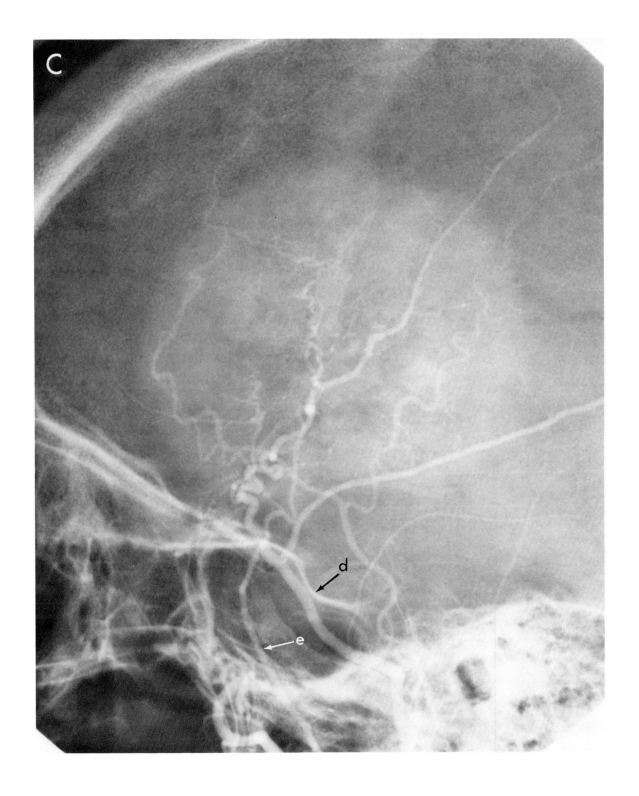

Figure 131 · Pterion Meningioma / 441

Figure 132.—Lateral Sylvian meningioma (meningeal sarcoma).

A 34-year-old woman had a six-year history of right-sided focal seizures. Six weeks before admission she began to have severe left temporal headaches and a right central field palsy developed. The original plain skull radiographs were normal.

Removal of the tumor was accomplished, but in its deepest portion the tumor was believed to be invading the brain. Histologic diagnosis was meningeal sarcoma, and radiation therapy to a dose of 5000 r in six weeks was given. One year and nine months later a recurrent tumor was nearly as large as the original one. Resection led to improvement, but nine months later further resection was required; seven months after that a third recurrent tumor was removed. This was thought to be invading the thalamus. Six months later a fourth operation was required.

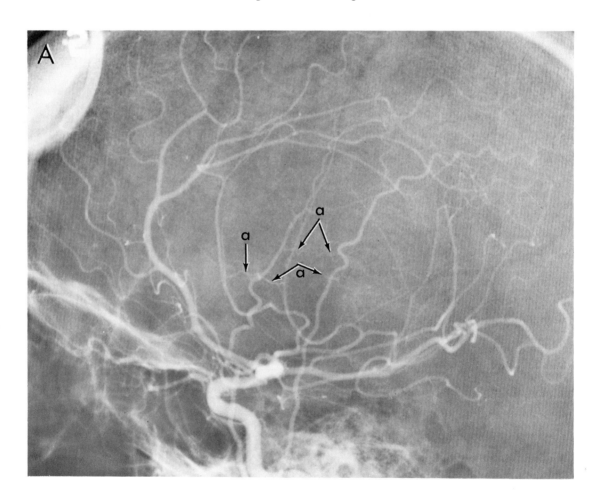

A, left carotid arteriogram, lateral view, arterial phase: There are marked stretching and bowing of arteries in the lower convexity and pronounced depression of the Sylvian triangle. The pericallosal artery is slightly elevated. Small tortuous branches (**a**) of the middle meningeal artery and superficial temporal artery supply the tumor.

B, left carotid arteriogram, frontal view, arterial phase: This shows striking displacement of the Sylvian vessels. The angiographic Sylvian point is markedly displaced downward as well. Anterior branches (**b**) of the middle cerebral artery in the frontoparietal operculum are stretched and are displaced medially away from the inner table of bone. There is moderate midline shift of the anterior cerebral artery and its branches.

(*Continued.*)

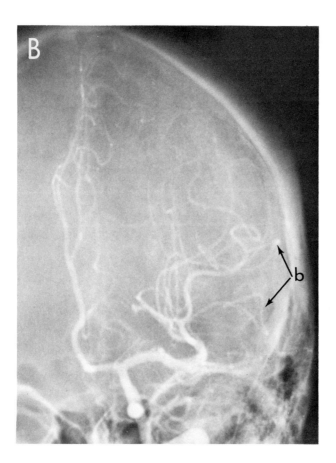

Figure 132 · Lateral Sylvian Meningioma (Sarcoma) / 443

Figure 132 (cont.).—Lateral Sylvian meningioma (meningeal sarcoma).

C, left carotid arteriogram, lateral view, later arterial phase: Patchy areas of tumor stain are evident in the central portion of the tumor.

D, left carotid arteriogram, lateral view, one year and nine months after original study: This demonstrates deformity of the vessels similar to that observed on original examination. This was believed to be due to recurrence.

E, left carotid arteriogram, frontal view: Compared with the original studies, this too shows a very similar but slightly less pronounced displacement of the Sylvian vessels and anterior cerebral artery branches.

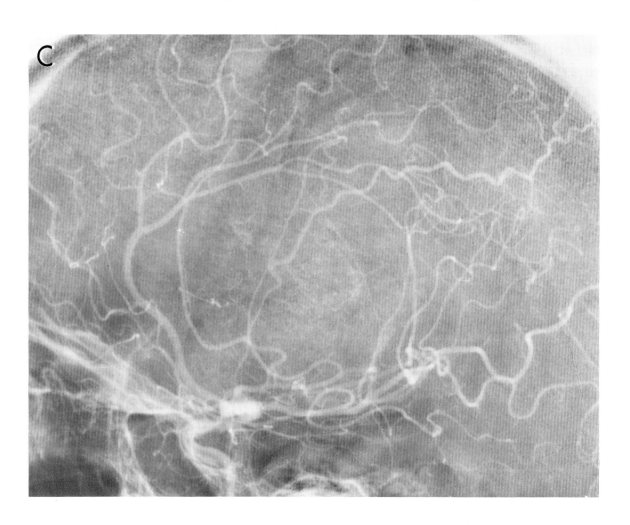

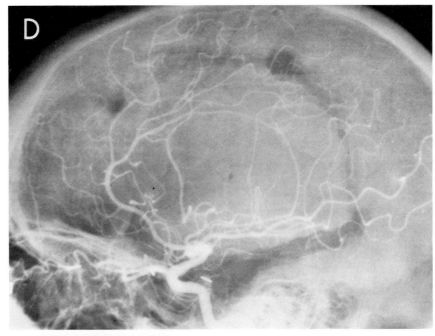

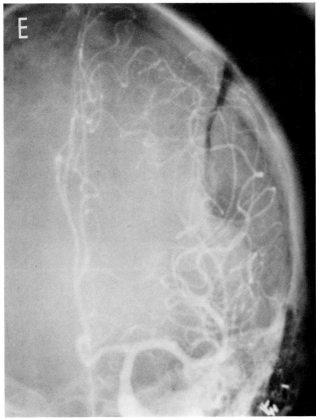

Figure 132 · Lateral Sylvian Meningioma (Sarcoma) / 445

Figure 133.—Left temporal angioblastic meningioma arising from tentorium and transverse sinus.

A 60-year-old man was seen four years before definitive diagnosis because of blackouts which were evaluated with echoencephalography, skull radiography, lumbar puncture and left carotid arteriography, all of which were reported to show no abnormality. The electroencephalogram was mildly and diffusely abnormal. Four years later he was admitted with progressive memory difficulty, impairment in word finding, left temporal headaches and right homonymous hemianopia. Operation revealed a soft tumor involving the transverse sinus and containing a 24-cc cyst with yellowish brown fluid within it. After postoperative radiotherapy he did well until four years later when he was re-admitted with increasing fatigability and difficulty with memory. Pneumoencephalography and arteriography at this time showed no evidence of tumor recurrence, but the presence of communicating

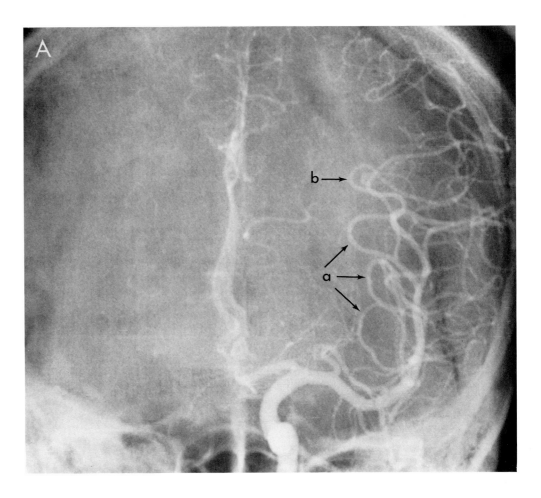

hydrocephalus. A ventriculoatrial shunt was followed by improvement.

A, left common carotid arteriogram, frontal view, arterial phase: The anterior cerebral artery is shifted left to right. The magnitude of shift is equally distributed except for the distal step, which is slightly larger than the rest of the shift. The insular loops (**a**) are displaced medially and the Sylvian point (**b**) is also elevated.

B, left common carotid arteriogram, lateral view, arterial phase: The anterior choroidal artery (**c**) is accordioned forward. Flash filling of a temporal branch (**d**) of the posterior cerebral artery showed marked arcuate stretching. The Sylvian triangle is elevated, particularly posteriorly. Note the thin vascular groove (**e**) posterior to the mastoid bones and slight mottled lucencies (**f**) in the region of the transverse sinus.

(Continued.)

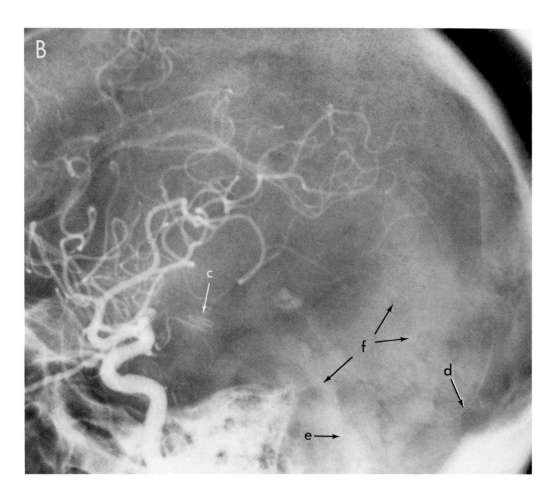

Figure 133 · Temporal Angioblastic Meningioma / 447

Figure 133 (cont.).—Left temporal angioblastic meningioma arising from tentorium and transverse sinus.

C, left common carotid arteriogram, lateral view, late arterial phase: Stretching of the posterior temporal branches (**g**) of the middle cerebral artery is evident. The distal portion of the posterior division (**h**) of the middle meningeal artery enlarges and gives off several fine tumor vessels. In addition the posterior auricular branch (**i**) of the external occipital artery is seen to fill the groove previously mentioned and end as a large ectatic tumor vessel. The external occipital (**j**) artery more posteriorly also is involved in the blood supply to the tumor.

D, left common carotid arteriogram, frontal view, venous phase: Marked medial displacement of the basal vein of Rosenthal is evident. The internal cerebral vein is shifted along with the pineal gland from left to right. Several straightened and compressed veins (**k**) are seen laterally in the region of the angular gyrus.

E, left common carotid arteriogram, lateral view, venous phase: A very faint tumor stain (**l**) is seen in the region of the transverse sinus. The posterior temporal and occipital areas are avascular and the gyri (**k**) of the angular gyrus and posterior parietal area are compressed. The internal cerebral vein and basal vein of Rosenthal are distorted secondary to the transtentorial herniation.

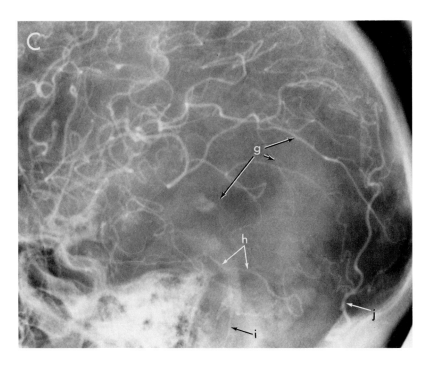

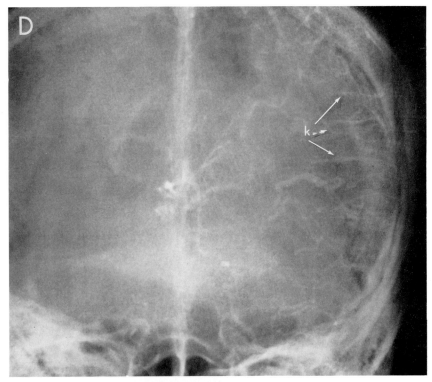

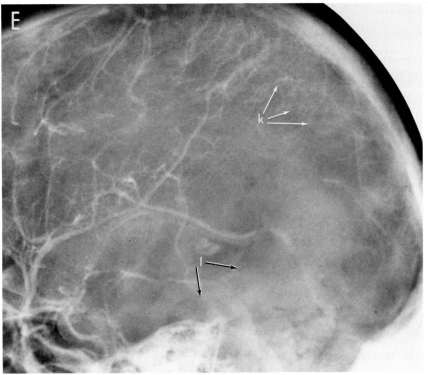

Figure 133 · Temporal Angioblastic Meningioma / 449

Figure 134.—Intraventricular meningioma of the proximal left temporal horn.

A 33-year-old man had a seven-month history of a change in personality with severe emotional swings. Initial electroconvulsive therapy gave no improvement. Examination revealed weakness of the right side, including the face. A Babinski sign was present on the right. Early papilledema was noted. Affect was labile and he expressed delusional thinking about his body. At surgery an intraventricular meningioma of the left temporal horn was grossly totally removed.

A, left common carotid arteriogram, frontal view, arterial phase: The anterior cerebral artery is shifted left to right. The distal insular loops and Sylvian point of the middle cerebral vessels are displaced laterally. The anterior choroidal artery is displaced medially (**a**) and is enlarged distally with a tuft of vessels (**b**) extending from its terminal portion.

B, left common carotid arteriogram, lateral view, arterial phase: The anterior choroidal artery is enlarged and its cisternal portion (**a**) displaced downward. The anterior choroidal artery turns upward again within the choroid fissure of the temporal horn and ends in numerous fine vessels (**b**) which begin to outline a homogeneous stain within a tumor. The floor of the Sylvian triangle is elevated.

(*Continued.*)

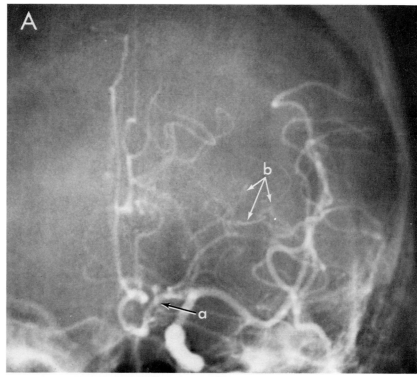

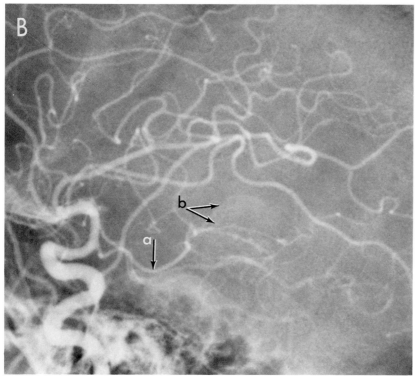

Figure 134 · Intraventricular Meningioma / 451

Figure 134 (cont.).—Intraventricular meningioma of the proximal left temporal horn.

C, left common carotid arteriogram, frontal view, intermediate arterial phase: A homogeneous tumor stain (**c**) outlines all but the inferomedial aspect of the tumor, which is probably being fed by posterior choroidal vessels which have not been opacified.

D, left common carotid arteriogram, lateral view, late arterial phase: This shows more complete outlining of the tumor (**c**) within the proximal

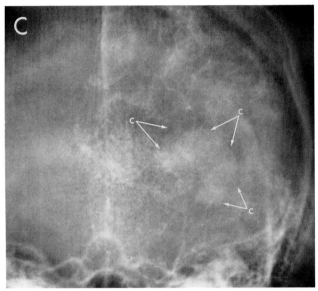

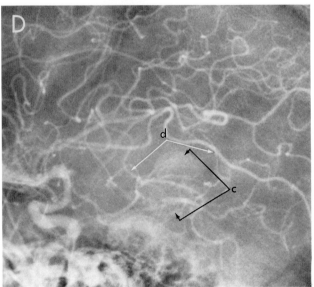

portion of the temporal horn. Some stretching and separation of the temporal branches (**d**) of the middle cerebral artery are also evident.

E, frontal, and **F,** lateral views, left common carotid arteriogram, venous phase: A faint homogeneous tumor stain (**c**) persists. The internal cerebral vein (**e**) is displaced approximately 1 cm from left to right. There is also mild medial displacement of the basal vein of Rosenthal (**f**). Small venous structures (**g**) outline the surface of the tumor within the temporal horn.

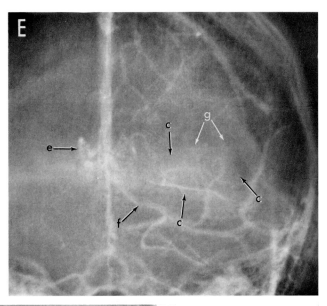

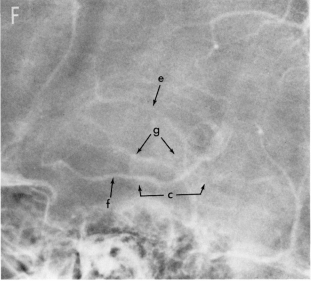

Figure 134 · Intraventricular Meningioma / 453

Figure 135.—Posterior fossa meningioma, heavily calcified.

A 62-year-old man was admitted with progressive weakness of the left upper extremity and occipital pain. Examination revealed diffuse muscle weakness of the left upper extremity and atrophy of the proximal shoulder muscles. At operation the mass was found situated ventrolaterally on the left from the C-2/C-3 level inferiorly to approximately the level of the ponto-medullary junction superiorly. The meningioma was arising from the dura along the anterior margin of the foramen magnum.

A, laminagram during pneumoencephalography, lateral view: The fourth ventricle (**a**) is elevated and displaced posteriorly. The cervical cord (**b**) is displaced posteriorly by tumor, accounting for the soft tissue mass seen between the foramen magnum and C-1.

B, laminagram at the level of the jugular tubercles and clivus at the time of pneumoencephalography, frontal view: The heavily calcified meningioma (**c**) is centered to the left of the midline but extends across the midline. The fourth ventricle (**a**) is displaced to the right. However, there is very little rotation of the fourth ventricle, the lateral recesses and superior medullary velum being practically horizontal (there is only slight upward tilt of the left side of the superior medullary velum).

(*Continued.*)

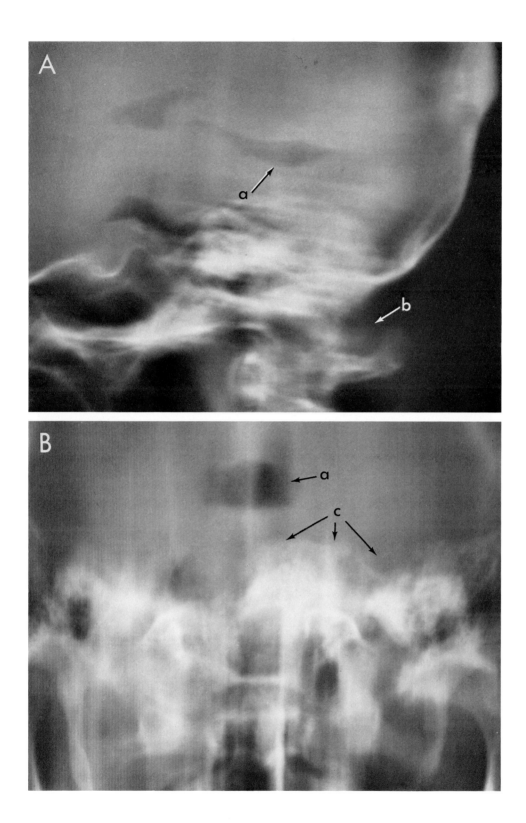

Figure 135 · Posterior Fossa Meningioma / 455

Figure 135 (cont.).—Posterior fossa meningioma, heavily calcified.

C, left vertebral arteriogram, frontal view, arterial phase: The left posterior inferior cerebellar artery (**d**) is quite large and is displaced to the right in its course around the brain stem. After reaching the back of the stem (**e**) the vessel returns to the midline. The proximal portion of the basilar artery and distal portion of the left vertebral artery are also displaced to the right.

D, left vertebral arteriogram, lateral view, arterial phase: The left posterior inferior cerebellar artery has a low origin. The ascending limb (**f**) of the choroidal loop is displaced posteriorly along with the brain stem. The top (**g**) of the choroidal loop is elevated. The descending limb (**h**) of the choroidal loop, particularly where the loop of the inferior vermian artery branch begins, is quite close to the initial segment of the ascending loop. The compression of the loop is characteristic of ventral extra-axial or brain stem lesions. The artery seen anterior to the left posterior inferior cerebellar artery is a branch of the large right-sided anterior inferior cerebellar artery (**i**).

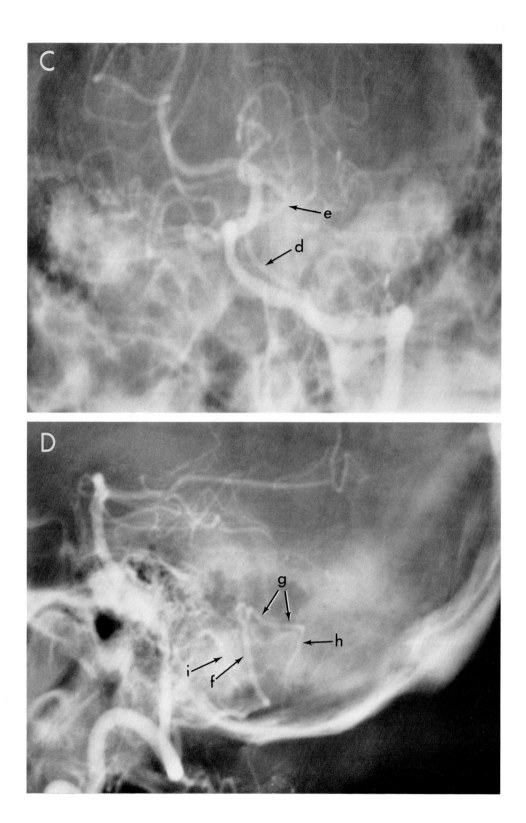

Figure 135 · Posterior Fossa Meningioma / 457

PART 14

Tumors of the Eye and the Orbit

Types and Diagnosis

TUMORS OF THE ORBIT are extremely rare, occurring in less than 1% of patients admitted to an active eye service. About 90% of the patients have unilateral exophthalmos when first seen. However, other, non-neoplastic conditions are manifested in this fashion, the leading one being thyroid ophthalmopathy. Of almost equal incidence is the combination of chronic granuloma (pseudotumor) and inflammatory masses often secondary to adjacent sinus disease. According to Reese's series, approximately one-fifth of the neoplasms arising in the orbit are angiomas; approximately one-sixth are malignant lymphomas; and retinoblastomas, neurinomas, dermoids and lacrimal gland epithelial tumors account for about one-fifteenth each. Melanomas had a similar incidence, but few of these were primary, most of them being extensions from the globe, conjunctiva or lid. Meningiomas accounted for about 4% and optic gliomas for about 3%. Primary carcinomas accounted for about 3%, although some were probably of lacrimal gland origin. Rhabdomyosarcomas are seen primarily in childhood, and the orbit is actually the second most common site of these muscle tumors; they comprised about 4% of the orbital tumors.

The hemangioma is the commonest primary tumor in the orbit. It is composed of vascular elements which may vary in cell type, maturity and formation of vascular channels. The hypertrophic hemangioma of infancy is composed primarily of primitive endothelial cells found prior to the development of true vascular channels. For this reason they are avascular tumors angiographically. Hemangiomas of capillary, cavernous and racemose types represent further stages of development of true vascular channels. It is common, however, to find different elements in any given hemangioma. Hemangiomas may undergo sclerosis, and if this process of thrombosis and fibrosis is rapid it may cause a sudden increase in orbital volume and occur as an acute event and so may be mistaken for a pseudotumor.

Malignant lymphomas are found most often in the orbit, lacrimal apparatus and conjunctiva. The most common cell types are lymphocytic and reticulum. As the lymphoid tissue around the eyes is found subconjunctivally and in the lacrimal gland, these sites are understandably the most common site of origin of the lymphocytic cell type. Although the lymphocytic and reticulum cell types are found in nearly equal numbers within the orbit the primary retrobulbar tumor is usually of the reticulum cell type as there is no lymphoid tissue behind the anterior septum of the eye.

Retinoblastoma is a malignant tumor of the nuclear layers of the retina which has a propensity to develop from multiple foci in one or both eyes. The incidence of bilaterality is recorded in the literature as anywhere from 25–75%. The tumor is usually manifested at about 1 year of age and is inheritable, as a single autosomal gene of high but incomplete penetrance.

Neurofibromas may cause orbital changes because of the presence of the tumor or because of dysplastic changes involving the sphenoid bone. We will be concerned with the changes secondary to the neoplasm. The lesion may be single and localized or multiple and associated with thickening and tortuosity of the nerves usually referred to as a plexiform neurofibroma. The latter involves primarily the orbital roof, but its presence on the orbital floor has also been documented. Malignant Schwannomas may also occur; approximately one-half of these arise in patients with von Recklinghausen's disease.

The dermoid cyst is an epithelial lesion developing from inclusions of epidermoid or deeper dermal structures. The former is known as an epidermoid cyst and the latter as a dermoid cyst. Because transitional types occur, the differentiation is of little importance. This cyst is congenital but often does not appear until young adulthood when the lesion has expanded sufficiently to cause changes of the eyeball. The diploe of the bone is most often involved, with expansion of both inner and outer tables and the formation of sharply demarcated erosive defects. Cysts are most common in the frontal bone but may occur in any bone adjacent to the orbit.

Tumors of the lacrimal gland fall into two main categories, mixed tumors and carcinomas, of approximately equal incidence. The mixed tumor with both epithelial and mesenchymal elements is in the vast majority a benign lesion. The most common carcinoma is the adenoid cystic type similar to a cylindroma. Granulomas, malignant lymphomas and dermoid cysts may also be found in the region of the lacrimal gland. Most patients with mixed tumors are in the 40–50 year age range. Because of the position of all of these tumors in the bony lacrimal fossa there is ready access to bone, and evidence of local invasion should be carefully looked for radiographically.

Meningiomas arising from the meninges covering the optic nerve have a very much lower incidence than meningiomas arising from the coverings of the brain and spinal cord. Consequently most of the meningiomas encountered in the orbit have their primary site in adjacent cranial structures. The meningiomas arising from the optic nerve sheath may be primary in the orbit or may follow the optic nerve in its intracanalicular and intracranial portions. The bone changes of these tumors then may be manifested as optic foramen enlargement. Secondary orbital meningiomas most often arise from the sphenoid bone; they are described in Part 13, on meningiomas.

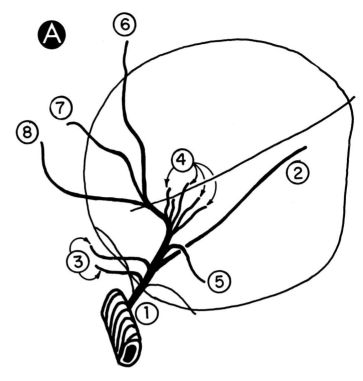

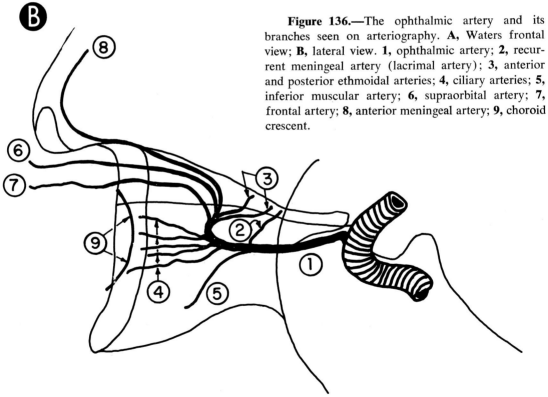

Figure 136.—The ophthalmic artery and its branches seen on arteriography. **A,** Waters frontal view; **B,** lateral view. **1,** ophthalmic artery; **2,** recurrent meningeal artery (lacrimal artery); **3,** anterior and posterior ethmoidal arteries; **4,** ciliary arteries; **5,** inferior muscular artery; **6,** supraorbital artery; **7,** frontal artery; **8,** anterior meningeal artery; **9,** choroid crescent.

Optic nerve glioma is primarily a tumor of childhood, 75% occurring in the first 10 years of life. The tumors are usually unilateral, but involvement of both optic nerves either from spread via the chiasm or from multiple origins may occur. The lesions are classified according to anatomic locations as orbital, intracanalicular, intracranial or involving the chiasm. The possibility of surgical intervention and the type of approach used obviously depend on the anatomic site of the tumor.

Orbital tumors may cause exophthalmos, vision loss (clinically defined by changes in both visual acuity and visual fields) and motility disturbances. When exophthalmos is present it is important to detect changes of the osseous structures formed in the orbit to determine if there is intracranial involvement as well. The classic localization of vision loss as prechiasmal, chiasmal or postchiasmal will also point to the type of anatomic involvement. Motility disturbances can usually also be differentiated as of intraorbital or intracranial origin. Examination of the orbit and adjacent cranial structures with contrast agents is usually done by venography, arteriography or pneumoencephalography. Ultrasonic localization of orbital masses can be extremely effective in competent hands. Although orbital venography is a very safe method of contrast examination, arteriography has a higher information yield regarding the vascular architecture of the tumor, its possible involvement of adjacent temporal lobe or parasellar structures, and local ischemic changes caused by the mass lesion and also outlines a larger portion of the orbit than does venography. In addition, the back of the globe is outlined by the choroid crescent; this is an invariable happening, contrary to what is stated in earlier literature. Magnification angiography as well as subtraction techniques combined with the increasing safety of the examination have led to widespread acceptance. Pertinent ophthalmic artery branches seen on arteriography are shown in Figure 136.

Computerized axial tomography has been able to demonstrate many noncalcified structures within the orbit that are not visible in plain films. The position of the globe, the course of the optic nerve, particularly its retrobulbar and muscle cone portions, as well as the appearance of the muscles forming the cone have been worked out by this technique.

Figure 137.—Hemangioma of the left orbit.

A 3-year-old girl was first noted to have bulging of the left eye at age 1 month. Several red birthmarks present on the child's body slowly regressed. Examination under anesthesia revealed marked enlargement of the left orbit on palpation. The eyelids on the left side were full, particularly the lower lid. On eversion of the lids a vascular mass was seen in the lower fornix, and some abnormal telangiectatic vessels were present on the lower bulbar conjunctiva. A 4-mm exophthalmos was measured. Both globes were of normal size and the fundi were also normal.

A, orbital radiograph, Caldwell projection: Enlargement of the left orbit is generalized. No hyperostosis or calcification is evident.

B, orbital radiograph, lateral view: The entire left orbital roof (**arrows**) is elevated and thinned. No phleboliths are evident.

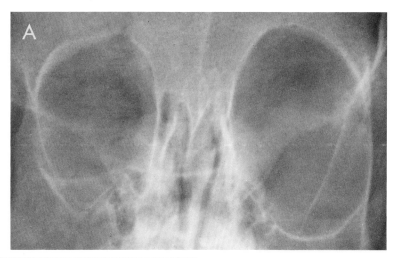

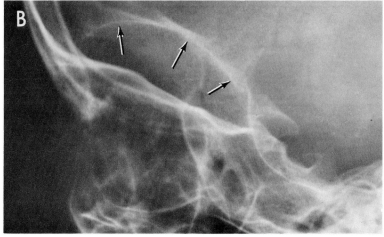

Figure 137 · Hemangioma / 465

Figure 138.—Lymphosarcoma.

In a 9-year-old girl, slight swelling of the right eye was noted four months prior to examination. Since then there had been a slow painless progressive proptosis of the right globe. There was never a sign of inflammation. On examination the right eye was displaced laterally, downward and forward. There was limitation of motion on upward gaze. Beneath the right superior nasal orbital rim was a firm palpable mass having the consistency of hard rubber. The mass extended from the region of the medial canthal ligament laterally to the junction of the middle and lateral thirds of the orbital rim. Results of blood studies were normal. At operation the tumor appeared to infiltrate the anterior ocular tissue, but was fairly well isolated posteriorly in the orbit.

A, orbital radiograph, Caldwell projection: A soft tissue density is seen throughout the right orbit. The orbit is enlarged in a generalized fashion, indicating increased intraorbital pressure. A soft tissue mass produced by the proptotic right globe is seen extending beyond the lateral confines of the orbit.

B, orbital radiograph, lateral view: The roof of the right orbit (**arrows**) is thinned and ballooned by the increased intraorbital pressure.

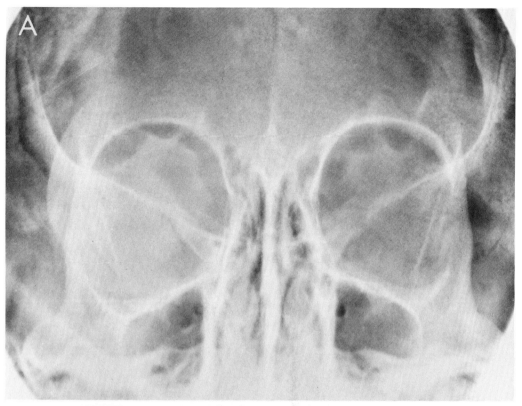

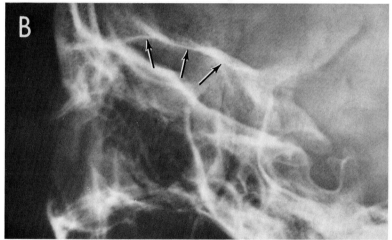

Figure 138 · Lymphosarcoma / 467

Figure 139.—Bilateral retinoblastoma.

A 13-month-old boy was examined because the mother noted a yellow reflex from the left eye at approximately age 7 months and a similar yellow reflex from the right eye at age 12 months. Examination under anesthesia revealed the retina to be completely detached on the right. Temporal to the disc a yellowish ill-defined tumor could be seen. No calcium was evident on the retina of the right eye. A detachment of the retina was also present on the left, and numerous areas of calcium were noted on the detached retina. Whitish yellow tumor tissue was seen temporal to the disc. Glaucoma eventually developed in both eyes, necessitating removal of both globes.

Orbital radiograph, Caldwell projection: Granular deposits of calcium are seen within both orbits, which are otherwise normal.

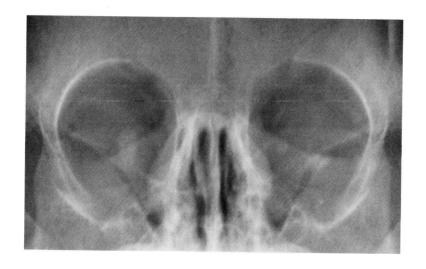

Figure 139 · Bilateral Retinoblastoma / 469

Figure 140.—Epidermoid of the floor of the orbit and antrum.

A 3½-year-old boy's parents noted a head tilt and drooping of the left lower eyelid. Examination revealed the left cornea approximately 2 mm above a corresponding point of the right cornea. The palpebral fissure was narrowed with the eyes looking straight ahead or down. The greatest ptosis was with the eyes looking down.

A, skull radiograph, Caldwell projection: A large lytic area involves the floor of the orbit and antrum; its superior margin has a fine sclerotic rim (**a**). The superior orbital fissure and foramen rotundum are seen through the lesion and are not involved. The inferior orbital foramen and contiguous anterior margins of the orbital floor are obviously destroyed.

B, skull radiograph, Waters projection: The lesion extends into the left nasal fossa up to the midline (**b**). The anterolateral border of the antrum is no longer visible, only a more posterior portion of the lateral wall of the antrum being seen. The lobulated nature of the lesion is more evident here, and its finely sclerotic margin (**a**) is seen to better advantage. The floor of the orbit in its medial two-thirds appears to be completely involved.

C, skull radiograph, lateral view: The large involvement of the floor of the orbit is demonstrated, with extension practically to the orbital apex. There is ballooning posteriorly of the posterior wall of the antrum (**c**).

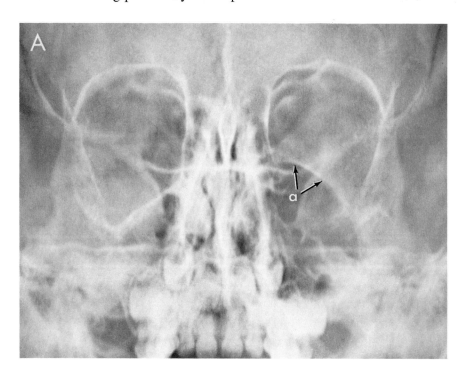

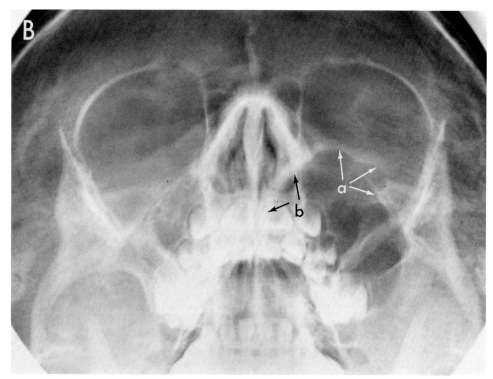

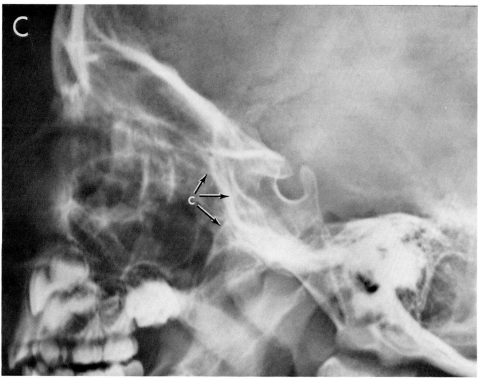

Figure 140 · Epidermoid / 471

Figure 141.—Epidermoid of the left orbit.

A 50-year-old woman had a long history of prominence of the left eye. On examination a 3-mm exophthalmos was measurable. Excursion of the left globe was good. No mass was palpable.

A, orbital radiograph, Caldwell projection: A mildly lobulated lytic lesion with a fine sclerotic rim occupies the superolateral aspect of the left orbit. The mass extends anteriorly on the roof of the orbit to the region of the lacrimal fossa, where the sclerotic border of the orbit is no longer visible. The mass does not extend anteriorly to involve the palpable margin of the orbit. A few fine flecks of calcium (**a**) are evident in the superomedial aspect of the cyst.

B, optic foramen view: The position of the cyst on the superolateral aspect of the orbit is evident. The cyst does not involve the zygomatic portion of the orbit.

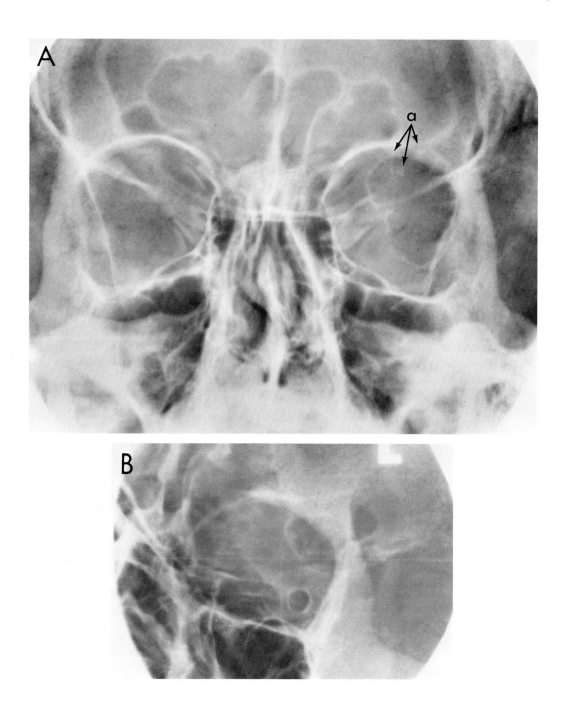

Figure 141 · Epidermoid / 473

Figure 142.—Left optic nerve glioma.

This 9-month-old child was born with a prominent left eye. The family history was notable as the father had café-au-lait spots and neurofibromas on the trunk and arms. The patient had a nevus of the forehead and multiple large café-au-lait spots on the torso. The left eye was exophthalmic, and light response was diminished. No other focal neurologic deficit was found. Pneumoencephalography revealed no evidence of involvement of the optic chiasm. On left frontal craniotomy the optic chiasm and distal left optic nerve were found to be normal, with enlargement only of the intracranial portion of the left optic nerve immediately beyond the optic canal. The left orbit and canal were unroofed, disclosing a discolored enlarged optic nerve. The nerve was excised at the intraorbital half and approximately 5 mm from the optic chiasm at the intracranial end. When last seen four years after surgery the patient was doing well.

Laminagram during pneumoencephalography, base view: At the level of the optic foramina there is widening of the entire extent of the left optic canal with erosive changes seen on both the lateral and medial walls of the canal. The difference in all diameters measures slightly over 2 mm. A small area of soft tissue prominence is seen on the immediate intracranial portion of the nerve (**a**) which then tapers toward normal (**b**) in the region of the chiasm.

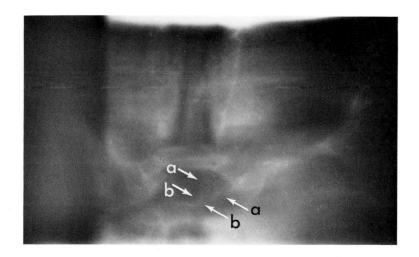

Figure 142 · Optic Nerve Glioma / 475

Figure 143.—Meningioma of the left optic nerve.

A 15-year-old girl noted prominence of the left eye at age 6 and progressive vision loss which became complete at age 13. Although at operation it was thought that the tumor had been completely removed, there was radiographic evidence of involvement of the lesser wing of the sphenoid bone, including the left optic foramen, on a follow-up examination three years later.

A, orbital radiograph, frontal view: Increased intraorbital pressure changes are manifested by increased soft tissue density, and enlargement of the orbit, particularly on the medial aspect where the lamina papyracea is bowed inward. A calcific density extends from the inferior medial aspect of the orbit to the center of the orbit. A lucency in the midportion of the calcium represents the optic nerve.

B, orbital radiograph, lateral view, slightly oblique projection: The roof of the left orbit (the higher roof) shows evidence of thinning because of the increased mass caused by the meningioma in the apex of the orbit. The anterior portion of the tumor is rather sharply defined as it is apposed to the back portion of the globe. The tumor is rather uniform in height until the apex of the orbit is reached, where it narrows in conformity with the conical shape of the orbital apex.

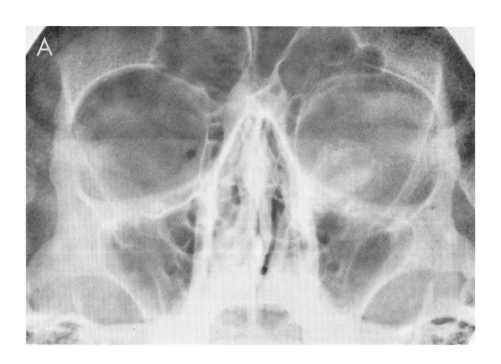

C, and **D,** radiographs of the optic foramina: The right orbit is normal. The left orbit shows psammomatous deposition of calcium within the meningioma, with relative sparing of the midportion, which contains the optic nerve. The outline of the optic foramen is obliterated by the calcified meningioma.

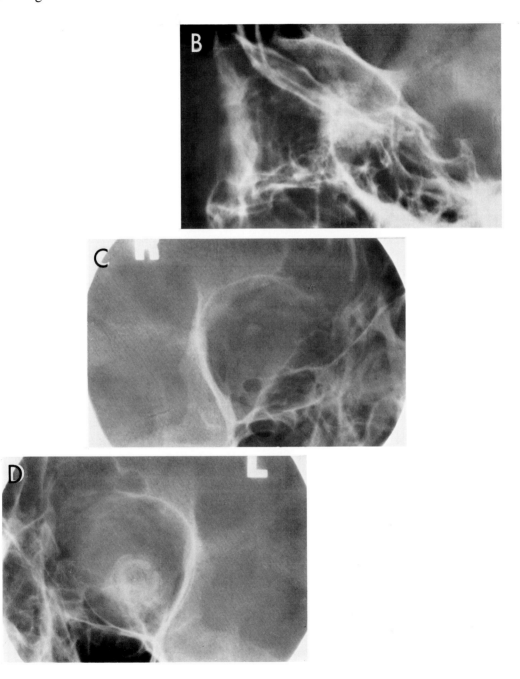

Figure 143 · Optic Nerve Meningioma / 477

Figure 144.—Benign mixed cell tumor of the lacrimal gland.

This patient was first seen at age 48 because of prominence and blindness of the left eye. Examination revealed extreme exophthalmos with fair motility and a palpable mass in the region of the lacrimal gland. At operation a solid encapsulated spherical mass the size of a golf ball was removed. Pathologic study indicated that the tumor was somewhat aggressive in that it tended to extend through the capsule. The patient was seen 12 years later with recurrence. At operation the anterior three-fourths of the tumor was amputated, with the residual tumor stump left in the orbital apex.

A, orbital radiograph, Caldwell projection: An increased soft tissue density is visible in the left orbit, the volume of which is mildly increased. Marked sharpening and erosion of the region of the lacrimal gland extend from the inferior third of the left zygoma into the palpable roof of the orbit to approximately its midportion.

B, radiographs of the optic foramina: The erosive changes involving the zygoma and superolateral aspect of the left orbital are seen in profile.

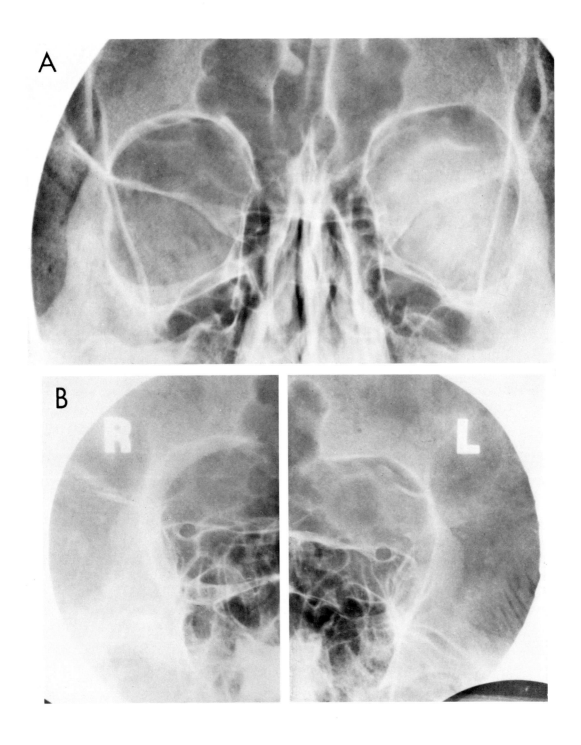

Figure 144 · Mixed Cell Tumor of Lacrimal Gland / 479

Figure 145.—Optic nerve glioma.

A 3-year-old girl was seen after an upper respiratory infection with mild proptosis of the right eye. Examination revealed early papilledema in that eye. Numerous café-au-lait spots were evident on her trunk. At craniotomy the optic chiasm and nerve were inspected, and dilatation of the right optic nerve at its distal portion was seen intracranially. The nerve was sectioned at the chiasm, leaving about 1 cm of normal-appearing nerve.

A and **B,** optic canal radiographs: There is enlargement of the right optic canal (**B**) with erosion of the superolateral cortical border resulting in an abnormal width horizontally.

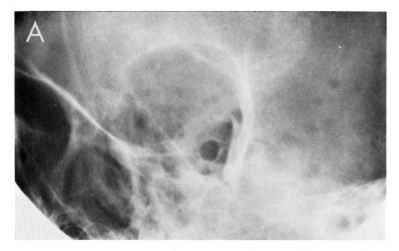

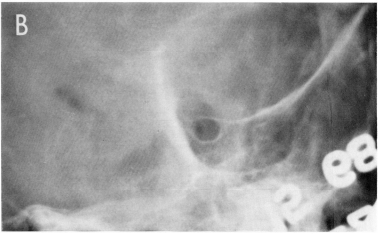

C, tomogram during pneumoencephalography, frontal view: The enlarged optic nerve (**a**) on the right tapers to normal size (**b**) as it blends with the shadow of the optic chiasm. The anterior portion of the third ventricle is normal.

D, pneumoencephalogram, lateral view, brow-up position: The drumstick-shaped appearance of the right optic nerve demonstrates the abnormal enlargement (**a**) of the intracranial portion of the nerve. The nerve returns to normal size (**b**) at the distal portion and chiasm. The recesses of the anterior portion of the third ventricle are normal.

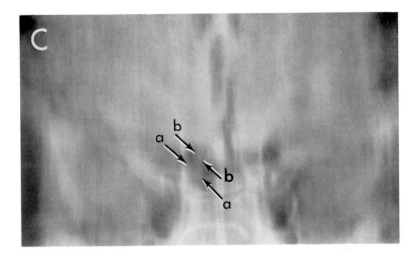

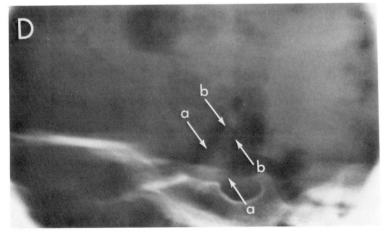

Figure 145 · Optic Nerve Glioma / 481

Figure 146.—Bilateral optic nerve glioma with chiasmal involvement.

This 14-month-old girl was well until age 9 months when she stopped crawling and refused to stand. The parents noted that she began turning the eyes up and had oscillatory motions of both eyes. Examination revealed truncal and distal ataxia. A horizontal nystagmus with slow component to the left was present. The pupils were dilated and hardly reacted to light. The fundi showed extremely pale discs bilaterally. Radiotherapy, to 5000 rads in five weeks, was given.

A, right carotid arteriogram, frontal view, Caldwell projection, arterial phase: The ophthalmic artery is stretched, and there is marked elongation as it passes from the undersurface to the top of the optic nerve. The internal carotid artery is slightly flattened on its medial surface, and there is definite lateral displacement of the posterior communicating and anterior choroidal arteries. There is slight elevation of the horizontal portion of the anterior cerebral artery.

B, right carotid arteriogram, lateral subtracted view, arterial phase: The ophthalmic artery is attenuated almost immediately as it enters the optic canal. The increase in the radius of the curvature as it passes around the markedly enlarged optic nerve intraorbitally is striking. Enlarged stretched perforating thalamic vessels (**a**) from the posterior communicating artery indicate extension toward the chiasm and hypothalamus.

C, pneumoencephalogram, lateral view, exaggerated brow-up position: Marked erosion (**b**) of the chiasmatic groove of the sella turcica is seen. Fragments of air outline the suprasellar portion (**c**) of the tumor. There is a definite cut-off of the anterior recesses of the third ventricle (**d**). A tumor lobule in the region of the tuber cinareum of the third ventricle (**e**) indicates involvement into the optic tract.

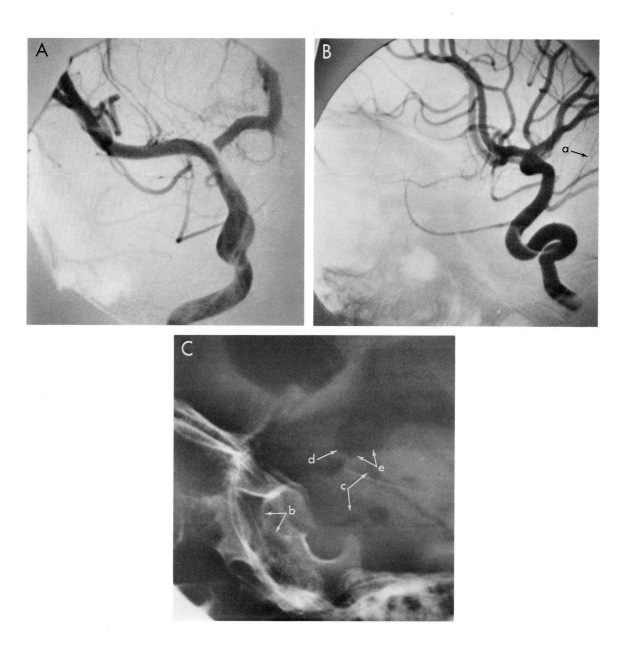

Figure 146 · Bilateral Optic Nerve Glioma / 483

Figure 147.—Optic nerve glioma.

A 14-year-old girl had a two-year history of progressive proptosis and vision loss on the right. A Krönlein procedure was done initially and biopsy revealed the presence of an astrocytoma. This was followed by a right frontal craniotomy with section of the right optic nerve at the chiasm and transorbital resection of the nerve at the back of the globe. Serial pathologic sections of the specimen showed no evidence of tumor extension to the chiasmal end of the nerve, so no radiotherapy was given postoperatively.

A, radiographs of the optic foramina: There is a 1-mm difference between the two optic canals, the right being larger than the left. This is within normal limits. However, laminagrams showed a significant enlargement of the orbital portion of the right canal.

B, right carotid arteriogram, subtracted base view, arterial phase: The ophthalmic artery is displaced medially (**a**) within its intracanalicular portion and shows numerous stretched branches with a small tumor stain (**b**) in the muscle cone portion. There is no evidence of intracranial extension.

C, right carotid arteriogram, subtracted lateral view: The ophthalmic artery is taut and displaced upward within the canal (**a**). Intraorbitally the lowest long ciliary vessel is dilated and displaced downward. Numerous smaller ciliary vessels are separated and give rise to a small tumor stain (**b**). The middle cerebral vessels coursing over the tip of the temporal pole show no evidence of backward displacement.

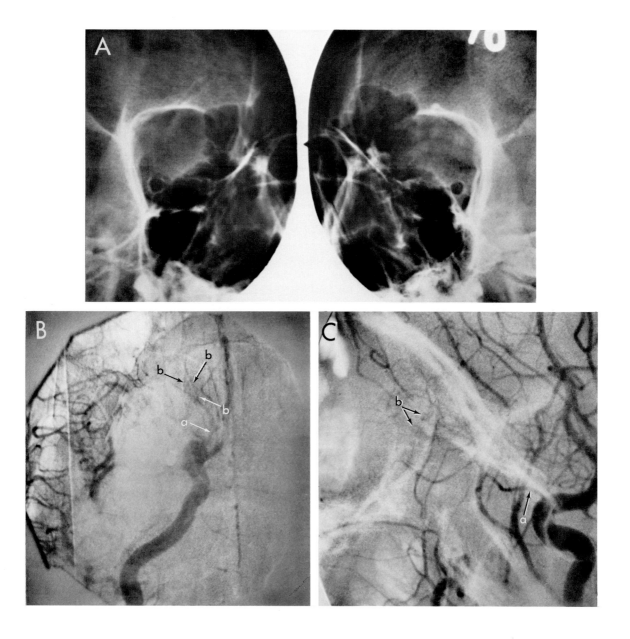

Figure 147 · Optic Nerve Glioma / 485

Figure 148.—Carcinoma of the puncta.

A 50-year-old man was seen because of intermittent tearing. On examination, the punctum of the lower lid appeared to be full and felt firm.

Dacrocystogram, lateral view: A lobulated filling defect (**arrows**) is present in the posterior portion of contrast medium within the upper lacrimal sac. Contrast material is able to descend into the nasal cavity.

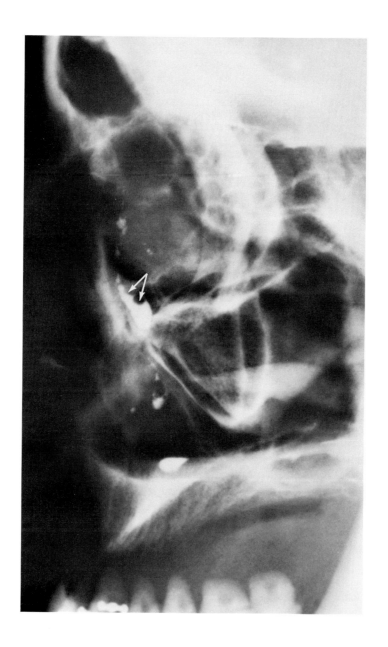

Figure 148 · Carcinoma of Puncta / 487

Figure 149.—Neurofibroma of the left orbit.

A 25-year-old man had a four-year history of swelling of the lids, proptosis and occasional pain. Examination revealed a small palpable mass in the superior portion of the left orbit. Ten months earlier he had undergone a Krönlein orbitotomy for biopsy, which was not diagnostic. At a second operation the left orbit was unroofed and a neurofibroma of the orbital roof removed.

A, plain radiograph, Caldwell projection: Enlargement of the left foramen rotundum (**a**) is seen. Slight fossa formation (**b**) is evident on the roof of the left orbit. Absence of the left zygoma is secondary to the Krönlein operation.

B, plain radiograph, Towne projection: There is definite widening of the left inferior orbital fissure (**c**) as compared with the right. This in conjunction with the finding of the large foramen rotundum presumably represents a neurofibroma of the second division of the fifth nerve in addition to the roof lesion.

C, orbital phlebogram: There is definite downward displacement of the trochlear point (**d**). The point at which the superior ophthalmic vein enters the muscle cone (**e**) is also displaced. However, the vein enters the superior orbital fissure and outlines the cavernous sinus without obvious mass effect. These findings are consistent with a mass on the orbital roof somewhat medially located but in the same plane as the anterior portion of the superior ophthalmic vein.

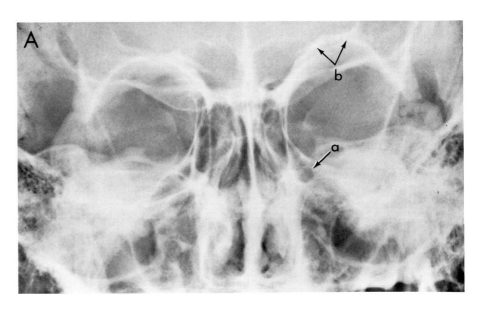

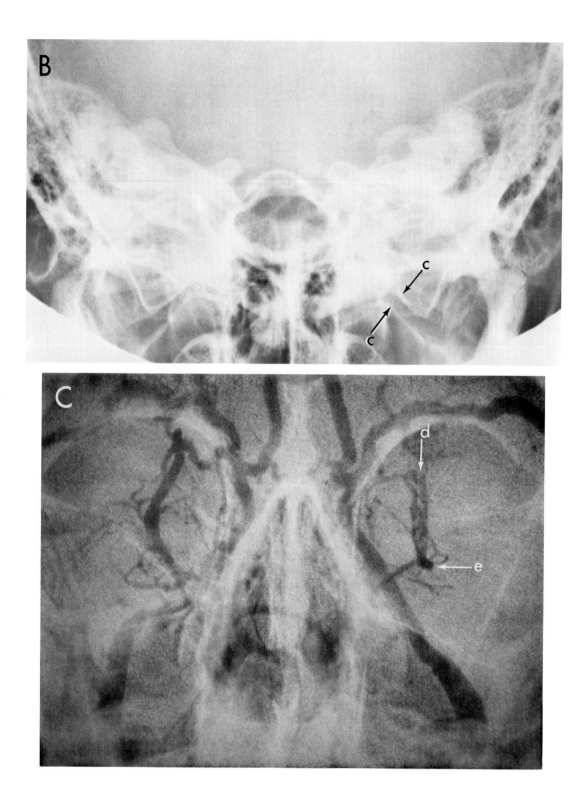

Figure 149 · Neurofibroma of Orbit / 489

Figure 150.—Optic nerve sheath meningioma.

A 41-year-old man had a nine-year history of progressive proptosis of the right eye that was painless and without visual symptoms. He underwent a transcranial orbital exploration with gross total removal of the meningioma from within the muscle cone of the orbit. Unfortunately it was necessary to sacrifice the ophthalmic artery because of its major blood supply to the tumor, so that postoperatively the patient had complete visual loss.

A, right internal carotid arteriogram, subtracted Caldwell view, arterial phase: The ophthalmic artery is conspicuously enlarged, and numerous ciliary branches are seen supplying a large area of rather homogeneous neovascularity.

B, right internal carotid arteriogram, subtracted Caldwell view, intermediate phase: A dense homogeneous stain fills the region of the right orbit.

(*Continued.*)

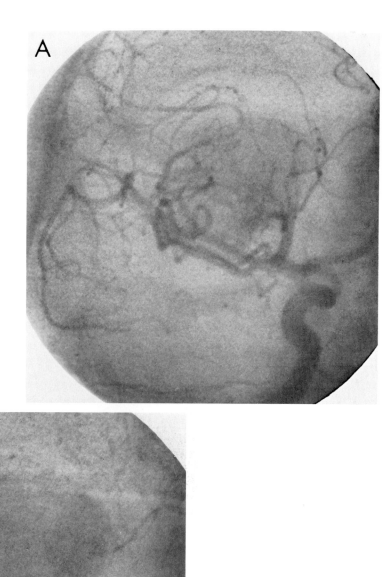

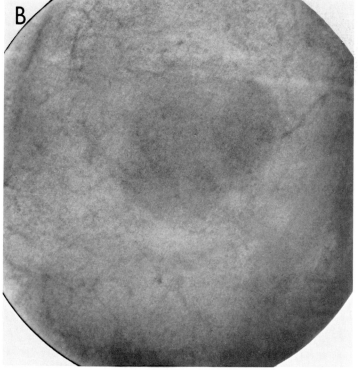

Figure 150 · Optic Nerve Sheath Meningioma / 491

Figure 150 (cont.).—Optic nerve sheath meningioma.

C, internal carotid arteriogram, subtracted lateral view: An enlarged ophthalmic artery gives off numerous branches from the ciliary arteries which encircle a large tumor.

D, right internal carotid arteriogram, subtracted lateral view, intermediate phase: The tumor stain rather completely outlines a meningioma which extends posteriorly to the orbital apex and anteriorly to just behind the globe (**a**), which is markedly displaced forward.

E, selective right external carotid arteriogram, subtracted lateral view: A small area of neovascularity (**b**) is seen in the inferior aspect of the anterior portion of the orbit which is supplied by the internal maxillary artery.

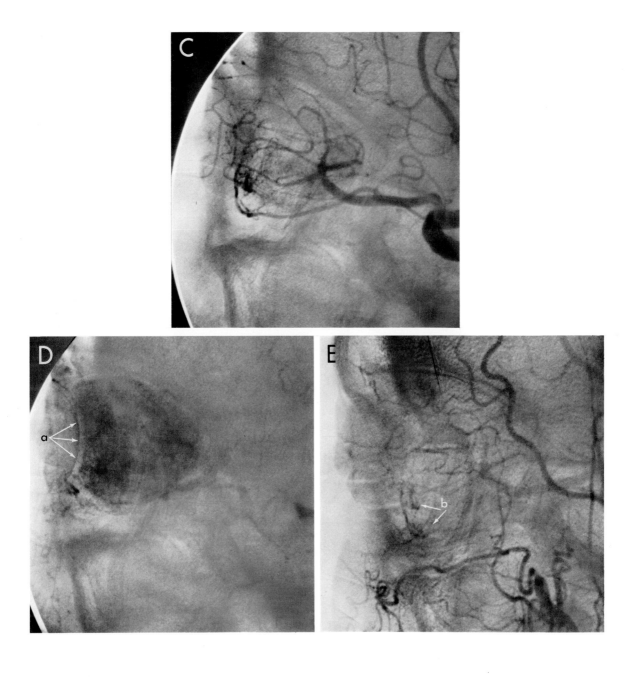

Figure 150 · Optic Nerve Sheath Meningioma / 493

Figure 151.—Recurrent meningioma of the right orbit.

A 14-year-old boy, a year before our study, had unilateral right-sided proptosis. At that time a Krönlein procedure was done and removal of a mass around the optic nerve was accomplished. Approximately seven months later he had recurrent proptosis. At a second operation a recurrent meningioma extending from just behind the globe to the apex of the orbit was removed.

A, right carotid arteriogram, subtracted lateral view, arterial phase: The ophthalmic artery is normal within the optic canal. As it courses around the optic nerve numerous enlarged ciliary vessels (**a**) are seen extending into the region of the muscle cone. The cutaneous branches (**b**) pass above the muscle cone and are not involved. Slight staining is seen from the region of the apex of the orbit where the ophthalmic artery appears to enlarge and extends in a spotty fashion to the region of the choroid crescent (**c**). Temporal lobe branches (**d**) show no evidence of backward displacement to suggest intracranial extension.

B, right carotid arteriogram, lateral view, intermediate phase: Numerous splotchy areas of homogeneous staining (**e**) are seen from the apex of the orbit to the region of the muscle cone. The choroid crescent is displaced forward, and several areas of indentation (**f**) are present due to adjacent tumor, particularly on the posteroinferior surface of the choroid crescent.

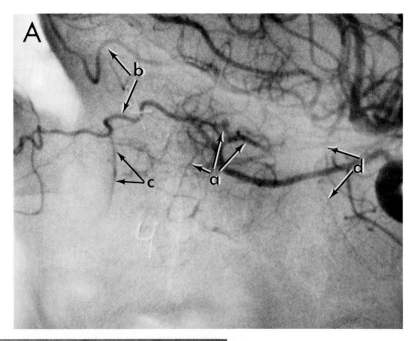

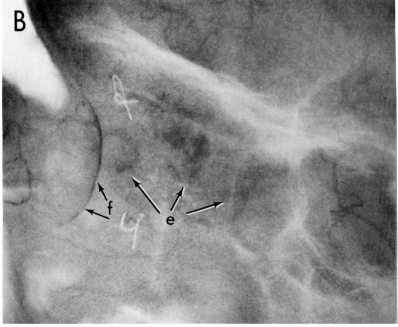

Figure 151 · Recurrent Orbital Meningioma / 495

Figure 152.—Reticulum cell sarcoma of the left orbit.

A 24-year-old man noted progressive enlargement of a lump that began under the medial aspect of the left upper lid. It became painful during the two weeks before examination, which revealed an orange-sized mass extruding from the left orbit and completely engulfing the globe. Otherwise the physical examination revealed no abnormality. He received 4500 rads in six weeks of cobalt teletherapy with bolus covering the lesion, with very little regression.

A, skull radiograph, frontal view, Waters projection: A very large soft tissue mass extends from the left orbit superiorly. A portion of the tumor extends into the left antrum. An incidental finding is a small osteoma in the frontal sinus.

B, skull radiograph, frontal view, Caldwell projection: The volume of the left orbit is greatly increased, with expansion and thinning of the superior and medial margins of the orbit in particular. The floor of the orbit has been eroded away by a lobular mass extending beneath it.

(Continued.)

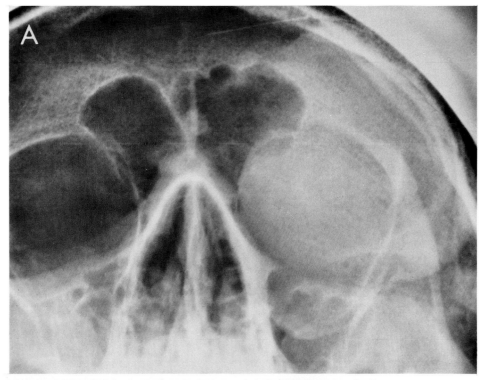

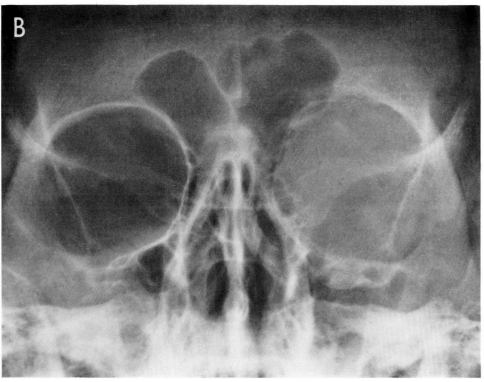

Figure 152 · Reticulum Cell Sarcoma / 497

Figure 152 (cont.).—Reticulum cell sarcoma of the left orbit.

C, left internal carotid arteriogram, frontal view, early arterial phase: Numerous vascular channels arise from the ophthalmic artery coursing toward the middle portion of the orbit and depositing contrast material within small necrotic pools (**a**) in the tumor bed as well as in a more homogeneous fashion.

D, left internal carotid arteriogram, frontal view, early venous phase: The tumor stain (**b**) is still visible, and numerous venous channels are seen draining this vascular tumor within the orbit.

E, left external carotid arteriogram, lateral view, arterial phase: There is a small contribution to the tumor's vascular supply from the internal maxillary artery. In particular note that the inferior portion of the tumor, which is extending into the left antrum, receives the bulk of its supply from the branch of the internal maxillary artery (**c**) displaced in an arcuate fashion beneath it.

(Continued.)

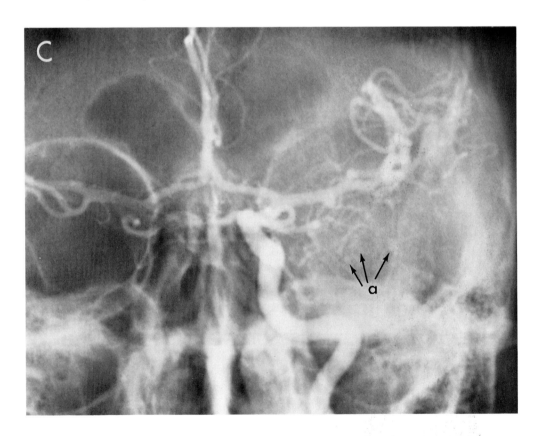

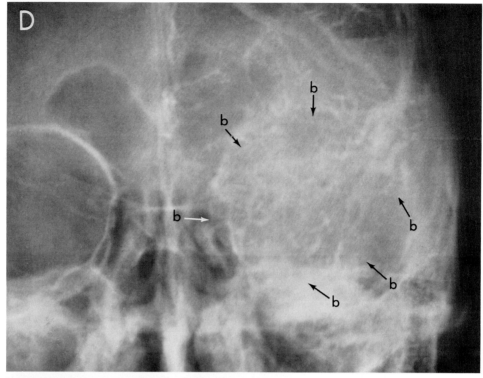

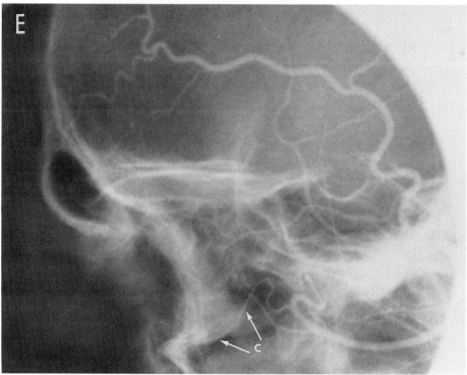

Figure 152 · Reticulum Cell Sarcoma / 499

Figure 152 (cont.).—Reticulum cell sarcoma of the left orbit.

F, left internal carotid arteriogram, lateral view, arterial phase: A large leash of vessels is seen arising from the ophthalmic artery extending into the tumor, which occupies practically the entire orbit. Numerous areas of deposition of small pools (**a**) of contrast material are visible within the tumor. The most inferior portion of the tumor extending into the antrum receives its blood supply from the external carotid artery, which normally supplies the floor of the orbit.

G, left internal carotid arteriogram, lateral view, late arterial phase: Numerous small veins are distributed throughout the tumor; staining of a portion of the tumor (**d**) extruding beyond the confines of the orbit can also be seen.

H, left internal carotid arteriogram, lateral view, venous phase: There is retention of contrast material in the tumor. The lack of early filling of either the superior or the inferior ophthalmic vein is probably due to compression of these structures by the greatly increased intraorbital pressure caused by the tumor.

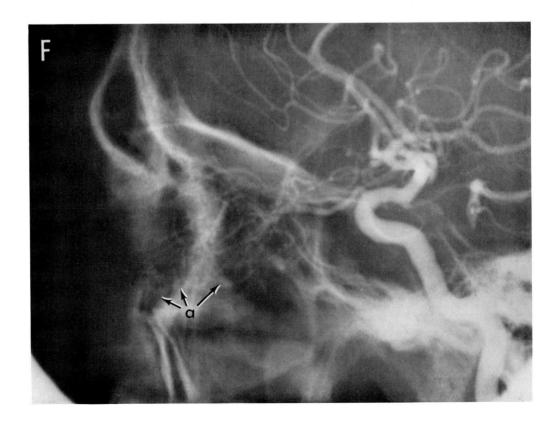

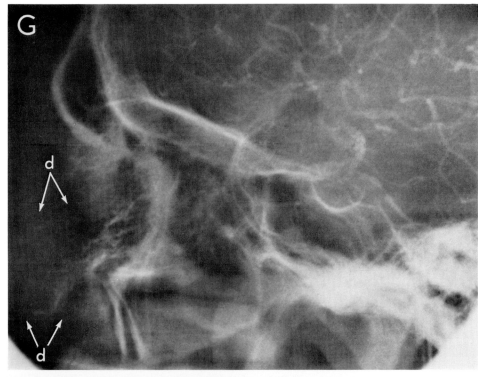

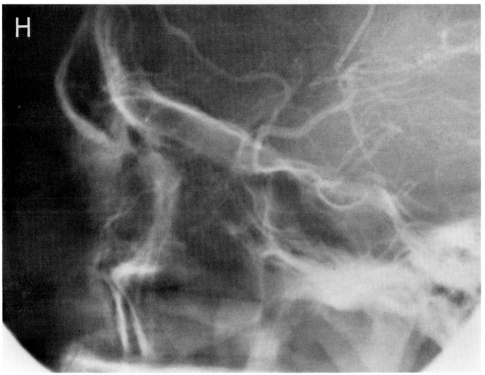

Figure 152 · Reticulum Cell Sarcoma / 501

Figure 153.—Metastasis to the left orbit from carcinoma of the breast.

A 72-year-old woman had had a left mastectomy 17 years previously for carcinoma. A year before our examination a lytic lesion was found in the right rib cage and another in the upper third of the left femur. Several months before admission she had intermittent swelling of the left eye with numbness in the left eyebrow. A month before this study she rather precipitously lost vision of the left eye. On examination the left eye was blind. The pupil reacted consensually to light but not directly. Both pupils reacted in accommodation. The left eye was proptotic with significant swelling of the periorbital area. The left lid was ptotic. Movements of the left eye were severely limited in all directions. Decreased sensation to touch and pain in the first and second divisions of the left trigeminal nerve was evident.

A, left common carotid arteriogram, subtracted lateral magnification view, arterial phase: Several branches (**a**) of the internal maxillary artery are enlarged and course toward the region of the orbital roof and orbital apex. In these areas irregular tumor vessels (**b**) are visible. The middle meningeal artery (**c**) is enlarged and via the recurrent meningeal artery (**d**) gives off a collection of tumor vessels (**e**) in the apex of the orbit more superiorly. The ophthalmic artery is displaced downward (**f**), is slightly enlarged and also gives off small tumor vessels (**g**) as the artery courses superiorly around the optic nerve.

B, left common carotid arteriogram, Caldwell projection, subtracted magnification study, arterial phase: The ophthalmic artery is displaced laterally (**f**) throughout its course until it reaches the anterior portion of the orbit to course toward the supraorbital region. The recurrent meningeal branch (**d**) of the middle meningeal artery (**c**) is seen as the large medially directed continuation of the latter vessel. Several areas of neovascularity (**h**) are delineated in the orbital apex projected into the maxillary antrum. In addition, areas of neovascularity are superimposed on the ophthalmic artery and along the medial aspect of the orbit.

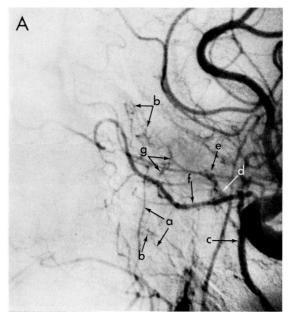

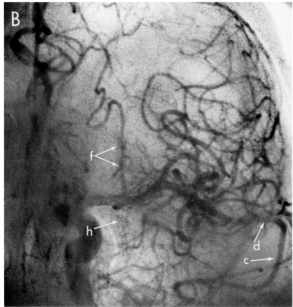

Figure 153 · Metastasis from the Breast / 503

Figure 154.—Fibrosarcoma of the left orbit.

An 11-year-old boy had the right eye enucleated for retinoblastoma during his first year of life. At age 5 a large temporally located tumor of the left eye with vitreous seeds up to 2–3 mm in diameter was treated by irradiation; total dosage calculated to the lateral aspect of the left orbit was in the neighborhood of 10,000 rads. A soft tissue mass was noted on the lateral aspect of the left orbit just prior to his last admission.

A, plain radiograph, frontal view: The lateral wall of the left orbit is missing. An ill-defined area (**a**) of amorphous calcification is seen in conjunction with destructive changes along the greater and lesser wings of the sphenoid bone involving a portion of the orbital roof as it extends toward the linea innominata.

B, laminagram obtained during pneumoencephalography in brow-up position, frontal view: The destruction of the lesser and greater wings of the sphenoid bone on the left is better appreciated, extending from the region of the orbital apex with preservation of the anterior clinoid process and extending laterally toward the linea innominata. There is mild compression of the left side of the suprasellar cistern (**b**). The left frontal horn is displaced upward and compressed. There is significant left-to-right displacement of the septum pellucidum.

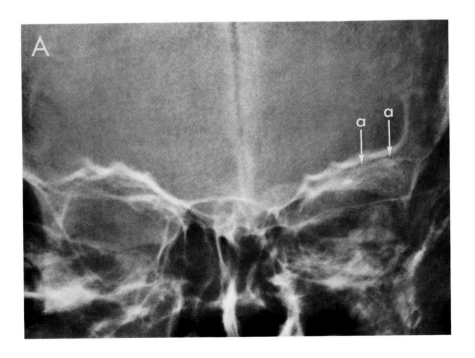

C, autotomogram, lateral view, brow-up position of the pneumoencephalogram: The frontal horn is truncated (**c**) due to the local mass effect extending into the frontal lobe. The third ventricle is normal.

(Continued.)

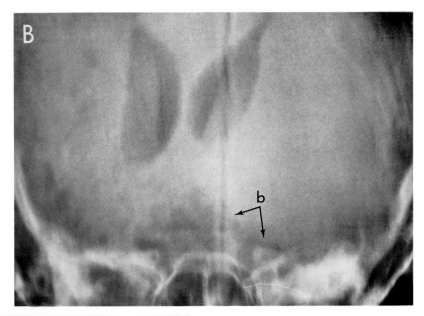

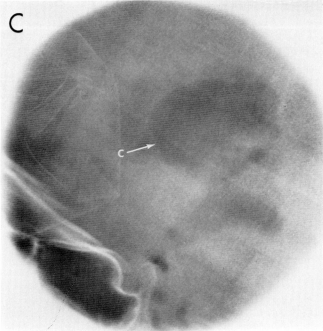

Figure 154 · Fibrosarcoma / 505

Figure 154 (cont.).—Fibrosarcoma of the left orbit.

D, left common carotid arteriogram, subtracted frontal view, arterial phase: The distal internal carotid artery (**d**) is straightened as it is displaced laterally. Local mass effect is evident on the branches (**e**) of the middle cerebral artery as they course through the proximal portion of the opercular lips of the Sylvian fissure. The genu of the middle cerebral artery is also displaced slightly inward. The middle meningeal artery widens (**f**) as it courses upward toward the pterion and divides into several small vessels and is associated with a slight but definite stain (**g**). A large accessory middle meningeal artery (**h**) coursing to the middle meningeal artery also supplies the tumor.

E, left common carotid arteriogram, subtracted lateral view, arterial phase: The horizontal portion of the middle cerebral artery (**i**) is displaced slightly posteriorly. Attenuation of the orbitofrontal branch (**j**) of the middle cerebral artery is seen just above the numerous abnormal dural vessels (**g**) of the middle meningeal artery. The accessory meningeal (**h**) and more posteriorly positioned middle meningeal (**f**) arteries are enlarged and give off numerous dural branches that supply the sarcoma.

(Continued.)

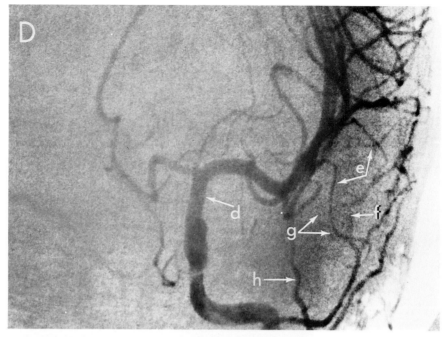

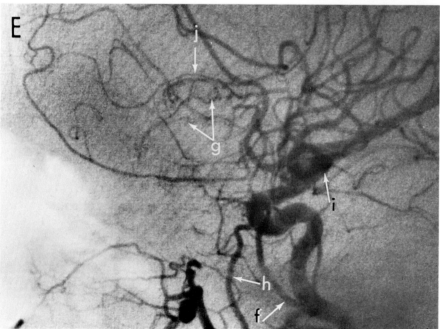

Figure 154 · Fibrosarcoma / 507

Figure 154 (cont.).—Fibrosarcoma of the left orbit.

F, left common carotid arteriogram, subtracted lateral view, intermediate phase: The tumor stain (**g**) extends from the region of the pterion superiorly to the midconvexity region of the frontal pole and inferiorly into the middle fossa.

G and **H,** left common carotid arteriogram, subtracted frontal and lateral views, venous phase: The middle cerebral vein (**k**) as it exits from the Sylvian fissure toward the sphenoparietal sinus is displaced posteriorly. In the frontal view (**G**) it is seen to be elevated and displaced medially. The uncal vein (**l**) is slightly displaced posteriorly in the lateral view (**H**) and medially in the frontal view (**G**). A stretched cortical vein (**m**) in the midconvexity area of the frontal pole is locally thinned by the tumor.

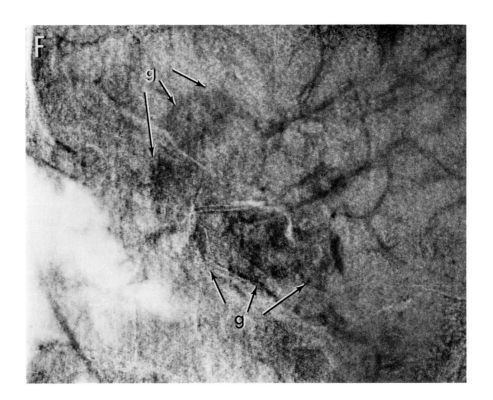

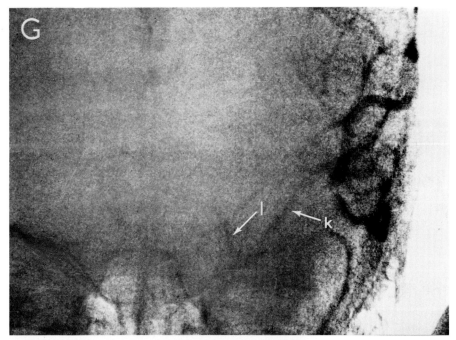

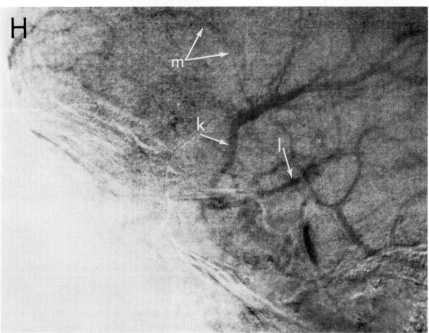

Figure 154 · Fibrosarcoma / 509

Figure 155.—Malignant fibrous histiocytoma involving primarily the right sphenoid bone.

A 6½-year-old boy had enucleation of the right eye for retinoblastoma at about age 7 weeks, followed by pneumococcic type II meningitis and subdural effusions which cleared postoperatively. At age 6 months a retinoblastoma was found in the left eye; this was successfully treated with triethyleneamine and betatron radiation to a dosage of 4,000 rads. Small tumor nodules noted in the retina of the left eye three years later were treated with light coagulation. At age 6 he had a grand mal seizure, complained of pain in the right suboccipital region and right side of the face and had a left hemiparesis. In addition, right-sided preauricular zygomatic swelling was noted. Autopsy disclosed an extensive neoplasm destroying the right sphenoid bone, invading the walls of the sella turcica and pituitary gland and growing out through the squamous portion of the temporal bone on the right. A diagnosis of malignant histiocytoma was based on the morphology of the cells and their behavior in tissue culture. It is of interest that the amount of radiation is quite small in comparison with other cases of radiation-induced sarcoma and also that it involved the side opposite to the irradiation. Death was attributed to a terminal incisural herniation of the temporal lobe with compression of the right posterior cerebral artery and a large hemorrhagic infarct in the area of its supply.

A, skull radiograph, frontal view, Caldwell projection: The linea innominata on the right is destroyed. The right superior orbital fissure cannot be made out, whereas the lateral margin of the left superior orbital fissure remains. The region of the planum sphenoidale and sella turcica floor cannot be seen.

B, skull radiograph, base view: Marked destruction of the greater wing of the sphenoid is demonstrated. The medial aspects of the posterior walls of the right antrum and orbit are destroyed. A soft tissue mass (**a**) extends into the region of the body of the sphenoid. There is obliteration of the right medial and lateral pterygoid. On the right, the foramen ovale and foramen spinosum are affected as the tumor involves the floor of the middle fossa to a marked extent.

(Continued.)

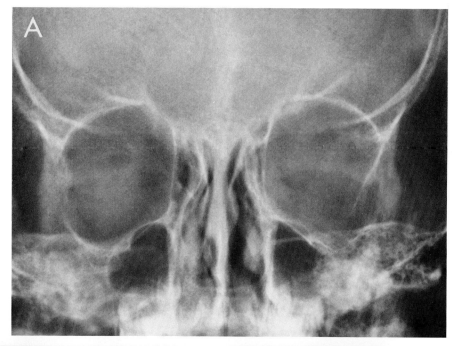

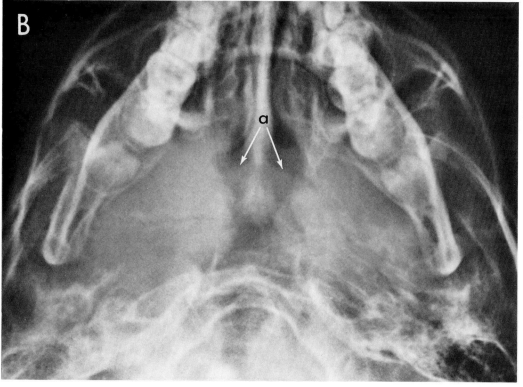

Figure 155 · Malignant Fibrous Histiocytoma / 511

Figure 155 (cont.).—Malignant fibrous histiocytoma involving primarily the right sphenoid bone.

C and **D,** radiographs of the optic foramina: there is marked destruction of the greater wing of the sphenoid and the planum sphenoidale with involvement of both optic canals.

E, skull radiograph, lateral view: A massive area of destruction is demonstrated. The single cortical density representing the greater wing of the sphenoid is on the left side. The right one has been destroyed, and the extension to and across the midline has involved the floor of the middle fossa, body of the sphenoid and both anterior clinoid processes as well as the planum sphenoidale.

F, pneumoencephalogram, frontal view, brow-up position: There has been no shift of the midline structures because the tumor is primarily extradural as well as being bilateral. No mass is seen within the air in the suprasellar cisterns.

(Continued.)

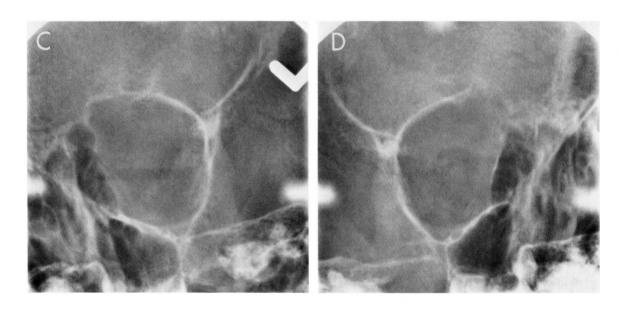

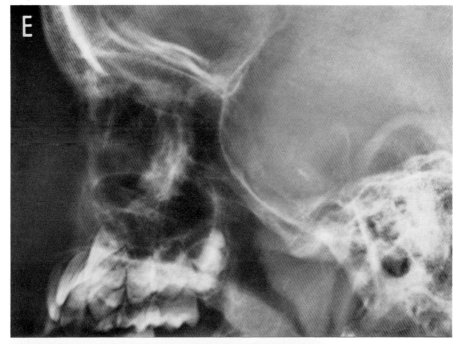

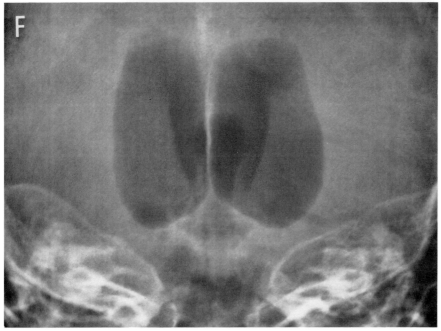

Figure 155 · Malignant Fibrous Histiocytoma / 513

Figure 155 (cont.).—Malignant fibrous histiocytoma involving primarily the right sphenoid bone.

G, pneumoencephalogram, lateral view, brow-up position: Moderate hydrocephalus is apparent. Air in the interpeduncular fossa behind the membrane of Lilliquist and air within the suprasellar cistern shows no evidence of impingement by a mass. The optic nerve is seen clearly within the suprasellar air. This confirms the basic extradural position of the sarcoma.

H, pneumoencephalogram, frontal view, brow-up position following a forward somersault: The right temporal horn (**b**) is deformed and displaced posteriorly. There is also very slight medial displacement with straightening of the anterior aspect of the temporal horn.

I, laminagram during pneumoencephalography with air in the suprasellar lateral and Sylvian fissures, frontal view: There is upward and slight medial displacement of these cisterns (**c**) by the mass, which has obviously eroded the floor of the middle fossa and body of the sphenoid bone.

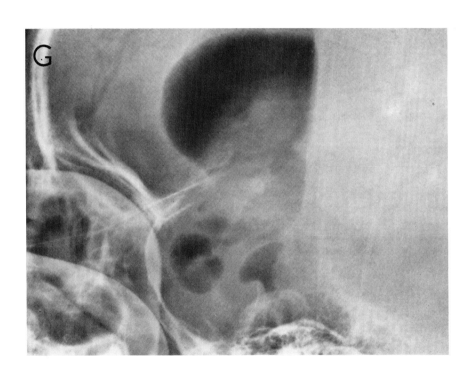

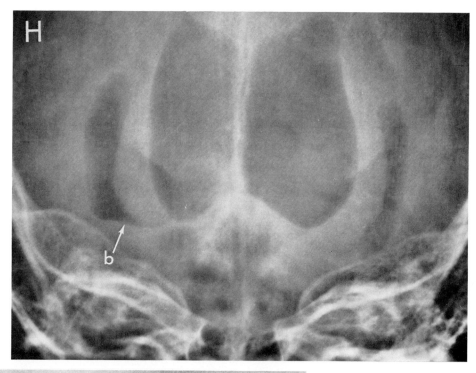

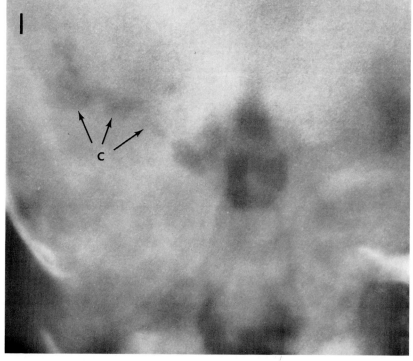

Figure 155 · Malignant Fibrous Histiocytoma / 515

Index